PSYCHOPATHOLOGY OF
CHILDREN AND YOUTH:
A CROSS-CULTURAL PERSPECTIVE

RECENT MACY
PUBLICATIONS

Edited by
Elizabeth F. Purcell

PSYCHOPATHOLOGY OF CHILDREN AND YOUTH: A CROSS-CULTURAL PERSPECTIVE

Report of a Conference

JOSIAH MACY, JR. FOUNDATION
One Rockefeller Plaza, New York, New York 10020

CONTENTS

FOREWORD

The Macy Foundation has taken an active interest in all aspects of psychiatry during the fifty years of its existence, and it is currently sponsoring a commission to study the present status and future prospects of academic psychiatry in the United States.

In view of the fact that 1979 was the International Year of the Child, on 14 to 16 November 1979 the foundation joined with the International Children's Center in Paris to convene a conference on aspects of psychiatric problems in childhood and adolescence.

An important impetus to this collaborative effort was the fact that the late Professor Robert Debré, founder of the Children's Center, was active in the field of child psychiatry for most of his distinguished career. This volume is therefore dedicated to the memory of Professor Debré.

In drawing up the program and in selecting the participants we are indebted to Leon Eisenberg, M.D., Maude and Lillian Presley Professor of Psychiatry, Harvard Medical School, for those from the United States, and to Cyrille Koupernik, M.D., associate professor at the College of Medicine of the Hospitals of Paris, for the Europeans. We wish to express our gratitude to all the participants for the excellent presentations that comprise this volume.

John Z. Bowers, M.D.
President

3 September 1980

ix

I. EPIDEMIOLOGY

EPIDEMIOLOGICAL CHILD PSYCHIATRY: AN AMERICAN PERSPECTIVE

Felton Earls*

In American child psychiatry the word epidemiology does not immediately inspire confidence that an understanding of the causes and cures of emotional disorders in children will be enhanced. Having made that statement I must decide how vigorously to defend it. On reflection the statement may be as much as four or five years out of date, for in that brief period several American epidemiological investigations in child psychiatry have been published, and others, including my own work, have begun.

At the same time, Americans have become more aware of epidemiological studies conducted in other English-speaking countries, primarily those of M. Rutter and coworkers in Great Britain.[1] These studies have provided, perhaps for the first time in America, a range of epidemiological approaches to analyze and compare. Epidemiological concepts and methods are currently being rapidly integrated into the mainstream of American child psychiatry, to an extent that epidemiology may yet become a basic science in this field.

It is perhaps curious that epidemiological strategies have been so slow to come to American child psychiatry. The mental hygiene movement at the beginning of this century, with its concern over the increasing incidence

* This investigation is being supported by grants MH-28266 and MH-00165 (RSDA) of the National Institute of Mental Health, and in part by core grant HD-06276 of the Mental Retardation Center.

Reprints may be requested from the author at the John Enders Pediatric Research Center, Children's Hospital Medical Center, 320 Longwood Avenue, Boston, Massachusetts 02115.

3

of juvenile delinquency, encouraged a few epidemiological ventures.[2] More recently, the community mental health movement has addressed policy and service delivery issues in an epidemiological framework, but it has not inspired much research in child psychiatry. Although outstanding contributions to child psychiatry epidemiology have of course been made by Americans for over fifty years,[3] they have been singular studies not integrated into a tradition of research in this field. As impressive is the fact that, after World War II, Americans made great strides in the epidemiological study of adult psychiatric disorders.[4,5]

The empirical tradition in American psychology introduced by J.B. Watson, C. Spearman, L.L. Thurstone, R.B. Cattell, and others might also have been thought to provide a natural medium for epidemiological thinking in psychiatry because of its basis in quantitative measurement. It is worth asking how child psychiatry remained impermeable to these influences. One answer may lie in the ascendancy of psychoanalysis into the mainstream of American child psychiatry; this influence may have compartmentalized the growth of ideas in the field. Certainly, concern for categorization, quantitative measurement, and statistical treatment of psychiatric phenomena is not encouraged by the more intuitive approaches of the depth psychologies such as psychoanalysis.

It is against this background that the issue of what impact epidemiological research is currently having in American child psychiatry is addressed. Three studies are selected for review, which, taken together, give a cross-section of current activities. They are the Chicago-based, Woodlawn Program of Assessment, Early Intervention, and Evaluation of Sheppard G. Kellam and coworkers; the New York-based Family Research Project of Thomas S. Langner and his group; and the Martha's Vineyard Child Health Survey directed by the author. Each will be analyzed in terms of its rationale, methods, and major findings. The influence these studies have on the practice of child psychiatry will be briefly discussed, as will some current developments in the field that are likely to sustain the present trend of ascendancy of epidemiological child psychiatry.

THE WOODLAWN PROGRAM

Kellam's project was in part a response to the community mental health movement of the 1960s.[6] This research unit evolved its rationale and methods in the context of a newly established mental health center in a disadvantaged, predominantly black urban area in Chicago.[7] The subjects were children entering the first year of school between 1964 and 1969. Six cohorts were formed, one of which was tracked over a nine-year period. Representation of the total population of children living in this urban area was achieved through sampling children from the twelve schools in the area, both private and public. Because of the intimate association of the research endeavor with the mental health center, a decision was made to evaluate the effectiveness of school psychiatric consultation services as part of the larger study. For that purpose the schools were randomly divided into intervention and nonintervention groups. This purpose coexisted with other epidemiological objectives during the first few years of the project.

Sample

About 1,700 children a year are included in each of the six cohorts. In work published to date the main emphasis has been placed on the 1966—67 cohort of about 1,240 children.[8] Refusal rates at initial assessment were low, on the order of 5-6 percent. The nine-year follow up was successful in reinterviewing about 75 percent of the original population, no simple task given the fact that nearly three-quarters of the families had moved from the study area. Not all the children in these families agreed to a follow-up interview, which resulted in an additional increment in the attrition rate. This was an appreciable loss, and, since many of the children could not be located or were institutionalized, it is probable that their loss contributed to significantly decreasing the rate of psychiatric disorders in the sample. Throughout the many combinations of concurrent and longitudinal data analysis, many different subsamples within and between cohorts were used. The value of this work would have been enhanced if characteristics of the various cohorts at different points in the longitudinal study had been described more thoroughly.

Rationale and Methods

Kellam derived a theoretical framework from the social psychology litera- ture to define the developmental transition of entering first grade as a critical phase in emotional growth, possibly linked to the onset of mental disorders in children.[9] Two spheres of mental health adaptation were measured within this framework: social adaptational status, a measure of the adjustment of the person to the social demands of the environment; and psychological well-being, a measure of emotional adjustment. Community members serving on the board of the mental health center and teachers at the local schools assisted the project staff in generating definitions of mental health disorders.

Social adaptational status is defined by six rating scales derived from a wide range of social tasks originally described by the local teachers. The six scales shown in Table 1 are meant to describe a universe of specific expectations ascribed to children living in Woodlawn. Each scale defines a range of adaptive and maladaptive behaviors. The validity of the scales is discussed in a variety of ways, but the more rigorous view relates to the ability of teacher ratings of social adaptation to predict independent measures of performance such as IQ, achievement scores, and school grades. In general, correlations of the variables are in the range of .20 to .50 for measures taken in the first grade. Lower correlations were achieved when first-grade teacher ratings were compared with outcome variables in the third grade. Inter-rater reliability of the teacher ratings was not carried out, but repeatability of the ratings proved satisfactory. This limitation in reporting reliability is of some significance because there is no compelling evidence that the teachers agreed in their perceptions of well-adjusted or maladjusted children. Moreover, the degree to which teachers acted as independent raters of maladjustment is not clear. It appears that teachers may have rated some children on both the social task scales and on some outcome measures such as school grades.

The other domain of mental health measured is termed psychological well-being. It is done in three ways: 1) classroom observations conducted by psychiatrists; 2) symptom-inventory questionnaires completed by mothers; and 3) self-reports. Each of these techniques was exploratory in design in that none had been used in a previous work or preliminary study.

TABLE 1. SOCIAL TASKS AND EXAMPLES OF ASSOCIATED MALADAPTIVE
BEHAVIORS INCLUDED IN TEACHER RATINGS:
WOODLAWN PROGRAM OF ASSESSMENT, EARLY INTERVENTION, AND EVALUATION

Categories of Social Tasks	Maladaptive Behaviors
Social contact	Shy, timid, isolated
Authority acceptance	Resists authority, lies, steals
Maturation	Cries often, has tantrums, enuretic
Cognitive achievement	Lazy, lacks effort
Concentration	Fidgety, restless

Furthermore, the six cohorts were not treated similarly in regard to which measures of psychological well-being were used. The reliability and validity of the measures are not mentioned, except for the fact that the mothers' symptomatic ratings agreed well with the results of normal children rated, using another scale of demonstrated validity.

Findings

Tables 2 and 3 indicate that a high percentage of children are rated as maladjusted by their teachers. Table 2 gives results based on the original categories of social maladaptation, showing that two-thirds of the children are considered maladaptive at least to a mild degree; of these, one-third are maladaptive to a moderate-to-severe degree. In a subsequent analysis of the same items a new typology of maladaptation was derived. This reclassification (Table 3) applies more clinically germane labels to the types of maladjustments observed. Shy children were observed to be anxious and flat in affective expression, and were reported by their mothers to have psychophysiological symptoms. Aggressive children were observed to be anxious and hyperkinetic in the classroom and were reported by their

TABLE 2. PREVALENCE OF MALADAPTIVE BEHAVIOR BASED ON TEACHER RATINGS: WOODLAWN PROGRAM OF ASSESSMENT, EARLY INTERVENTION, AND EVALUATION— COHORT 1, N = 944
(PERCENTAGES)

| | Teacher Ratings | | |
Social Tasks	Adapting 0	Maladapting 1	Moderately and Severely Maladapting 2 + 3
Social contact	71.4	10.7	17.9
Authority acceptance	68.3	15.9	15.8
Maturation	57.6	16.7	25.7
Cognitive achievement	56.8	18.3	24.9
Concentration	52.0	25.4	22.6
GLOBAL: Rating of 2 or more on any one social task	31.0	36.5	32.4

TABLE 3. PREVALENCE OF MALADAPTIVE BEHAVIOR CLUSTERS
BASED ON TEACHER RATINGS:
WOODLAWN PROGRAM OF ASSESSMENT, EARLY INTERVENTION, AND EVALUATION—
COHORT 1, N = 2,010

Maladaptive Clusters	Percent of Sample
Shy	20.5
Aggressive	15.7
Shy-aggressive	13.9
Neither shy nor aggressive	18.7
Total sample rated maladaptive	68.8

mothers to be immature, nervous, and enuretic. These are the most strongly positive associations found; several others with weaker correlations are reported. The main patterns of behavior adjustment appear to agree in general with externalizing and internalizing dimensions found in numerous clinical samples.[10]

The intervention program, in which a psychiatrist conducted group therapy sessions in a classroom with children who had been previously identified as maladaptive on teacher scales, produced results that are difficult to interpret. There were short-range, positive effects in changing teacher ratings within the same year of schooling, but longer-term results— between first and third grades—were inconsistent among cohorts. For example, in examining the correlation between teacher ratings and IQ and school grades, modestly positive effects appear in some cohorts, but not in others. Indeed for many of the analyses the children from the intervention and nonintervention schools were combined after no differences were demonstrated between them on the variable being measured.

One of the more impressive and easily interpreted findings of this large study relates to demonstrating the association between family constellation and the mental health of young children. Eighty-six family types are described, based on configurations of adults present in the homes.[11] Among these, the single-parent families constitute the greatest risk to the development of poor social and emotional status. It is interesting to note that families in which at least two adults are present (mother/father or mother/grandmother) represent comparatively low risks of maladaptation. Families in which a mother and stepfather are present represent nearly as high a risk of maladaptation as single-parent families.

A nine-year follow up of the 1966–67 cohort was completed in 1978.[12]

The dependent variables were designed to measure the same two domains of mental health measured in first-graders: adaptational status and psychological well-being. Attainment of normally expected grade level and drug use were indices of social adaptational status, and psychiatric symptoms served as an index of well-being. Social adaptational status as measured in first-graders proved to work well in predicting adolescent status.

Seventy-three percent of the adaptive children were at grade level, compared to 47 percent of maladaptive children. Males rated aggressive in first grade were found to experience greater drug use than males rated shy. For example, approximately 90 percent of the moderate-to-severe aggressive boys smoked marijuana, compared to 35 percent of the moderate-to-severe shy boys. Males rated as shy in first grade also were found to have more symptoms in adolescence $(r = 0.66)$. First-grade social adaptational status was not predictive of adaptation or symptoms in female adolescents.

Measures of first-grade psychological well-being did not work well in predicting drug use and symptoms in males, but parental reports of symptoms—sad, worried, trouble expressing feelings, muscular tension, and speech problems—did relate to teenage symptoms in girls. Some changes in the family environment, such as parental separations and remarriages, and geographic mobility did not appear to make an independent contribution to the risk of drug use or symptoms in children of either sex. Other measures of the family environment, however, did appear to affect females in particular. Mothers who reported low expectations for the children and who reported having psychiatric symptoms themselves contributed to the increasing frequency of symptoms in their daughters.

These findings suggest that from middle childhood to adolescence the prediction of drug use and psychological symptoms in males is primarily influenced by the extrafamilial social environment; females may be more directly influenced by aspects of the family environment. In fact a major contribution of this study is the demonstration of how important it is, in measuring mental health, to take into account both adaptation to societal demands and emotional status.

A more detailed analysis of the Woodlawn study reveals several limitations that primarily relate to low validity, and, in some instances, to undemonstrated reliability of measures. At times the investigators used quite liberal definitions of mental disorder, which might have further compromised the validity and reliability of the measures.

The most difficult task faced in summarizing the findings of this study is the pattern of continuities and changes in mental health status charted longitudinally. For at least one of the six cohorts included in the initial assessment phase of the study, measurements of social adaptational status and psychological well-being were made at four separate periods: early first grade; late first grade; third grade; and midadolescence. Some compelling patterns have already been reported by the authors: for example, social adaptive status measures taken at the end of first grade, but not at the beginning, are predictive of a high rate of drug usage in male teenagers.[13] It may be expected that correlations between third-grade social adaptational status measures and teenage measures would be even stronger, but these are not reported. By the third grade, weak associations between these measures in females might even appear.

In such an undertaking, of course, it takes a very persistent research team to exhaust all possibilities in data analyses. In such a complicated venture, however, in which many measurements are being taken under poorly controlled conditions and in different cohorts over long periods of time, a determined effort is needed to show, as clearly as possible, change in stability of measurements. The most clinically important finding to emerge from this project is the long-term, predictive validity of teacher ratings in forecasting quite different adolescent mental health outcomes. Unfortunately the authors do not discuss the limitations and drawbacks of their methodology, and this, along with a lack of clarity about sample size and attrition rates and their possible effects on the findings, detracts from the scientific merits of an otherwise herculean enterprise.

THE FAMILY RESEARCH PROJECT

The New York-based Family Research Project is an epidemiological study that combines a cross-sectional sample and longitudinal designs.[14] Representative samples of children between the ages of six and eighteen living in a defined area of New York City were examined twice over a five-year period. The definition of psychiatric disorder was based on responses to a detailed, structured interview with mothers of the children. The objectives of the study were to find the prevalence, environmental correlates, and stability of psychiatric disorder in children. In addition, the need for intervention and the effects of intervention were investigated.

Sample

The sample consisted of 1,034 children representing a cross-section of the general population in the delineated area, and another 1,000 disadvantaged children whose parents were dependents of the state—known as the welfare sample. The children were interviewed on two occasions, which on average were separated by a five-year period: the first (Time 1) occurring in 1967, and the second (Time 2) in 1972. Analysis of cross-sectional data examines the entire sample at either Time 1, when the children were age six to eighteen, or Time 2, when they were age eleven to twenty-three. The longitudinal data analysis follows children within age cohorts over the five-year follow-up period.

The refusal rate for the initial assessment was 15 percent; the rate of attrition over the five-year interval between interviews was 29 percent. By the end of the survey, then, less than 60 percent of the sample initially defined had been included in both phases of the study. This is one index of the mobility of the urban population in the United States, which poses a limitation for longitudinal research, generally, as previously discussed in the Woodlawn Program.

Rationale and Methods

The structured interview developed for the project contains over 800 items, most of which concern aspects of child behavior; others measure various dimensions of the social and emotional environment of the family. Psychiatrists were assigned the task of making impairment ratings on edited summaries of the data that contained only responses to questions dealing with child behavior. As one test of validity, 26 percent of the cross-sectional sample and 9 percent of the welfare sample were directly interviewed by two project psychiatrists.[15] Correlation of impairment ratings with interview ratings is .48, indicating a modest level of validity. The reliability of the psychiatrists' impairment ratings based on the questionnaire data is .80, but a substantially lower inter-rater reliability was reached based on interview data. As a source of external validity, then, observational and interview data as measured in this situation is of quite limited value.[16] In addition to this clinical approach, the study relied on statistical methods to determine the types of behavioral adjustments experienced by children, and the association between these types of adjustments and social factors.

Findings

Based on the impairment ratings alone, the prevalence of psychiatric disorder was judged to be 13.5 percent for the cross-sectional sample and 23 percent for the welfare sample.[17] Table 4 shows the distribution of impairment ratings. Definitions of the ratings are not given except to state

TABLE 4. DISTRIBUTION OF IMPAIRMENT RATINGS ACROSS TWO SAMPLES:
NEW YORK FAMILY RESEARCH PROJECT
(PERCENTAGES)

Impairment Rating	Cross-Sectional Sample	Welfare Sample
Well or minimal	5.9	9.9
Mild	36.8	33.5
Moderate	43.8	33.5
Marked	12.1	19.1
Severe	1.4	4.0

that children in the marked and severe categories were considered to be in need of treatment. Why so few children were considered minimally impaired or what meaning is to be assigned to the mild and moderate levels of impairment is unclear. About one in two of the markedly or severely impaired children had been referred to treatment by a mental health professional, but most of the treatments and interventions were for periods of less than six months.

In the several publications available on the Family Research Project, a primary investment has been made in factor analysis and cluster analysis as methods to reduce the large number of items in the parent interviews to a manageable but representative size.[18,19] Factor analysis of a large item pool is viewed as a means to derive independent dimensions of child behavior and parent factors, rather than relying on unidimensional scales, which may merge several unique dimensions into a single scale. Eighteen child behavior factors, eight parental factors, and five parent-child factors were derived with factor analysis. The seven child behavior factors found to correlate most highly with impairment ratings, and all of the parental and parent-child factors, are listed in Table 5.

While factor analysis demonstrates the degree to which certain behaviors tend to be closely associated within the entire population, cluster analysis examines the similarity of the behavioral problems of individual children. Based on the latter technique, six types of behavioral adjustments are reported (Table 6).

Other major findings from the project can be grouped into three broad categories: 1) the development of a screening instrument; 2) the association of social factors with child behavioral adjustment; and 3) changes in behavioral adjustment over time. One product of the Family Research

TABLE 5. TYPES OF CHILD BEHAVIOR, PARENTAL, AND PARENT-CHILD FACTORS
DERIVED FROM FACTOR ANALYSIS: NEW YORK FAMILY RESEARCH PROJECT

CHILD BEHAVIOR FACTORS

Self-destructive tendencies
Mentation problems
Conflict with parents
Regressive anxiety
Fighting
Delinquency
Isolation

PARENTAL FACTORS

Mother's physical and emotional illness
Unhappy marriage
Isolated parents
Mother's economic dissatisfaction
Unleisurely parents
Parental quarrels
Husband ill or withdrawn
Traditional marriage

PARENT-CHILD FACTORS

Parents cold
Parents punitive
Mother traditional/restrictive
Mother excitable/rejecting
Mother supportive/directing

Project was a shortened interview form focusing on child behavioral symptoms.[20] The screening instrument is composed of seven of the eighteen child factors originally obtained from the factor analysis of all child behavior items included in the long interview form. These factors (Table 5) were chosen because of their relatively high correlations with impairment ratings. Five questions comprise each factor, yielding a screening inventory of thirty-five questions requiring no more than twenty minutes to complete. Correlation between the screening inventory and total impairment rating is .69; correlation between the screening scores and external criteria of

TABLE 6. BEHAVIORAL CLUSTERS IN THE TOTAL POPULATION SAMPLE,
AND THE RELATIONSHIP OF BEHAVIORAL CLUSTERS TO IMPAIRMENT
IN THE WELFARE SAMPLE ONLY: NEW YORK FAMILY RESEARCH PROJECT
(PERCENTAGES)

Child Behavioral Clusters	Total Population	Impairment Ratings: 4 or 5
Mildly dependent	51.2	4.2
Aggressive, backward, isolated	24.0	44.5
Competitive, independent	13.8	12.3
Delinquent, aggressive	5.7	73.6
Self- and other-destructive	1.6	81.2
Delusional	2.0	70.0

validity, such as direct examination or referral to treatment, is, as with the unabridged form, low.

Two things should be noted about the screening instrument. First, it is a derivative of a large-scale study of the general population. This is not the more usual strategy in epidemiology, in which the validity and reliability of a screening inventory is typically derived from a case-control study in a clinical context prior to launching a general population study. In fact the investigators suggest that by avoiding clinical concepts in the design of this study they eliminated an important source of bias.

Second, the low validity of the questionnaire may in part be due to the wide age span of the children for whom it is intended—six to eighteen years. Considering the pronounced developmental trends in individual behavioral items reported for this sample, as well as others, it taxes rather heavily any single set of items to perform equally well at all ages. As an empirically derived screening inventory, however, it represents a notable contribution to compare with other instruments similar in design.[21]

The first step in examining the role of social factors in child behavior status was a comparison of families in the general population with welfare families. Children in the cross-sectional sample were characterized by intrafamilial problems—delinquency and weak group membership—and dependency. Welfare parents reported more illness, marital dissatisfaction, and economic problems than the cross-sectional parents, and were seen as more restrictive and cold toward their children.[22]

Other demographic, parental, and parent-child factors were examined in relationship to specific kinds of child behavioral adjustments. Parental coldness, for example, was associated with conflict with parents, peers, and siblings, and with delinquency. In general, parent-child factors, such as punitive or cold parents, and membership in a racial minority group carry the greatest predictive power at both Time 1 and Time 2. Table 7 summarizes the predictive capacity of five of the most powerful factors, chosen on the basis of the number of child behavior factors with which they are uniquely correlated, that is, on partial correlation coefficients, at either or both times of measurement. Comparison of racial and social class variables reveal that race is significantly associated with delinquent behavior and mentation problems, and that social class is more closely associated with symptoms of anxiety and depression.

In another report this research group challenged the hypothesis that life events, as transient fluctuations of stress, contribute significantly to behavioral problems in children because they are confounded with many ongoing difficulties or sociocultural problems of families.[23] Interpreted in another way, their data suggest that the status of being on welfare or being a member of a disadvantaged minority group in New York City constitutes such a major contributing factor to the development of behavioral disorders in children as to obscure or minimize the role of transiently stressful conditions.

The final group of findings to discuss from this project relates to stability and change of behavioral characteristics in children.[24] Six factors that had the highest correlation with impairment ratings were the focus of analysis; separate comparisons of cross-sectional and longitudinal data were made. In nearly half the comparisons made, however, these two approaches produced discrepant results. Decreasing symptoms of anxiety, increasing delinquent behavior, and increasing conflict with parents, as

TABLE 7. RANK ORDER OF ENVIRONMENTAL PREDICTORS OF BEHAVIOR PROBLEMS AT TWO POINTS IN TIME: NEW YORK FAMILY RESEARCH PROJECT

Predictors	Time 1	Time 2	Times 1+2
Spanish speaking	3	1	4
Punitive parents	4	2	6
Cold parents	2	4	6
Black	6	3	9
Mother excitable/rejecting	1	9	10

demonstrated by the cross-sectional data, were confirmed in the longitudinal analysis. On the other hand, discrepant findings were observed in comparing results on changes in symptoms of isolation, fighting, and mentation problems. When ages beyond midadolescence are examined, the stability of anxiety symptoms parallel the well-established stability of delinquent behavior, indicating that onset of affective disorders after age fourteen or fifteen may have a much longer duration than symptoms of this type occurring in younger children. It would be of interest to know to what extent improvements and deterioration in the home environment accompany changes in behavior.

The limitations of this work relate to the high attrition rate in the longitudinal study, modest validity of methods, and some difficulty in interpreting results clinically. These are essentially the same limitations as described for the Woodlawn Program. The importance of the project is that it represents a successful application of strict empiricism and sophisticated analytical techniques to epidemiological studies in child psychiatry. Both empiricism and an extensive body of statistical methods for social science research are uniquely American products exerting important contemporary influence on the field. The work of the Family Research Project is most significant in demonstrating the influence of environmental sources of variance in child behavior disorders, particularly the paramount importance of racial and cultural factors.[25] In a closing statement of one paper, Langner states that when all demographic, parental, and parent-child factors are taken into account, over 60 percent of the variance in child behavior outcomes are explained.[26]

MARTHA'S VINEYARD CHILD HEALTH SURVEY

The Martha's Vineyard Child Health Survey has a more recent history than the other two studies discussed; it began in 1977. Its objectives are also more limited, in that it covers a smaller sample, in a more restrictive age range, and has a much shorter term of follow up. In the first stage of this project, our purpose was to improve the validity of methods used to determine behavioral variations in young children.

The background for the study evolved from an interest in the influence of early childhood experiences on emotional development. While early childhood development has become a popular area of research in the United States, studies on cognitive development exceed by several-fold those on emotional development. Furthermore, epidemiological studies on the emotional development of preschoolchildren are still quite rare, primarily due to the difficulty in finding suitable sampling frames. The work of Naomi

Richman and colleagues at the Hospital for Sick Children in London represents a milestone in the study of emotional adjustment in children of preschool age from a population perspective.[27] While training as an epidemiologist I had the good fortune to spend a period of apprenticeship with these investigators, and certainly their approach influenced my own.

Sample

Martha's Vineyard is a rural island community off the coast of Massachusetts. This population base was chosen because of its relative stability and because it had been previously involved in an epidemiological study of adult psychiatric disorder.[28] It is an island of low density habitation that seeks to preserve a traditional New England lifestyle; this results in a unique degree of social cohesiveness among islanders.[29] Good housing and well-developed health and social services are characteristics of the community. In recent years the economic base of the island has turned away from the main industries of farming and fishing toward tourism and housing construction. The social changes brought about by this transition represent a major source of community tension. Social class and racial differences are, however, less distinct here than they are in most parts of the United States.

The sample was selected from a register of all families with preschool-age children living as permanent residents of the island. Beginning in 1978 a preliminary study was conducted to determine the prevalance of behavioral problems in the total population of three-year-olds. One hundred of the 110 families selected from the register who had a child approaching age three were successfully interviewed.

These families are similar in most demographic characteristics to families with children in the same age range living in other rural communities in this region of the country, except for one characteristic: 40 percent of the families reported they had moved within the past three years, and 18 percent had moved within the twelve-month period preceding our interviews. The majority of these relocations were on the island, in response to the pressure on housing created by seasonal demands of tourism or by general improvements in the living circumstances of young families.

Rationale and Methods

The project began with a two-year preliminary study in which methods of selecting three-year-olds with behavioral problems from the general population were rigorously examined. The preliminary work has now been completed and two longitudinal studies are underway. The first study will follow the total population sample of three-year-olds involved in the preliminary study; the second will examine the causative role of stressful life events and temperamental characteristics of infants in predicting behavioral status by the age of three. To date, only the results of the preliminary study are available.

In most previous efforts to define behavioral problems in very young children, data have been obtained solely from mothers.[30] In this study we wished to extend the data collection procedures to include interviews with fathers, as well as to carry out a direct assessment of the children's emotional adjustment. The small sample size permitted us a bit more indulgence in data collection than would be the case in a larger-scale study. As a final objective of the preliminary study, the complete data set was reduced to proportions suitable for review by a panel of child mental health professionals.

The methods consist of interviews with parents and a play session with the child, both conducted in the family's home. The parent interview includes questions about family health, social supports, stressful events, and the quality of marital and sibling interactions in the home. A section of the interview contains a series of questions concerning the health and behavior of the three-year-olds; these questions comprise the Behavior Screening Questionnaire (BSQ) of Richman and P. Graham,[31] which is of previously reported validity and reliability, and represents the central measure of behavioral status in the child. The fact that the BSQ has been used in a sample of different national origin and demographic characteristics provides the opportunity to compare our results with those from another population. The questionnaire is based on a symptom-loading technique, which derives a total behavior score by summing across twelve unweighted items of behavior, each rated on a three-point ordinal scale of increasing severity. The possible range of behavior scores is 0 to 24; a score of 10 is arbitrarily set as a cutoff score, at or above which a behavioral problem is defined.

Both parents were interviewed separately and as close in time as possible. Following the interview, 89 percent of the mothers and 74 percent of the fathers completed a questionnaire dealing with the child's temperament. This questionnaire is based on the longitudinal studies of S. Chess and A. Thomas, who have conducted original work on the conceptualization and measurement of temperament.[32]

Following the parents' interviews, a home-based play session with the child was scheduled by two examiners who were unaware of the content of the interviews. The play apparatus used during the session has been adapted for field work from a laboratory study of personality development,[33] and consists of a portable sandbox and a collection of miniature toys. The child was invited to play spontaneously with the toys in the sandbox for twenty minutes. To observe the child making a transition to a more structured situation, a brief developmental assessment was added to this period of free play. Immediately following the session, both observers independently rated the child's play in terms of the quality of the relationship established, expression of emotions, use of language, and the configuration of toys the child played with. In addition to quantitative coding of variables in each of these categories, a detailed narrative of the play session was completed.

This summary and a summary of each parent's interview were prepared for each child. The summaries, consisting of about six pages of information organized in a standard and carefully edited style, represented the material for clinical judgment. A panel of clinical judges rated the protocols. In addition, a complete statistical analysis was performed; only the procedure involving the use of clinical judgment as a criterion of validity for the BSQ will be reported here, however.

Findings

Clinical judgment was made in three separate exercises.[34] In the first two preliminary exercises, six judges rated about one-third of the entire sample of 100 children and then met to discuss their ratings. Satisfactory reliability (greater than .90) and validity (greater than .70) were reached in both exercises, even though a more complex rating scale was derived following the initial exercise. The final clinical rating scale derived from the preliminary exercises is composed of three distinct components—severity; need for intervention; and prognosis (Table 8).

Two of the six judges were assigned to read through protocols for the entire sample. Figure 1 shows results obtained when the ratings of the two judges were averaged. Bars extending above the abscissa represent the frequency of children rated "noncases" at different behavior scores; bars below the line represent children rated "cases." The definition of "caseness" required both judges to agree on assigning the child to a moderate-to-severe degree of impairment.

The BSQ appears to function well in distinguishing cases from noncases along the dimensions of severity and need for intervention, but not so satisfactorily on the dimension of prognosis. Visualizing the distribution of cases and noncases in this way is more informative than stating

TABLE 8. REVISED CLINICAL RATING PROCEDURE:
MARTHA'S VINEYARD CHILD HEALTH SURVEY

SEVERITY RATING (5 Points)

Based on the degree to which the problem reflects emotional suffering in the child or interferes with significant interpersonal relations.

INTERVENTION RATING (3 Points)

Based on the need for extrafamilial help in reducing the severity of behavioral problem in the child.

PROGNOSIS RATING (3 Points)

Based on the degree that the child's behavioral problem and social environment predict mental status by school age.

---

the relationship as a correlation coefficient, since it can be more clearly seen that judges were using the same information in somewhat different ways in assessing the three separate components of the rating scale.

The validity of the BSQ as a screening instrument can also be represented in the form of sensitivity and specificity, two familiar epidemiological concepts. Table 9 gives sensitivity and specificity values and their formulae for the BSQ at three different thresholds along the distribution of behavior scores. Several other commonly employed expressions of validity used by epidemiologists are also shown in the table.

The accuracy of the BSQ as a measure of the clinical severity of behavioral adjustment is a function of the cutoff point chosen. In a clinical context the choice of the lower threshold (most sensitive) is recommended, as it is desirable to reduce the number of false negative cases to a minimum. The resulting higher number of false positives would be eliminated in the diagnostic process. As a screening instrument for study in general population groups, the higher threshold (most specific) is recommended as it decreases the probability of false positives, but increases the number of false negative cases. No matter which threshold is used, however, the number of children found to have behavioral problems in this population is high. The most accurate prevalence estimate is based on those cases in the entire population whom both judges agreed had a moderate-to-severe behavioral problem. Based on this criterion, the burden of emotional problems in three-year-olds living in this community is 14 percent.

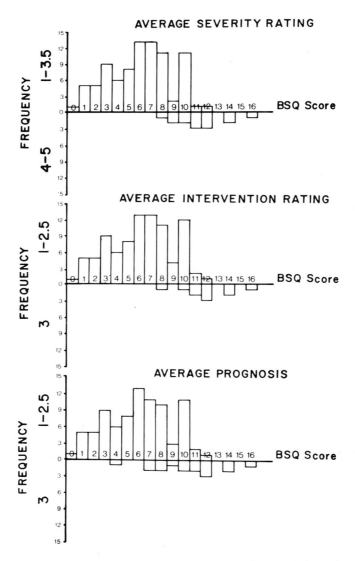

Figure 1. Distribution of averaged clinical ratings by two judges of mothers' BSQ scores in the Martha's Vineyard Child Health Survey. N =100. The horizontal legends represent the range of BSQ scores; the vertical axis, the three clinical ratings: severity, need for intervention, and prognosis. Bars extending above the horizontal axis show the frequency of "noncases"; those below the line, the frequency of "cases."

TABLE 9. MEASUREMENT CHARACTERISTICS OF THE
BEHAVIOR SCREENING QUESTIONNAIRE AT THREE THRESHOLD LEVELS:
MARTHA'S VINEYARD CHILD HEALTH SURVEY
(PERCENTAGES)

Characteristic	Formula	T 1 (BSQ = 8)	T 2 (BSQ = 10)	T 3 (BSQ = 11)
Sensitivity	$\dfrac{TP}{TP+FN}$	100	78	64
Specificity	$\dfrac{TN}{TN+FP}$	70	85	98
Predictive value positive	$\dfrac{TP}{TP+FP}$	35	46	82
Predictive value negative	$\dfrac{TN}{TN+FN}$	100	96	94
False positive rate	$\dfrac{FP}{TN+FP}$	30	15	2
False negative rate	$\dfrac{FN}{TP+FN}$	0	12	36

NOTE: TP = true positive; TN = true negative; FP = false positive; FN = false negative.

The fact that so many children at such an early age are experiencing serious degrees of emotional distress is a disturbing finding, but it is similar to findings reported in the London study.[35,36] These prevalence estimates are also strikingly similar to figures reported for older children and adults.[37-39] It may be that the majority of the problems are of relatively short duration, and if that is the case the incidence of behavioral problems between early and middle childhood must be quite high in order to maintain such prevalence rates.

Now that the selection of children with behavioral problems has been convincingly achieved in our work, the association of social, temperamental, and observational play variables is underway. At present we are limited to the concurrent association of these variables with behavioral problems, although our prospective, longitudinal study is designed to make inferences about causation. Thus far in our data analysis we have been impressed with the dominant influences of certain temperamental variables in children with behavioral problems. Two clusters of traits, "low distractability," an index of stubbornness, and "high intensity" of emotional expression, are the major temperamental characteristics associated with behavioral problems.

It is perhaps not surprising that a poor or disruptive marriage is the major social variable associated with behavioral problems. When the quality of the parents' marriage and the two temperamental variables are taken into account, the remaining contributions of parent-child interaction, stressful life events, social supports, and other temperamental variables add very little to the level of explained variance in our measures of behavioral adjustment.

The particular power of the temperamental variables in predicting mental health status over long intervals in childhood has been pointed out by E. Werner and R. Smith in a summary of another important American epidemiological study on the island of Kauai.[40] These investigators interpret their findings to mean that psychiatric disorders in children are greatly influenced by a biological contribution to behavior represented in the measurement of temperament.

We are hesitant to draw a similar conclusion from our work for two reasons. First, there is an unresolved conceptual issue involving the extent to which the temperament questionnaire used is valid. Here validity is taken to mean the extent to which the questionnaire actually provides an estimate of a biological component of behavior. In the Kauai study perinatal stress strongly interacted with maternally related features of the early child-caring environment. The second problem is a methodological one: the measurement of behavioral problems and temperamental characteristics are based on parents' reports, and therefore may be influenced by the same kinds of biases.

In our future work we hope to more clearly separate social and temperamental variables as predictors of emotional status in children, on the measurement of emotional adjustment per se, by using a prospective, longitudinal design. At this point, we are convinced that very young children in general population groups have as high a prevalence of behavioral problems as older children. The predictive meaning of this can only be determined in longitudinal studies that ask not only what goes wrong in emotional development, but how competence is achieved. It is in this sense that we believe our work is relevant to the primary prevention of psychiatric disorders in children. Behavioral problems as measured in our study can be used as a means of evaluating children's emotional adjustment quite early in life in a systematic and inexpensive way.

It must be stressed, however, that behavioral problems in this age group are not the same as psychiatric disorder in older children. Children at age three still possess the resiliency to respond quickly and positively to improvements in their circumstances. Our objective in this preliminary phase has been to demonstrate that a simple measurement approach such as the BSQ is a valid indicator of emotional maladjustment, and that its application can be successfully replicated in different geographic, cultural, and national settings.[41]

Our next goal is to isolate causes for differences measured by the BSQ and to suggest preventive trials that decrease the incidence of behavioral problems in young children. This work should lead to important new dimensions in stimulating an international perspective in preventive child psychiatry.

CONCLUSIONS

These three studies represent epidemiological approaches to the study of psychiatric disorder, or the risk of psychiatric disorder, in children from a general population perspective. Together they suggest that the prevalence of behavioral problems is uniformly quite high throughout childhood. They say very little about the incidence of psychiatric problems during childhood, however, although the first two, as completed longitudinal studies, might well have had this as a major objective. Measures of incidence and duration are more important than prevalence, as they can more clearly be used to document causal and sustaining influences in the course of psychiatric disorder. The incidence and duration of various types of psychiatric disorders may be quite different from one population group to another, although the prevalence of all types of disorders measured at one point in time may be similar. Moreover, similar types of behavior problems might be caused by different kinds of agents, or different combinations of explanatory variables.

Much work remains to be done on validity and reliability of psychiatric disorders in children before causal theories will have much scientific value. All three investigations have been plagued with the problems of validity and reliability, which have limited their efforts to demonstrate the influence of associated social and biological factors.[42] What is of most interest in comparing the three studies is their very different approaches to the measurement of behavioral problems. While using quite different concepts and techniques for children of different ages, it is striking that the Family Research Project reported a prevalence of 13.5 percent, and the Martha's Vineyard study a prevalence of 14 percent. Whether these findings are artifacts of the methods used or accurate reflections of the level of suffering among children in these communities is unknown. Resolution of this dilemma is not feasible as long as major differences exist in defining psychiatric disorder.

I suggest that a major handicap in epidemiological child psychiatry in the United States is the desire of each investigator to create a new and therefore untested assessment technique to measure behavioral adjustment. The time has come to develop an attitude that encourages and promotes replication of a few well-established interviewing and questionnaire methods, not only for the purpose of investigating behavioral disorders in different settings, but because there is a need to know how the same techniques work when used by different research teams. Few well-standardized methods have been translated into languages other than English,[43] and this too is a primary need in stimulating cross-cultural and cross-national research in epidemiological child psychiatry. In the United States, the introduction of a new diagnostic manual that attempts to delineate disorders through a multiaxial framework is a promising development[44] that I believe will stimulate a continuation of the present ascendency of epidemiology as a basic science in child psychiatry.

NOTES

1. M. Rutter, J. Tizard, and K. Whitmore, *Education, Health and Behaviour* (London: Longmans, 1970).

2. C. Shaw and H. McKay, *Juvenile Delinquency and Urban Areas* (Chicago: University of Chicago Press, 1942).

3. F. Earls, "Epidemiology and Child Psychiatry: Historical and Conceptual Development," *Comprehensive Psychiatry* 20 (1979): 256-69

4. L. Srole, T.S. Langner, S.T. Michael, et al., *Mental Health in the Metropolis: The Midtown Manhattan Study* (New York: McGraw-Hill Book Publishing Co. 1962).

5. D.C. Leighton, J.S. Harding, D.B. Macklin, et al., *The Character of Danger—Psychiatric Symptoms in Selected Communities. The Stirling County Study of Psychiatric Disorder and Sociocultural Environment*, vol. 3 (New York: Basic Books, 1963).

6. S.G. Kellam, J.D. Branch, K.C. Agrawal, et al., *Mental Health and Going to School: The Woodlawn Program of Assessment, Early Intervention and Evaluation* (Chicago: University of Chicago Press, 1975): 3-24.

7. S.G. Kellam and J.D. Branch, "An Approach to Community Mental Health: An Analysis of Basic Problems" *Seminars in Psychiatry* 3 (1971): 207-25.

8. S.G. Kellam, M.E. Ensminger, and M.B. Simon, "First-Grade Antecedents of Teenage Drug Use and Psychological Well-Being: A Ten-Year, Community-Wide Prospective Study," in *Origins of Psychopathology: Research and Policy*, ed. D. Ricks and B. Dohrenwend (Cambridge: University of Cambridge Press, forthcoming).

9. S.G. Kellam, "Stressful Life Events and Illness: A Research Area in Need of Conceptual Development," in *Stressful Life Events: Their Nature and Effects*, ed. B.S. Dohrenwend and B.P. Dohrenwend (New York: John Wiley, 1974).

10. Kellam, Branch, Agrawal, et al., *Going to School* (See note 6).

11. S.G. Kellam, M.E. Ensminger, and J. Turner, "Family Structure and the Mental Health of Children: Concurrent and Longitudinal Community-Wide Studies," *Archives of General Psychiatry* 34 (1977): 1012-22.

12. Kellam, Ensminger, and Simon, "Teenage Drug Use" (See note 8).

13. Ibid.

14. T.S. Langner, E.D. McCarthy, J.C. Gersten, et al., "Factors in Children's Behavior and Mental Health Over Time: The Family Research Project," in *Research in Community Mental Health*, vol. 1, ed. Robert Simmons (Greenwich, Connecticut: Jai Press, 1979).

15. E.L. Greene, T.S. Langner, J.H. Herson, et al., "Some Methods of Evaluating Behavioral Variations in Children 6 to 18," *Journal of the American Academy of Child Psychiatry* 12 (1973): 531-53.

16. T.S. Langner, J.C. Gersten, E.L. Greene, et al., "Treatment of Psychological Disorders among Urban Children," *Journal of Consulting and Clinical Psychology* 42 (1974): 170-79.

17. Ibid.

18. J.G. Eisenberg, T.S. Langner, and J.C. Gersten, "Differences in the Behavior of Welfare and Non-Welfare Children in Relation to Parental Characteristics," *Archives of the Behavioral Sciences* 48 (1975): 1-33.

19. J.G. Eisenberg, J.C. Gersten, T.S. Langner, et al., "A Behavioral Classification of Welfare Children from Survey Data," *American Journal of Orthopsychiatry* 46, no. 3 (1976): 447-63.

20. T.S. Langner, J.C. Gersten, E.D. McCarthy, et al., "A Screening Inventory for Assessing Psychiatric Impairment in Children 6 to 18," *Journal of Consulting and Clinical Psychology* 44 (1976): 286-96.

21. T. Achenbach, "The Child Behavior Profile: An Empirically Based System for Assessing Children's Behavioral Problems and Competencies," *International Journal of Mental Health* 7 (1979): 24-42.

22. Eisenberg, Langner, and Gersten, "Welfare and Non-Welfare Children" (See note 18).

23. J.C. Gersten, T.S. Langner, J.G. Eisenberg, et al., "An Evaluation of the Etiologic Role of Stressful Life-Change Events in Psychological Disorders," *Journal of Health and Social Behavior* 18 (1977): 228-44.

24. J.C. Gersten, T.S. Langner, J.G. Eisenberg, et al., "Stability and Change in Types of Behavioral Disturbance of Children and Adolescents," *Journal of Abnormal Child Psychology* 4 (1976): 111-27.

25. Langner, McCarthy, Gersten, et al., "Family Research Project" (See note 14).

26. T.S. Langner, J.C. Gersten, and J.G. Eisenberg, "The Epidemiology of Mental Disorders in Children: Implications for Community Psychiatry," in *New Trends in Psychiatry in the Community*, ed. G. Serben (Cambridge, Massachusetts: Ballinger Publishing Co., 1977).

27. N. Richman, J.E. Stevenson, and P. Graham, "Prevalence of Behavior Problems in Three-Year-Old Children: An Epidemiological Study in a London Borough," *Journal of Child Psychology and Psychiatry* 16 (1975): 277-87.

28. M. Mazer, *People and Predicament* (Cambridge: Harvard University Press, 1977).

29. Ibid.

30. F. Earls. "The Fathers (Not the Mothers): Their Importance and Influence with Infants and Young Children," *Psychiatry* 39 (1976): 209-26.

31. N. Richman and P. Graham, "A Behavioral Screening Questionnaire for Use with Three-Year-Old Children: Preliminary Findings," *Journal of Child Psychology and Psychiatry* 12 (1971): 5-33.

32. S. Chess and A. Thomas, *Temperament and Development* (New York: Brunner-Mazel, 1977).

33. J.H. Block and J. Block, "The Role of Ego-Resiliency in the Organization of Behavior," in *Minnesota Symposia on Child Psychology*, vol. 3, ed. W.A. Collins (New York: Lawrence Erlbaum, 1979).

34. F. Earls, G. Jacobs, P. Goldfein, et al., "Concurrent Validation of a Parent Questionnaire Used to Select Three-Year-Old Children with Behavior Problems," paper in preparation.

35. Richman, Stevenson, and Graham, "Study in a London Borough" (See note 27).

36. F. Earls and N. Richman, "The Prevalance of Behavior Problems in Three-Year-Old Children of West Indian-Born Parents," *Journal of Child Psychology and Psychiatry*, 21 (1980): 999-1070.

37. Langner, Gersten, Greene, et al., "Disorders among Urban Children" (See note 16).

38. M. Rutter, A. Cox, C. Tupling, et al., "Attainment and Adjustment in Two Geographic Areas: Prevalence of Psychiatric Disorder," *British Journal of Psychiatry* 126 (1975): 493-509.

39. A. Leighton, "Research Directions in Psychiatric Epidemiology," *Psychological Medicine* 9 (1979): 235-47.

40. E. Werner and R. Smith, "An Epidemiologic Perspective on Some Antecedents and Consequences of Childhood Mental Health Problems and Learning Disabilities," *Journal of the American Academy of Child Psychiatry* 18 (1979); 292-306.

41. F. Earls, "The Prevalence of Behavior Problems in Three-Year-Old Children; A Cross-National Replication," *Archives of General Psychiatry*, in press.

42. _____, "Epidemiological Methods for Research in Child Psychiatry," in *Studies of Children*, ed. F. Earls (New York: Neale Watson Academic Publications, forthcoming).

43. C. Zimmerman-Tansella, S. Minghetti, A. Tacconi, et al., "The Children's Behavior Questionnaire for Completion by Teachers in an Italian Sample: Preliminary Results," *Journal of Child Psychology and Psychiatry* 19 (1978): 167-73.

44. Task Force on Nomenclature and Statistics, *Diagnostic and Statistical Manual of Mental Disorders*, 3rd ed. (Washington: American Psychiatric Association, 1978).

EPIDEMIOLOGICAL APPROACHES TO CHILD MENTAL HEALTH IN DEVELOPING COUNTRIES

Philip J. Graham

INTRODUCTION

Over four-fifths of the world's children live in countries characterized by a level of economic development incapable of sustaining even an adequate standard of nutrition for a sizable proportion of their populations. In these so-called developing countries, although social disadvantage is recognized as an important adjunct of poor economic conditions, and has consequently been the focus of much attention, psychological well-being is not usually reckoned to be a matter of pressing importance. Among health professionals, especially those who work with children, the prevention of poverty, malnutrition, and infection by programs of agricultural and industrial development, together with specific mass immunization campaigns and family planning, are understandably placed at the top of the priority list for action. It is the purpose of this paper to suggest that even in the present circumstances, when so many other matters are demanding the attention of governments of developing countries, there is a need to consider the field of child mental health a great deal more seriously than is the case at the present time.

DEFINITION

First, how is mental health defined in a developing country? In Western Europe and North America the existence of specialized professional groups has resulted in a tendency to separate epilepsy from other manifestations of

28

brain dysfunction and damage, which are treated by pediatricians and pediatric neurologists; mental retardation, by psychologists and specialists in mental handicaps; and psychiatric disorders or emotional and behavioral problems, by child psychiatrists.

The scarcity of medical manpower in developing countries has prevented such specialization from emerging; all manifestations of disturbed functioning of mind and brain tend to be dealt with to a much greater degree by a single group of professionals. In this respect professional organization in developing countries tends to resemble that which still exists in parts of Eastern Europe. In passing it may perhaps be worth observing that this situation is not without its advantages, especially in the degree to which it encourages doctors who treat the mentally ill to value and retain their biological approach. For our purposes, however, we surely need to note that the term "child mental health," when used by most professionals working in developing countries, includes epilepsy, neurological and developmental disorders, mental retardation, and emotional and behavioral problems.

LINKS WITH MALNUTRITION

The case for the importance of these child mental health problems rests on two broad supports: their relevance to the major health problems of malnutrition and infection, and their need for attention as potent causes of suffering and disability in their own right. First, let us consider how child mental health is relevant to undernourishment and infection, the main causes of mortality in the developing world.

At times of a major national catastrophe, such as that currently overwhelming Cambodia, everyone who cannot escape the affected area tends to suffer. Most malnutrition is not, however, caused by such overwhelming misfortune; rather it occurs among populations chronically exposed to the hazards of a type of agricultural production sufficient to meet the needs of some but not all their members. Nutritional adequacy is further threatened by inappropriate dietary habits, which result in children suffering from malnutrition even when there is enough food to meet their needs. In these circumstances it has been demonstrated that cases of malnutrition in children largely occur in families exposed to poor standards of home care and a lack of stimulation.[1]

It is well recognized that the effects of nutritional disorders such as kwashiorkor include depression and apathy. These adverse physiological features inhibit the individual from fending adequately for himself, and thus available sources of food are not tapped and the vicious cycle persists. Programs of stimulation, however, speed the rate of recovery of the malnourished child.[2]

What has been less adequately studied is the primary effect of psychological factors such as maternal deprivation. It has been observed, for example, that the advent of a new baby who displaces the twelve- to eighteen-month-old toddler from the breast puts the older child at nutritional hazard. Less attention has been given to the possibly adverse psychological effect of handing the older child over to a grandmother at this point.* Toddlers in developed countries who are partially rejected by their mothers in this way may suffer psychologically, but they will become malnourished only in unusual instances.

In developing countries, where there is barely enough food anyway, stress of this type may set off a more devastating chain of events. Such factors operate at a personal level. At a social level one needs to consider the deskilling that takes place when the social change that occurs—for example, when a family migrates to a city—results in parents who are separated from their families losing the knowledge and means to maintain their children in the hygienic conditions available in their original homes.

In addition to their role in causation, the adverse physical, cognitive, psychological, and psychiatric sequelae of malnutrition and infection deserve attention. In developed countries the rate of cerebral palsy among children tends to be in the region of 2 per 1,000; epilepsy 8 per 1,000; and severe mental retardation 3 per 1,000.[3] Evidence of the rates of these conditions in developing countries, which is summarized later in this paper, is perhaps less secure, but it does indicate that they are generally higher.

Analyses of the health problems of children seen in clinics in developing countries suggest that the higher rates of brain damage and dysfunction are largely due to infectious diseases, resistence to which is undoubtedly lowered by inadequate nutrition and a lack of specific immunizations. H.G. Edgell and J.P. Stanfield, on the basis of their experience in a pediatric neurology clinic in Uganda, claim that the etiological significance of catastrophic infections is of greater importance than birth trauma in the causation of brain damage in children in that part of the world.[4]

The problem of estimating rates of severe mental retardation in developing countries will be discussed later, but the levels of acute and chronic infectious diseases affecting the brain that afflict their children make it certain that mental handicap is one outcome of malnutrition. The results of a number of controlled studies such as those of F.G. Monckeberg[5]

_____

* R. Giel: personal communication.

and L.F. Cobos and coworkers[6] support this contention. Further evidence exists from studies such as that of B. Ashem and M.D. Janes, who point to clear-cut deficits in cognitive function among malnourished Nigerian children, and to differences in patterns of functioning between well-nourished American and Nigerian preschoolchildren, probably attributable to different social experiences.[7] Although the degree to which deficits are produced by malnutrition or by the accompanying psychosocial disadvantage is a matter of controversy, it seems probable that nutritional deficiencies do contribute to chronic impairment of brain functioning (Figure 1).

Considering the possible behavioral sequelae of malnutrition in a West Indian population, S.A. Richardson and colleagues compared six- to ten-year-old boys who had been admitted to hospital in the first two years of life with kwashiorkor, marasmus, or marasmic kwashiorkor with their siblings and with classroom controls.[8] Compared to their classmates these early malnourished boys showed numerous deficits, especially in classroom behavior and in their peer relationships: they were less cooperative, had poorer memories, were easily distracted, and were less popular. There were, however, few differences between them and their siblings who may have been malnourished but who had not needed hospitalization, so it is

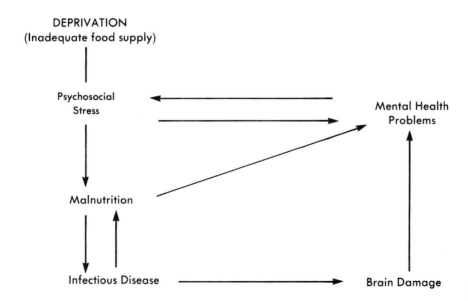

Figure 1. Links between inadequacy of food supply and mental health problems.

uncertain to what degree their deficiencies may have been produced by psychosocial disadvantage or by the direct effects of malnutrition.

In summary, then, it is clear that there are important links between malnutrition, infection, psychosocial disadvantages, and all aspects of child mental health, although how these are mediated is unclear at the present time. These links represent a significant claim for child mental health among those concerned about the scarce resources of developing countries.

CLAIMS OF CHILD MENTAL HEALTH

Child mental health problems are of importance in their own right, however. The well-nourished, fully immunized child who exhibits a severe emotional disorder or who has turned to delinquency as a means of obtaining gratification has a claim to attention that carries its own imperative; and there is reason to believe that such psychiatric disorders may, if consideration is not given to their prevention, rapidly replace the physical conditions of children that currently disturb health professionals in developing countries.

The industrial development acknowledged to be necessary for the economic growth of developing countries is resulting in a rapid trend toward urbanization. It has been estimated that the already vast Latin American cities and their accompanying poverty-stricken shanty towns will double in size every fourteen years. Although a form of dignified family life may be possible in the circumstances such cities provide, the appalling housing and the lack of opportunities for employment, which often result in the temporary or even permanent break up of the family, place stresses on family life that will quite inevitably lead to high rates of childhood behavioral and emotional disorders.

Traditional beliefs and practices, which have formed the matrix of family life and child rearing for centuries, are currently threatened, and, with nothing to replace them, the breakdown of family life becomes more probable. Even to the most sympathetic Western observer, many traditional practices, particularly female circumcision, seem abhorrent; but traditional practices give structure and meaning to life, are often physically harmless, and play a part of great importance in the culture of the peoples who practice them. The disappearence of strong sanctions against socially disapproved behavior, especially in the cities, while doubtless liberating to some degree, is also a potent factor in, for example, the rise in the rate of illegitimacy, the numbers of poverty-stricken, unsupported mothers, and, worse still, in the numbers of children totally abandoned and bereft of family life. It has been estimated that there are currently several million abandoned children in South America.

These factors have already stimulated professionals and lay people in developing countries to take initiatives relevant to mental health problems in children. In 1972, for example, the third Pan-African Psychiatric Congress was devoted to child psychiatry. In 1976 a World Health Organization (WHO) expert committee discussed child mental health and psychosocial development, and its report contained numerous recommendations, mostly relevant to or specifically concerned with the situation in developing countries.[9] The volume of professional attention the subject is receiving from psychiatrists and pediatricians practicing in such settings increases every year. It seems that the subject is therefore one that those who live and work in developing countries wish to establish on a firmer basis.

Although the natural wish of a caring profession when faced with a newly recognized problem is to set up diagnostic and treatment services on as wide a scale as practicable, this approach may not in the present case be so desirable. Lessons learned from Western child psychiatry should enable one to suggest that, when problems are common and not particularly linked to low social status, as is the case with child mental health, available services become rapidly swamped by demands from the middle social class. Treatment methods are readily established, and they become precious to those who practice them, despite lack of evidence of their effectiveness. Inappropriate methods of providing services come to be seen as pioneering achievements, even though they may be no more than sacred cows delivering the milk of human kindness, at considerable expense, to a privileged few. Increasingly, Western societies are realizing they cannot afford this luxury; how much more true is this likely to be for developing countries? In these circumstances, with a view toward prevention, it seems particularly desirable to take an epidemiological approach that will allow identification of the size of the problem and an examination of associated factors. Services may of course be set up at the same time, but experience suggests that planning is likely to be most beneficial if community surveys are undertaken at the same time as services are instituted.

ISSUES IN EPIDEMIOLOGICAL RESEARCH

The application of epidemiological methods to the study of child mental health in developing countries presents certain problems that may be grouped under three main headings: definition of a case; access to the population; and development of suitable methods.

The problem of defining a case is perhaps most relevant to the field of emotional and behavioral disorders. As we shall see later, most investigators have assumed that the same sort of behavior checklists—indeed, in general, exactly the same items in the checklists—can be used to detect emotional and behavioral disorders in developing countries as have been used in Scandinavia, the United Kingdom, and the United States. This approach may be appropriate, but it does seem important, first, to establish the nature of concepts of deviance, disorder, disability, and handicap in each society studied in order to be sure that behavior identified as problematic is indeed perceived as such by the community in question.

The pioneering work of J.H. Orley, who undertook just such a task among the Bagandan people of rural Uganda,[10] surely needs to be extended to other societies. In general, such information as we have suggests that even in isolated rural communities the types of behavior thought to be problematic, and which are brought to the attention of traditional healers, are rather similar to those in industrial societies; but such information cannot be taken for granted. B. Nurcombe and J.E. Cawte, for example, investigating behavioral disorders among the children of an aboriginal population living on an island off mainland Australia,[11] found it necessary to modify the Group for the Advancement of Psychiatry (GAP) classification[12] in order to take into account the types of disturbances they identified. This was because of their dissatisfaction with the applicability of the existing classification, however, rather than a discovery that the aboriginal parents had a different model of deviance than their own.

Access to such populations presents problems that differ from those in industrialized societies. In the United Kingdom, for example, general practitioner records provide a reasonably good coverage of the total population. Because schooling is compulsory from age five to sixteen, up until the last two years, when attendance rates begin to fall off, schoolchildren represent a ready source of total population data. It is not that population access is without its problems in developed countries—various questions such as the importance of confidentiality are often appropriately raised; there is no doubt, however, that the obstacles are harder to surmount and, incidentally, more expensive to surmount, where household surveys offer the only solution to population access.

Finally, the question of the development of appropriate methods to identify cases must be considered. A. Kiev has reviewed methods available to survey researchers in adult psychiatry in developing countries, but there is little information to guide those working with children.[13] Mailed questionnaires are clearly not applicable, and personally administered questionnaires, if adopted from existing checklists, need to be translated and then retranslated independently to check for accuracy. K.K. Minde has successfully achieved this with the questionnaires of Rutter and Conners, but the exercise is clearly not a straightforward one. He describes, for example, how the word "fidgety" has to be translated for use in Uganda as "moving the limbs pretty fast in a funny way like the Konga monkey."[14] The identification of epilepsy in community surveys is also likely to require a great deal of attention to language, particularly if partial seizures that do not involve total loss of consciousness are to be identified.

The use of intelligence tests to identify mental retardation in developing countries is controversial, but such tests seem an inevitable requirement if a serious attempt is to be made to quantify the extent of mental handicap and its associated or etiological features. There seems to be no reasonable objection to this, provided misleading attempts are not made to compare the intelligence of members of one society with that of another.

A more serious stumbling block lies in the lack of tests suitable for use in developing countries, which have been adequately standardized and for which population norms have been obtained. The translation of the Wechsler Intelligence Scale for Children in some parts of India, for example, where the content of the educational system is clearly based on that of industrialized societies, might produce a tool applicable for survey use, but it would be quite inappropriate to use the American or British norms. The standardization of intelligence tests on new populations is an expensive exercise, but the use of such tests in developing countries could have great value in providing a stimulus for scientific work in the area of mental retardation.

EXISTING EPIDEMIOLOGICAL KNOWLEDGE

Despite these obstacles to the advancement of knowledge, a significant amount of epidemiological work has already been carried out in developing countries to assess the dimensions of the problem they face. This work will now be summarized under three main headings: epilepsy; mental handicap; and psychiatric (emotional and behavioral) disorders.

Epilepsy

This condition is more difficult to identify than might be imagined because cultural beliefs surround it with shame. In African village societies, particularly, epilepsy is believed to be brought about by witchcraft; to be infectious; to result in inevitable lowering of intelligence; and to produce violence. Such beliefs help to account for the fact that, even in areas where education is fairly universal, only 25 percent of children with epilepsy are allowed to attend school.[15]

In Chile, using exactly the same survey methods as those employed in a study in the United States, minimum and maximum epilepsy prevalence rates of 21 and 31 per 1,000 nine-year-olds have been recorded—rates roughly double those found in the United States. Greater differences were found in afebrile convulsions.[16] A study in Guam in the Western Pacific, however, albeit in a rather small population, found lower rates, somewhat similar to those found in the United States—2.4 per 1,000 in five- to nine-year-olds and 1.8 per 1,000 in ten- to fourteen-year-olds.[17] In Enugu, Nigeria, in a study of a selected group of middle-class nonpatients, a rate of 14 per 1,000 recurrent or chronic nonfebrile seizures has been reported.[18]

Important differences between epilepsy in developed and developing countries may lie in the nature of the infections—in developing countries, for example, malaria and measles often lead to febrile convulsions—and to the higher risk of a child with febrile convulsions developing nonfebrile epilepsy. G.T. Izuora and J.C. Azubuike suggest that as many as 15 to 21 percent of children with febrile convulsions develop epilepsy in Enugu, but, on the evidence presented, this figure must be treated with caution.[19] It is perhaps worth noting that there appear to be no studies of the prevalence of cerebral palsy in total populations of children in developing countries, although Y. Asifiri has reported that this problem is twice as common in Nigeria as in developed countries.[20]

Mental Handicap

Although, as stated earlier, some psychological tests have been composed for use in developing countries, the lack of standardized data from the populations in which they are to be used means it is difficult to assess the value of prevalence figures sometimes quoted, such as those given by N. Lal and B.B. Sethi.[21] There is moreover a general dearth of epidemiological studies in this area. J.H. Axton and L.F. Levy, discussing their clinical experience of the problem among Rhodesian children, suggest that those with severe mental handicap tend to succumb at an early age.[22] This situation may change. Furthermore, one might expect diagnosed mild and moderate handicap to increase as education becomes more widely available.

The issues and requirements for action in developing countries are well summarized in a recent WHO publication.[23]

Psychiatric (Emotional and Behavioral) Disorders

Overall prevalence. Most of the studies on overall prevalence have been carried out on the African continent and in India. A. Verghese and coworkers conducted a survey in Vellore of 747 children age four to twelve using a three-stage procedure. They found a rate of disorder varying between 66.8 and 81.7 per 1,000 children.[24,25] This rate applied to all those children found to suffer from sleepwalking, enuresis, behavioral disturbance, and mental retardation. It is not possible to calculate from the data presented the rate of psychiatric disorders exclusive of mental retardation, but it is probably in the region of 50 per 1,000.

Lal and Sethi, in a smaller scale study of 272 children age up to twelve years from 109 families living in an urban community, found 11 percent to be suffering from "neurotic and allied disorders."[26] Again no clear-cut criteria are given for the presence or absence of disorders. The same problem exists in interpreting the findings of the study carried out by P.R. Gupta and coworkers of 600 normal preschoolchildren age one to five living in unsanitary conditions in a township in Jaipur. They found an unusually high rate (63.8 percent) of children with disorders, 48 percent of whom manifested pica.[27]

Finally, an interesting investigation of suicide among children living in Bangalore has been reported: there were forty-five deaths among children age fourteen and under over a seven-year period.[28] By comparison, D. Shaffer found thirty-one suicides among the child population of the United Kingdom, which is twenty to thirty times greater than that of Bangalore, also over a seven-year period.[29] Underreporting is a problem here, but one might well imagine that underreporting is more likely to occur in India, so the difference in rate is striking. The available evidence indicates that rates of psychiatric disorder in India are therefore at least no smaller than those in Europe and North America (Table 1).

A small number of surveys have also been carried out in Africa. M. Cederblad conducted a two-stage study of 1,716 children age three to fifteen living in three villages in the neighborhood of Khartoum. The children were initially screened for a variety of symptoms including encopresis, enuresis, sleepwalking, nighttime crying, and stuttering, and, on the basis of this procedure, 197 were selected for more intensive study. The rates obtained

TABLE 1. PREVALENCE OF BEHAVIORAL AND EMOTIONAL PROBLEMS
AMONG CHILDREN IN DEVELOPING COUNTRIES

Area	Age Range (Years)	Rate of Disorder (Percent)	Method of Study	Investigator(s)
Uganda	6-15	18 (Deviance)	Teacher questionnaire	K. Minde (34)
Mornington Island	2-14	10	Interview	B. Nurcombe and J.E. Cawte (11)
Vellore, India	4-12	8	Questionnaire & interview	A. Verghese and A. Beig (25)
Sudan	1-15	10	Questionnaire	T.A. Baasher and H.H.A. Ibrahim (31)
Ethiopian village	0-9	3	Questionnaire & interview	R. Giel, M. Bishaw, and J.N. Van Luijk (36)
	10-19	10		
Ethiopian town	0-9	4		
	10-19	6		

NOTE: Numbers in parentheses after authors' names refer to notes at the end of this chapter.

were compared with those of a similar study carried out on Stockholm children. About 28 percent of the Sudanese children were found to have moderate or severe symptoms. Enuresis and aggressive behavior were found to be somewhat common in Sudanese children; more common among Stockholm children were a larger number of symptoms, mainly neurotic in type—disturbed sleep, headache, tics, nailbiting and thumbsucking, and certain types of antisocial behavior. The data presented suggest that there were no sizable, consistent differences between the two groups of children studied.[30]

A later study of 270 one- to fifteen-year-old children living in another Sudanese village indicated that 10 percent of the children showed "pronounced psychiatric symptoms which may call for medical attention."[31] Minde has reported a series of thorough methodological studies examining rates of behavior and emotional disorders in seven- to fifteen-year-old Ugandan children. Children from three primary schools were screened, using the Rutter teacher questionnaire[32] and the Peterson-Quay questionnaire for parents and teachers; on the basis of Minde's findings, forty-eight potential problem children and thirty-six controls were selected for more intensive individual investigation. Deviance rates were higher than those found in the United Kingdom population, on which the questionnaire had originally been developed; 18 percent of Ugandan children, for example, scored over a predetermined cutoff point on the Rutter questionnaire, compared to 11 percent of boys and 3 percent of girls in the United Kingdom. Furthermore the validity of the questionnaire for use with Ugandan children was to some degree established by the demonstration that parents and teachers agreed to a greater degree than one might have expected on which children were showing disturbance.[33-35]

From the African continent one can quote also the work of Giel and colleagues in Ethiopia. They comment on the fact that children with behavioral disorders are very rarely admitted to clinics for inpatient or outpatient treatment, yet for children who live in towns they found a rate of 4.2 percent disturbance in those age zero to nine and 5.7 percent in ten- to nineteen-year-olds; the rates in villages were 3.1 percent and 10 percent.[36] The evidence from the African continent therefore supports that from India, but it provides additional knowledge in studies directly comparing rates of disorder in children from developing countries with those in industrialized societies.

Nurcombe and Cawte, in their study of aborigines on an island off the coast of Australia, reported a rate of 9.7 percent of children age two to fifteen who showed some form of psychogenic disorder—most commonly consisting either of a "tension-discharge" or an "anxiety-inhibition" syndrome.[37]

It is perhaps also worth commenting that "culture-bound disorders," such as *koro* and *latah*, are rarely reported as occurring in prepubertal children. Children can be, and indeed often are, the object of behavior related to culture-bound beliefs such as "evil eye." The explanation for the lack of culture-bound syndromes in children may reflect the fact that these disorders represent rather well-defined neuroses, anxiety states and hysterical disorders, for example, that appear to require a certain level of psychological and physiological maturity for their manifestation. Other syndromes, such as anorexia nervosa, which is relatively common in some Western societies, do not seem to occur among adolescents in developing countries; with increasing affluence, greater availability of food, access to higher education, and pressure from parents, however, one might expect this situation to change.

Childhood autism does occur in developing countries, although V. Lotter's study suggests that its appearance in African mentally handicapped children may be less frequent than in children of the same level of intelligence in industrialized societies.[38] Total population prevalence figures for this condition are not available for any developing country.

ASSOCIATED FACTORS

The various studies cited in the foregoing pages provide a good deal of evidence of features linked to the presence of psychiatric disorders in developing countries; these will now be summarized.

Sex. Most studies do not quote figures according to sex. In those that do, it seems that, as in Western societies, boys tend to predominate in the rates of "conduct disorder," whereas emotional symptoms are either more commonly present in girls[39] or are found roughly equally in both sexes.[40] In the Vellore study the reversal of sex ratio that occurs with age in the United Kingdom is replicated: under age twelve, boys outnumber girls by 1.3:1; between thirteen and twenty the ratio is 1:1; between twenty-one and thirty it is 1:1.3; and between thirty-one and forty-five it is 1:1.8.[41] From the data provided it seems highly likely that the predominance of boys in the prepubertal period is produced by their higher rate of conduct disorder, and that, as in the United Kingdom, the later preponderance in girls can be attributed to an excess of affective disorders such as anxiety and depressive states.

Social Class. Most studies have been carried out in socially homogeneous groups, but in those where a possible link with socioeconomic status has been investigated either no association has been found,[42] or there has been a slight excess of psychiatric disturbances in children in low socioeconomic groups.[43]

Family Factors. In general, most investigators have not found it possible to study the quality of family relationships, except to examine the relatively crude indicators provided by the presence or absence of a "broken home." If anything, broken homes appear to have a lesser effect on children in developing countries than in Western society; this is most likely due to the higher mortality and lower divorce rates in developing countries. Rutter, reviewing a large number of Western studies, reported a much higher rate of disturbance among children from homes broken by divorce or family break up than among bereaved children.[44] Giel and J.N. Van Luijk found no effect of a broken home on the rate of disorders in Ethiopian children, where parents' deaths are more common (22 percent) than divorce (15 percent).[45] On the other hand, Minde reported more broken and "disorganized" homes among Ugandan problem children than in his control group.[46]

Large family size has also been linked with the presence of a higher rate of disturbance.[47]

It is often suggested that the extended family pattern found in many developing countries, especially among people living in rural areas unaffected by industrialization, has a strong protective influence on child development. The opportunity to form warm and loving relationships with a wide circle of relatives, and the support provided by a large kinship if, for example, a parent is ill, are believed to result in lower rates of behavioral and emotional disturbance. This may be the case, but the evidence for this view is largely lacking.

First, some studies that report relatively high rates involve children living in "extended" families. Second, direct comparisons, such as those of Verghese and A. Beig,[48] have demonstrated either a slightly beneficial effect of living in a joint rather than a nuclear family or a positive disadvantage. In his Ugandan study Minde found polygamous households more related to disturbance than nuclear households.[49]

Finally, some workers, such as B.K. Ramanujam,[50] who have had the opportunity to conduct clinical studies of children from a variety of family types, have identified special problems in extended families related, for example, to the status of a wife, who upon her marriage comes to live with her husband's large family. Orley's experience in Uganda has led him to believe that, although extended family patterns may benefit the active elderly, they may result in the neglect of disturbed young adults, adolescents, and children, who may wander inconsequentially from one part of the family to another without anyone taking responsibility other than to feed them.[51] The subject is clearly ripe for further investigation in other societies.

Urbanization and Social Change. The effects of urbanization on the pattern of life in developing countries are obvious, and it is the impression of all who have studied the scene that urbanization is associated especially with rising rates of delinquency. Kiev, for example, states that:

> Rising delinquency rates in Africa have been attributed to the scattering of the extended family, changing attitudes towards industrialization, polygamy (with its partiality towards the children of favoured wives and the resultant neglect of other children), displacement of families by tribal conflict and political instability, the novelty of city life, child labour, unstable families, alcoholism and cruelty. Indeed it has been blamed at one time or another on all the social and cultural changes that are so characteristic of the developing countries.[52]

One might add to this list of possible causative factors the increase in the amount of personal property—driving a car away becomes a possible delinquent act only when there are cars around to drive away—and growing emphasis on educational achievement. While wider availability of schooling and a more literate population are clearly desirable aims, it has to be noted that educational failure, such a potent cause of disturbance in developed countries, is likely to become important as a stress only when most people are academically successful. The children of preliterate societies do not experience such a sense of failure.

ACTION NEEDED

Although it is customary to acknowledge the variety of situations existing in developing countries, this brief review seems to suggest that, as far as child mental health problems are concerned, the less industrialized countries share many characteristics. Their governments and people are preoccupied with social and economic problems to the understandable exclusion of psychological well-being. There is an assumption that improved economic conditions will bring better physical and mental health. While this may be the case as far as neurological disorders and severe mental retardation are concerned, the reverse may occur with milder mental retardation and with emotional and behavioral problems.

The existing epidemiological evidence presented here suggests that rates of child psychiatric disorders in developing countries, at least in the populations so far studied—and these investigations have been carried out in different types of settings in a variety of countries—are very similar to those in more highly industrialized societies. Further, associated biological and social factors, such as the sex of the child and disharmonious family relationships, appear to be linked rather consistently in most of the cultures studied.

The experience of industrialized societies in this field suggests that the answer to such problems does not lie in concentrating on setting up specialist treatment services. An alternative approach espoused by the WHO Expert Committee on Child Mental Health and Psychosocial Development involves greater emphasis on prevention and on the use of skilled professionals to train and counsel those engaged in the provision of primary health care.[53] To explore this approach further the WHO is now initiating a program in child mental health aimed at encouraging countries to make systematic studies of their own problems and existing resources so that action may be taken that is relevant to the needs of the entire population rather than to the needs of that minority of the middle class able to afford specialized treatment.

If this move toward a public health approach to child psychiatric and allied disorders is to be successful, it needs to be accompanied by an expansion of the types of enquiry described in this review. Topics that seem to require special consideration are the stresses that occur in different types of extended family life; the development of techniques for primary health care staff to use in counseling parents; and improvements in the training of primary health care workers based on the use of such effective methods.

But perhaps more important than any of these factors is the need for governments of, and those living in, developing countries to start to count the cost of the impact of uncontrolled social change on psychological well-being. Sufficient food, better hygiene, higher standards of education—these desirable ends will be worth a great deal less if they are attained by a population disturbed by broken family lives and confused by the loss of a sense of meaning to existence.

NOTES

1. J. Cravioto and E. Delicardie, "Environmental Correlation of Severe Clinical Malnutrition and Language Development in Survivors from Kwashiorkor or Marasmus," in *Nutrition, the Nervous System and Behavior*, (Washington: Pan American Health Organization/World Health Organization, 1972).

2. J. Cravioto and R. Arrieta, "Stimulation and Mental Development of Malnourished Infants," *Lancet* ii (1979): 899.

3. M. Rutter, J. Tizard, and K. Whitmore, *Education, Health and Behaviour* (London: Longmans, 1970).

4. H.G. Edgell and J.P. Stanfield, "Paediatric Neurology in Africa: A Ugandan Report," *British Medical Journal* 1 (1972): 548-52.

5. F.G. Monckeburg, "Effect of Marasmic Malnutrition on Subsequent Physical and Psychological Development," in *Malnutrition, Learning and Behavior*, ed. N.S. Scrimshaw and J.E. Gordin (Cambridge: Massachusetts Institute of Technology Press, 1968): 259-74.

6. L.F. Cobos, C. Latham, and F.J. Stare, "Will Improved Nutrition Help to Prevent Mental Retardation?", *Preventive Medicine* 1 (1972): 185-94.

7. B. Ashem and M.D. Janes, "Deleterious Effects of Chronic Undernutrition on Cognitive Abilities," *Journal of Child Psychology and Psychiatry* 19 (1978): 23-31.

8. S.A. Richardson, H.G. Birch, E. Grabie, et al., "The Behavior of Children in School Who Were Severely Malnourished in the First Two Years of Life," *Journal of Health and Social Behaviour* 13 (1972): 276-84.

9. *Child Mental Health and Psychosocial Development*, Technical Report Ser. 613 (Geneva: World Health Organization, 1977).

10. J.H. Orley, *Culture and Mental Illness*, East African Studies No. 36 (Nairobi: East African Publishing House, 1970).

11. B. Nurcombe and J.E. Cawte, "Patterns of Behaviour Disorder Amongst the Children of an Aboriginal Population," *Australian-New Zealand Journal of Psychiatry* 1 (1967): 119-33.

12. Committee on Child Psychiatry, *Psychopathological Disorders in Childhood: Theoretical Consideration and a Proposed Classification*, GAP Report No. 62 (New York: Group for the Advancement of Psychiatry, 1966).

13. A. Kiev, *Transcultural Psychiatry* (Harmondsworth, England: Penguin Books, 1972).

14. K.K. Minde, "Psychological Problems in Ugandan School Children: A Controlled Evaluation," *Journal of Child Psychology and Psychiatry* 16 (1975): 49-59.

15. J.R. Billingshurst, G.A. German, and J.H. Orley, "The Pattern of Epilepsy in Uganda," *Tropical and Geographical Medicine* 25 (1973): 226-32.

16. N. Chioialo, A. Kirschbaum, A. Fuentes, et al., "Prevalence of Epilepsy in Children of Melpilla," *Epilepsia* (Chile) 20 (1979): 261-66.

17. M.K. Mathai, D.P. Dunn, L.T. Kurland, et al., "Convulsion Disorders in the Mariana Islands," *Epilepsia* (Chile) 9 (1969): 77-85.

18. G.T. Izuora and J.C. Azubuike, "Prevalence of Seizure Disorders in Nigerian Children around Enugu," *East African Medical Journal* 54 (1977): 276-80.

19. Ibid.

20. Y. Asifiri, "Aetiology of Cerebral Palsy in Developing Countries," *Developmental Medicine and Child Neurology* 14 (1972): 230-32.

21. N. Lal and B.B. Sethi, "Estimate of Mental Ill Health in Children of an Urban Community," *Indian Journal of Pediatrics* 44 (1977): 55-64.

22. J.H. Axton and L.F. Levy, "Mental Handicap in Rhodesian African Children," *Developmental Medicine and Child Neurology* 16 (1974): 350-55.

23. *Inter-Country Workshop on Mental Retardation* (New Delhi: World Health Organization Regional Office, 1979).

24. A. Verghese, A. Beig, L.A. Senseman, et al., "A Social and Psychiatric Study of a Representative Group of Families in a Vellore Town," *Indian Journal of Medicine Research* 61 (1973): 608-20.

25. A. Verghese and A. Beig, "Psychiatric Disturbance in Children—An Epidemiological Study," *Indian Journal of Medical Research* 62 (1974): 1538-42.

26. Lal and Sethi, "Estimate of Mental Ill Health" (See note 21).

27. P.R. Gupta, A.K. Dutta, and P. Dutta, "Growth and Development. A Cross-Sectional Study of Pre-School Children," *Indian Journal of Pediatrics* 45 (1978): 189-95.

28. K. Sathyavathi, "Suicide among Children in Bangalore," *Indian Journal of Pediatrics* 42 (1975): 149-57.

29. D. Shaffer, "Suicide in Childhood and Early Adolescence," *Journal of Child Psychology and Psychiatry* 15 (1974): 275-92.

30. M. Cederblad, "A Child Psychiatry Study on Sudanese Arab Children," *Acta Psychiatrica Scandinavica*, suppl. 200 (1968).

31. T.A. Baasher and H.H.A. Ibrahim, "Childhood Psychiatric Disorders in the Sudan," *African Journal of Psychiatry* 1 (1976): 67-78.

32. M. Rutter, "A Children's Behaviour Questionnaire for Completion by Teachers," *Journal of Child Psychology and Psychiatry* 8 (1967): 1-11.

33. Minde, "Ugandan School Children" (See note 14).

34. _____, "Children in Uganda: Rates of Behavioural Deviations and Psychiatric Disorders in Various School and Clinic Populations," *Journal of Child Psychology and Psychiatry* 17 (1978): 23-27.

35. K.K. Minde and N. Cohen, "Hyperactive Children in Canada and Uganda: A Comparative Evaluation," *Journal of the American Academy of Child Psychiatry* 17 (1978): 476-87.

36. R. Giel, M. Bishaw, and J.N. Van Luijk, "Behaviour Disorders in Ethiopian Children," *Psychiatrica, Neurologica et Neurochirurgica* (Amsterdam) 72 (1969): 395-400.

37. Nurcombe and Cawte, "Aboriginal Population" (See note 11).

38. V. Lotter, "Childhood Autism in Africa," *Journal of Child Psychology and Psychiatry* 19 (1978): 231-44.

39. Cederblad, "Sudanese Arab Children" (See note 30).

40. Verghese and Beig, "Disturbance in Children" (See note 25).

41. Verghese, Beig, Senseman, et al., "Families in a Vellore Town" (See note 24).

42. Minde, "Ugandan School Children" (See note 14).

43. Verghese and Beig, "Disturbance in Children" (See note 25).

44. M. Rutter, *Maternal Deprivation Reassessed* (Harmondsworth, England: Penguin Books, 1972).

45. R. Giel and J.N. Van Luijk, "On the Significance of a Broken Home in Ethiopia," *British Journal of Psychiatry* 14 (1968): 957-61.

46. Minde, "Ugandan School Children" (See note 14).

47. Verghese and Beig, "Disturbance in Children" (See note 25).

48. Ibid.

49. Minde, "Ugandan School Children" (See note 14).

50. B.K. Ramanujam, "Psychiatric Problems of Children Seen in an Urban Centre of Western India," *American Journal of Orthopsychiatry* 45 (1975): 490-96.

51. Orley, *Culture and Mental Illness* (See note 10).

52. Kiev, *Transcultural Psychiatry* (See note 13).

53. *Psychosocial Development* (See note 9).

DISCUSSION

Effects of Malnutrition

In malnutrition the importance of one factor, psychosocial stress, should be emphasized. The well-known clinical symptomatology is apathy. The lack of interaction between children with relatively moderate malnutrition relates to a lack of stimulating interaction with their mothers that literally distorts the mother-child relationship.

The malnourished infant is a nonstimulating, nongratifying child, and hence the malnutrition can lead to mental retardation. It is also an important problem in terms of prevention and treatment, because in nutritional rehabilitation everything possible must be done to decrease the stress factor and to enrich the cultural milieu in which the child lives; otherwise nutritional recovery is frequently prolonged and less complete.

Parasitic Diseases

In the terminology of the World Health Organization, "communicable disease" is used in addition to infectious and parasite-induced disease. Parasitic disease in children is extremely prevalent in developing countries, and parasites have a direct effect on nutrition and circulation. In parasitic disease there is not only nutritional competition with the host, but continuous hemorrhage of the gut and intestinal malabsorption. We are all familiar with the neurological aspects of malaria in children.

Need for Epidemiological Research

We need valid epidemiological research in developing countries to help us understand the consequences of psychological abnormalities and disturbances that appear in those regions of the world. One or two factors might contribute to the increasing rate of disorders in traditional societies. Undoubtedly there are stresses associated with long-standing practices: it would be amazing, for example, if female circumcision were not associated with a great deal of mental suffering among those involved. The fact that such practices are of great importance because they give some meaning to those societies makes one suspect they are no less stressful, and they therefore bear examination for that reason.

From a selfish point of view, if better epidemiological data were available from developing countries, those working in socially and economically more fortunate circumstances might learn a great deal from an understanding of the mechanisms associated with social change.

Studies in Kenya

Professor Robert A. Levine at Harvard has been conducting studies using the interesting technique of showing Kenyan mothers videotapes of American mothers interacting with their infants, and inviting the Kenyan women to comment on what they thought they saw.

In one film an American mother playing with her baby on a table turns away to get a diaper and the baby begins to cry; in a matter of moments the mother returns with a clean diaper. The Kenyan women were outraged that the mother would let her baby cry like that; they felt one must hold the baby and talk to it when it cries.

In another sequence the baby is being played with by a grandmother, who draws very close and engages in vigorous interactive play; the Kenyan women who watched this scene thought the grandmother disliked the baby because she was much too rough.

When Levine asked the Kenyan mothers to describe problems among their two-year-old children, the worst problem was that a child would cry when its mother left it to go out and work in the fields; most American mothers would be distressed if the child did not protest when they went to work.

But the Kenyan economy requires women to return to work soon after the infant reaches age three or four months, and the child must learn to accept being cared for by older siblings or other children in the compound. A child who cries when the mother leaves is therefore exhibiting a behavior problem.

Child Rearing in Developing Countries

Most epidemiological studies on child-rearing practices in developing countries have been carried out in relative homogeneous populations where the opportunities to contrast the effects of different practices have not existed. Studies published in the 1950s on the effect of different child-rearing practices on personality development generally used a psychiatric or psychological framework, which is difficult to interpret in terms of later concepts of emotional and behavioral problems. Nevertheless it does seem as though particular types of child rearing could be correlated with certain kinds of later personality development.

Earlier fundamental social anthropologists such as Bronislaw Malinowski and Margaret Mead were not very preoccupied with psychological deviance. Consequently, although one may read occasional interesting anecdotes, they do not provide any really systematic information. It is a field wide open to further investigation.

Long-Term Predictors

One of the dilemmas in child mental health work and in longitudinal studies is how long an impact must an identified stress factor have before it is given credit for being significant; on the other hand, how radically is the child's personality formed by early events so as to be impervious to the future. The notion of looking for long-term predictors denies in some sense the validity of intervening experience; it is an epigenetic viewpoint.

Kellam's work is impressive in terms of the long-term predictability of first-grade teacher ratings of shy versus aggressive boys; the long-term prediction does not hold up as well for girls. Shy boys seem to be the worst off from an emotional point of view; on the other hand, in high school it is the aggressive boys who usually engage in drug use. From the perspective of psychiatric symptoms, however, they seem rather well adjusted.

So, in Kellam's study, whatever coupling there is between social adaptation and psychological well-being in the first grade is lost at follow up. Perhaps too much emphasis is placed on long-term follow up: the assumption should be that prevalence does not change.

No epidemiological research in child psychiatry has attempted to define incidence and duration from the very outset of the study. Assumedly one would find that in fact many disorders, particularly emotional disorders, are of short duration, but with much turnover in terms of who is being identified at certain points.

Criteria for Diagnosis

Researchers at the National Institute of Mental Health are trying to plan an epidemiological study of child mental health in order to find an instrument that might serve a large-scale survey. No one in the group has been brave enough to suggest that the time before age six be included in the criteria for making specific diagnoses of children. How does one categorize young children in terms of psychopathology?

In the study being conducted by Earls, the investigators try consciously not to use the term "psychiatric disorder" for children who are being defined with the questionnaire and interview techniques; it is assumed that having high scores on the questionnaire, or being defined by clinical judgment as having a problem, is a signal of stress or distress in a child, and that if it goes undetected it may result in psychiatric disorder. The significance of the project is in fact related to primary, not secondary, prevention; these children are not considered to be in need of traditional psychiatric treatment. At least that is the way the study started out.

As it unfolds, however, the types of children who are defined as having emotional problems by the clinical judges—roughly 14 percent of the population—are diagnosed by six psychiatrists as having a psychiatric disorder; so more than just parent education is needed. When factor analysis and cluster analysis are done on that small group, the classical dimensions of conduct and neurotic disorders are observed. Boys are primarily characterized as having temper tantrums, being aggressive outside the home, and having poor peer relationships; more girls than boys are characterized as having fears and worries. So the study suggests that these types of disorders are in fact being crystallized at a younger age than was believed when the project began. Although it may seem too soon, age three may in fact be a reasonable age at which to hazard a traditional psychiatric diagnosis.

Observations of Children at Play

Earls was asked if he had looked specifically at the play items in the interviews to see if they were useful in predicting specific behavior problems as identified by the adult raters; at age three a standardized interview should involve indirect rather than direct information.

That was a very interesting part of the study: in the home-based play interviews with a child the investigators observed big differences in the child's ability to adapt, that is, leaving the mother to engage in play, making a play construction, and then making the transition back to normal circumstances—given the fact that two strangers with lots of equipment, including videotape, were carrying out these activities in the home. Statistically, then, variables such as the child's relationship to the examiner and ability to adapt and cope in the play situation correlate strongly with the mother's reports of behavior problems.

The clinical judges, however, were wary of using that source of data in making their evaluations, and they also used the narrative description of what the child did in different ways. They weighted it, and those who were psychoanalytically inclined tended to weight the relationship to the examiner very heavily, as well as levels of anxiety as revealed in the child's behavior; those who were more eclectically inclined tended to use observations and not to infer states in the child.

They were therefore quite surprised when the statistical analysis produced good correlations. Both the psychoanalytically and nonpsychoanalytically inclined judges agreed in their ratings of the parents' reports of the children.

Minority Group Families

In his study, Langner did not handle the issue of correlation between demographic and parenting factors very well. If one reads his reports closely, however, there are correlations between certain child-rearing styles and identification as a minority group family. A distinction has to be made between black families and Spanish speaking families, however, because their child-rearing orientations are quite different. Of the four parenting factors listed, there was a correlation between punitiveness and being black; other correlations are less clear.

One point Langner makes is that transient stresses, that is, factors such as mothers being ill or hospitalized, are of no great significance in producing psychiatric disorders over time: the factors predicted are those that have to do with systematic difficulties, such as being in a disadvantaged minority group for long periods of time. Langner also makes the point that these factors have such a strong influence they tend to minimize, although correlate with, certain parent-child interactive factors. That certainly seems to be the spirit of the discussions in his report.

Early Identification of Disorders

Naomi Richman has followed a group of children from age three to eight, and it is quite clear that the disorders identified at three have very considerable significance to the later development of emotional and behavioral problems, at least at age eight. One measure, perhaps the most valid one, is that 60 percent of the problem group defined at age three were disturbed at age eight, compared with something like 22 percent at age three in the control group, consisting of children with no problems.

In Richman's study it was of course possible to look at the factors related to the development of disturbance in a group of hitherto undisturbed children, as it was in Rutter's Isle of Wight study, in which a group of children were studied from age ten to fourteen. It was possible to investigate how newly developed disorders differed from persisting ones. The way different stress factors are important at different ages is a very important area of work for the future; results are already being obtained that are relevant to its understanding.

One of the rationales epidemiologists should keep in mind is how changes are brought about in natural ways. Some interesting sources for epidemiological work are the political-economic changes occurring in many countries. We know very little, for example, about how definitions of disorders have changed in places such as China or Cuba. Certainly over the next ten to fifteen years it would be of interest to conduct studies on how, for example, Nicaragua is designing better preventive services, and whether or not they are having any effect on changing rates of disorders—or even on types of existing disorders.

II. MENTAL RETARDATION

AN EPIDEMIOLOGICAL STUDY OF SEVERE MENTAL DEFICIENCY IN CHILDREN

Roger Salbreux*

Mental deficiency causes impairment of social competence to varying extents in those afflicted. This is particularly obvious in children when they are faced with the need to come up to the standards required at school.

In an epidemiological approach to mental deficiency we believe, with Z.A. Stein and M. Susser, that there are three aspects to be taken into consideration: deficiency, disability, and handicap.[1] Biological *deficiency* originates from an anatomical lesion or an error of metabolism; functional *disability* is demonstrated in psychological terms of structure or efficiency; and a *handicap* is essentially of a social nature since it brings the individual face-to-face with her or his peer group. A study of these factors and their frequency of appearance at a given time (incidence) provides information on the chronological sequence of events and on their respective weightings, thus helping in etiological correlations; but it gives a poor assessment of disability and handicaps, which become apparent only as time passes. The ratio of the number of cases observed to the surviving population as a whole over a given period of time (prevalence) is of more interest to us, because it assesses the needs of mentally deficient as compared to healthy children, that is, it takes their handicap into consideration.

* For the completion of these extensive studies, the author is indebted to a team of physicians, psychologists, secretaries, statisticians, and a translator: M. Auriol, G. Auzoux, M. Bach, J.M. Chaaban, C. Chartier, J.M. Deniaud, M. Diaz, N. Diederich, N. Duplant, C. Gazard, J. Grancoin, C. Levy, M. Leterrier, V. Lochard, B. Rougier, N. Yankelevich, and M. Zafiropoulos. I am indebted, especially, to the statisticians for their patient and untiring labors.

Several surveys on this subject have recently been made in France: we shall first mention the work of C. Lévy in the Department of Seine et Marne,[2] and of F. Hatton and coworkers in the Department of Haute Vienne.[3] Later we shall refer particularly to the coordinated studies carried out in the Ile de France, in Auvergne, and in Meurthe et Moselle, by the author and his colleagues,[4] by C. Col and X. Bied-Charreton,[5] and by M. Manciaux and coworkers,[6] respectively. At various stages E. Zucman and S. Tomkiewicz have been closely associated with the studies.*

These studies reach the conclusion that it is misleading to try and establish the prevalence of mental deficiency when it is slight (IQ of 66-90) or even medium (IQ of 51-65) in form. Indeed in these types of mental deficiency, intellectual level appears closely correlated to success or failure in school and to the parents' social and cultural levels.[7] Moreover, nearly half of "maladjusted" schoolchildren have a normal intellectual performance, with IQs of over 80 or 90.[8,9] These "false" mentally impaired or pseudosubnormal children do not really seem to be basically different from youngsters with slight mental deficiency, or even from some cases of medium subnormality.

Whatever the level of their IQs, these maladjusted children show striking correlations with factors in their emotional and, particularly, cultural environment. Criteria of risk in the emotional field are more often found among "false" cases of mental impairment, and social determinants are frequently found in true cases of subnormality. This is only a question of degree, however, and it would not seem proper to separate the children merely on the basis of differences in their IQs. In both types of cases there is a serious risk in the educational field as a result of partial nonconformity to social requirements in the school system that are too selective; successful performance requires a high social and cultural background and a well-balanced family life. The label "handicapped" so often put on such children fails to take into account the dynamic nature of the underlying mental structure and the elementary rules of any kind of education.[10,11]

Such an analysis does not necessarily cast doubt on the heuristic value of the intelligence quotient as a means of locating and classifying mental deficiencies. The tests certainly prove workable and are convenient for the demarcation of intellectual capacity into wide areas. But surveys confirm how pertinent are the many criticisms made in the past few years of the use of collective tests, metric scales whose contents are concerned mainly with school, and, especially, the calculation of a precise figure and the interpre-

* E. Zucman, technical adviser, Centre Technique National d'Études et de Récherches sur les Handicaps et les Inadaptations (CTNERHI); S. Tomkiewicz, director, U.69 Institut National de la Santé et de la Récherche Médicale (INSERM).

tation given to it in terms of personal deficiency and biological constant. A psychometric approach assesses the present capabilities of a subject, but it cannot state what she/he is fundamentally, outside the constraints of time: it can determine what has become of the subject in comparison with her/his peers.[12]

For this reason the authors of the studies mentioned earlier have not managed, and have refused to attempt, to establish the prevalence of slight or even medium mental deficiency, whereas a study by the author demonstrates that there are available in France 300,000 places in specialized educational institutions for school-age children with slight mental handicaps.[13] Fortunately the number of places has very little connection with prevalence.[14]

These considerations explain why the majority of epidemiological surveys undertaken so far have dealt with severe mental deficiency (IQ $\leq$ 50), which actually raises far fewer theoretical and practical problems. Although cultural weighting is present, it is less important; the predominance of organic determinants is more obvious. We shall return to this later.

METHODOLOGY

The epidemiological survey of severe maladjustment in the juvenile population of the Paris area, made between 1972 and 1975, gave no priority to mental deficiency, although it did include it. Its object was to record, as exhaustively as possible, children born in the Paris Ile de France region—which consists of eight departments and accounts for one-sixth of the population of France—in 1965 and 1966 who had suffered from handicaps severe enough to lead to their *exclusion from the normal school system*. It was thus a retrospective study based on files, but with numerous sources of information that cross-checked and complemented one another, and that, once the data from these sources were compiled on a single record card, provided 4,236 observations, each consisting of fifty coded variables. It should be mentioned that all the authorities concerned with severe handicaps at any level—case finding, care, education, and administration—were consulted.

The epidemiological survey carried out in Auvergne, more or less during the same period, 1974–77, covered two rural departments, Cantal and Puy-de-Dôme. Its target, also, was children born in 1965 and 1966, and was based on the same methodology, using the same record card. Observations thus collected on 390 children who were unable to attend school were exactly comparable with the observations made in the Ile de France region.

The data were processed by computer and, for statistical analysis, classical techniques were used: contingency tables with chi-square test and factorial analysis.

RESULTS

Prevalence of Severe Mental Retardation

The survey in the Paris area provided a breakdown of children excluded from the normal school system in accordance with their intellectual levels (Table 1): 820 had IQs of ≤ 50, and, of these, 254 had IQs of ≤ 30. According to the Institut National de Statistiques et d'Études Économiques (INSEE), the number of survivors of the two age groups concerned was 303,839, thus prevalence was 2 percent for severe subnormality and 0.9 percent for severe retardation, that is, a total of 2.9 percent.

A similar calculation, made for purposes of comparison with the data from the survey in Auvergne, showed a prevalence of 3.5 percent for severe subnormality and 1.4 percent for severe retardation, a total prevalence of 4.9 percent.

An average established on the basis of fourteen surveys covering 945,113 children between age five and nine gave a rate of 2.85 percent, with a standard deviation of 0.71;[15] all the surveys made in rural areas give a figure in the neighborhood of 5 percent. This leads us to the conclusion that Puy-de-Dôme and Cantal account for the difference between the prevalence rates in Ile de France and in Auvergne, particularly since the influence of Cantal, the less urbanized of the two departments, predominates in the origin of this deviation.

The prevalence of trisomy was 1.1 percent, and 0.62 percent of these cases were of a level below 50; one mentally deficient child in five therefore had Down's syndrome.

No survey, however meticulous it may be, can claim to be absolutely exhaustive. Thus a critical review of the Auvergne survey has already been started[16] and will be continued. The few comparisons mentioned here, however, together with the trisomy rate, may be considered as reliability tests.

TABLE 1. DISTRIBUTION OF THE POPULATION IN EPIDEMIOLOGICAL SURVEY IN THE PARIS AREA ACCORDING TO INTELLECTUAL LEVEL.

	No Information	Not Susceptible to Testing	Vegetative	IQ ≤30	IQ 31-50	IQ 51-65	IQ 66-90	IQ ≥91
Numbers	302	284	54	200	566	773	1,301	756
Reduced percentage[1]	—	7.22	1.37	5.08	14.39	19.65	33.07	19.22

820 = 20.84% (Vegetative, ≤30, 31-50)

2,057 = 52.29% (66-90, ≥91)

NOTE: 1) The reduced percentage is calculated after exclusion of those on whom there was "no information," and assumes that the breakdown for the latter is the same as for the rest of the population.

SOURCE: R. Salbreux, J.M. Deniaud, S. Tomkiewicz, et al., "Typologie et Prévalence des Handicaps Sévères et Multiples dans une Population d'Enfants. Premiers Résultats de l'Enquête Épidémiologique sur les Inadaptations Sévères dans la Population Juvénile de la Région Parisienne," *Revue de Neuropsychiatrie de l'Enfance et de l'Adolescence* (Paris) 27 (1979): 9.

The Place of Mental Deficiency

In the Paris survey only 20.84 percent of the children with severe mental deficiency had serious maladjustment problems; the 52.29 percent of those with IQs over 66 were the ones who were excluded from school attendance. These children, who theoretically should be able to go to school, need to be checked for the causes of their nonattendance in order to better understand the place of mental deficiency in the group of youngsters with severe handicaps and maladjustments who constitute the population covered by the survey.

As shown in Table 2, behavioral disorders—whether in isolation (IQ ≥ 91) or associated with slight mental deficiency (IQ 66-90)—head the list, with a total of 1,244 cases, or more than half of all causes. But exclusion from school may also be due to physical handicaps, which even in isolation—IQ ≥ 91 and with no behavioral disorders—lead, though less frequently, to the same result.

The total number who could not be accepted in school represented 13.94 percent of the children in the Paris area, and 17.53 percent in

TABLE 2. EPIDEMIOLOGICAL SURVEY IN THE PARIS AREA.
CAUSES OF NONATTENDANCE AT SCHOOL OF CHILDREN WITH
SLIGHT DISABILITY OR OF NORMAL INTELLIGENCE (IQ ≥ 66)

	Number	Percentage
Behavior disorders	1,244	60.5
Hypacusia or deafness	281	13.7
Cerebral palsy	187	9.1
Amblyopia or blindness	139	6.8
Severe epilepsy	111	5.4
Child psychosis	102	5.0
Noncerebral motor disability	93	4.5
Heart disease	83	4.0
Total	2,240	109.0

SOURCE: R. Salbreux, J.M. Deniaud, S. Tomkiewicz, et al., "Typologie et Préva-lence des Handicaps Sévères et Multiples dans une Population d'Enfants. Premiers Résultats de l'Enquête Épidémiologique sur les Inadaptations Sévères dans la Population Juvénile de la Région Parisienne," *Revue de Neuropsychiatrie de l'Enfance et de l'Adolescence* (Paris) 27 (1979): 9.

Auvergne; 1.5 percent would therefore seem to be an acceptable figure, and cases of severe mental deficiency were only one-fifth of these.

Associations and Multiple Causes

Mental deficiency very rarely occurs in isolation, and we shall now describe its most important associations in accordance with intellectual level.

BEHAVIOR DISORDERS

Children with severe subnormality and retardation are assumed to show fewer psychopathic disorders than the population as a whole. As the level rises the proportion of behavioral disorders increases, reaching a patently high level: IQ between 65 and 90. We therefore find that behavior disorders play a fundamental role in the process of exclusion from school of children whose IQs are above 50, and, particularly, in the 65-90 group; perhaps more tolerance is shown toward cases of severe abnormality for the very reason that their deficiency is so serious (Figure 1).

With regard to psychotic manifestations, we should note, first, that since they are found at all levels they have no connection with IQ, although there is a definite decrease for those with IQs of over 66 (Figure 2). Furthermore, a very high proportion of psychotic states is found among children who are not susceptible to testing, a fact obviously linked to the very nature of their behavior.

The 414 psychotics* make it possible to calculate a prevalence of mental deficiency of 1.37 percent. This figure may clarify certain variations in prevalence according to different conceptions of the boundary between child psychosis and deficiency.

PHYSICAL IMPAIRMENTS

The presence of an isolated cardiopathy is found in children with IQs of between 30 and 50, a level at which many cases of trisomy are detected (Figure 3).

There is also a very significant correlation between mental deficiency and short stature of over 3 standard deviations (SDs) (Figure 4). This

---

* The 388 children for whom psychometric assessment was attempted (Figure 2), and twenty-six about whom we have no information in this connection.

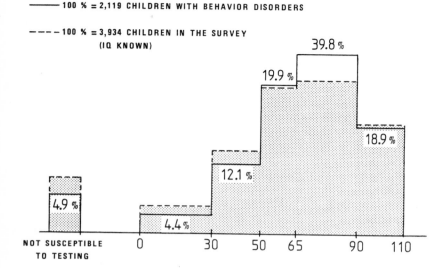

Figure 1. Histogram of behavior disorders by IQ groups.
SOURCE: R. Salbreux, J.M. Deniaud, and B. Rougier, "Étude de la Déficience Mentale dans la Région Parisienne. Á Partir des Premiers Résultats d'une Enquête Épidémiologique," *Revue de Pédiatrie* (Paris) 14 (1978): 389-400.

histogram shows particularly clearly the opposition that exists between IQs of ≤ 65, often accompanied by a decrease in height of at least 3 SDs, and IQs of ≥ 66, where the absence of organic impairment is manifest in all spheres, but chiefly in terms of development of height.

In cases of severe subnormality and retardation, a study of weight as compared to height shows very clearly a high proportion of excess weight of at least 3 SDs. Thus, in addition to the well-known picture of small stature and low weight, we find small stature with obesity in cases of severe mental deficiency.

MOTOR IMPAIRMENT

Two-thirds of the severely retarded and 23.7 percent of the severely subnormal have a motor impairment, compared to only 12.6 percent of subjects with IQs ≥ 91. A statistically significant link is found between intelligence quotient and the severity of motor impairment. But there is also a link with the form of motor impairment, which is much more

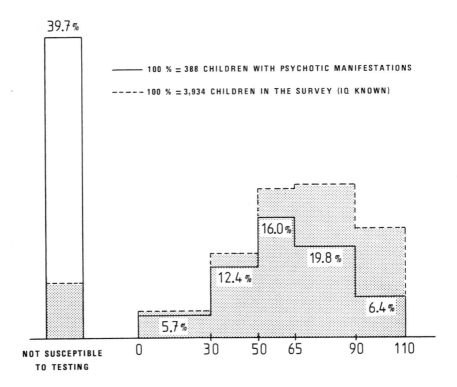

Figure 2. Histogram of psychotic manifestations by IQ groups.
SOURCE: R. Salbreux, J.M. Deniaud, and B. Rougier, "Étude de la Déficience Mentale dans la Région Parisienne. Á Partir des Premiers Résultats d'une Enquête Épidémiologique," *Revue de Pédiatrie* (Paris) 14 (1978): 389-400.

frequently quadriplegic in cases of severe subnormality and retardation, and, more often, hemiplegic in cases of medium subnormality.

As a consequence of these phenomena, cerebral palsy patients with IQs of ≥66 represent less than one-third of those with motor impairment of cerebral origin (Figure 5).

EPILEPSY

Epilepsy is much more prevalent among the severely subnormal, and is even found more frequently among the severely retarded than among the other children in the survey. Thus epilepsy was found in 54.2 percent of the

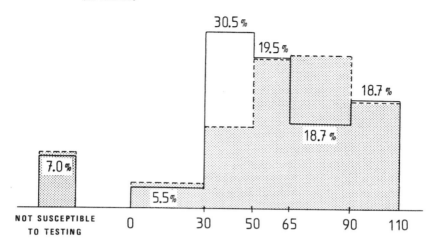

Figure 3. Histogram of the presence of an isolated cardiopathy according to IQ.
SOURCE: R. Salbreux, J.M. Deniaud, and B. Rougier, "Étude de la Déficience
Mentale dans la Région Parisienne. Á Partir des Premiers Résultats d'une Enquête
Épidémiologique," *Revue de Pédiatrie* (Paris) 14 (1978): 389-400.

severely retarded and 26.7 percent of the severely subnormal, compared to
5.8 percent of the subjects with a level of ≥ 91. The significant link between
the severity of epilepsy and level of intelligence is shown in Figure 6.

SENSORY DISORDERS

Visual anomalies. Blindness is closely linked to mental deficiency, particularly
to severe retardation, whereas amblyopia has a bimodal distribution: very
slight in cases of severe retardation; more marked in normal subjects.

Defective hearing. Deafness does not seem to have any connection with
mental deficiency. A moderately high proportion of hypacusia is observed
only in children with IQs of ≥66, and a very high proportion of deafness in
subjects with normal intelligence.

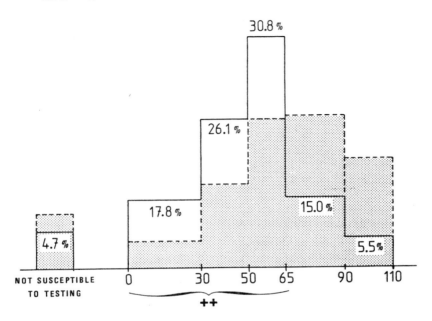

Figure 4. Histogram of heights at least 3 standard deviations below average according to IQ groups.
SOURCE: R. Salbreux, J.M. Deniaud, and B. Rougier, "Étude de la Déficience Mentale dans la Région Parisienne. A Partir des Premiers Résultats d'une Enquête Épidémiologique," *Revue de Pédiatrie* (Paris) 14 (1978): 389-400.

Importance of the Concept of Multiple Handicaps

The various handicaps in Table 2 total 2,240, which is higher than the corresponding fraction of the 2,057 children in the survey with IQs of ≥ 66 (Table 1); this is due to the existence of multiple handicaps in some subjects. The complexity of multiple handicaps, however, is revealed only by an overall analysis of the epidemiological survey and, particularly, in two instances:

• When, for example, we try to summarize various categories of handicaps into a single variable in order to study the influence of the categories on another variable, such as the organization of care.

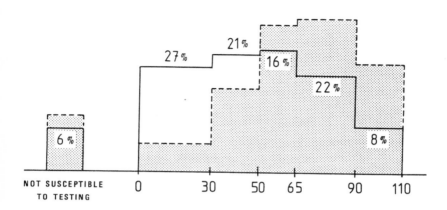

Figure 5. Histogram of cerebral palsy patients by IQ groups.
SOURCE: R. Salbreux, J.M. Deniaud, S. Tomkiewicz, et al., "Typologie et Préva-
lence des Handicaps Sévères et Multiples dans une Population d'Enfants. Premiers
Résultats de l'Enquête Épidémiologique sur les Inadaptations Sévères dans la
Population Juvénile de la Région Parisienne," *Revue du Neuropsychiatrie de l'Enfance et
de l'Adolescence* (Paris) 27 (1979): 5-28.

• When we attempt to work out a separate prevalence for each
disability or maladjustment.

In such cases we find ourselves faced with numerous handicaps
superimposed on one another. Because of the frequency of associations
present in the population, the number of handicaps exceeds the number of
handicapped persons by 41 percent, so that the crude prevalence of a
handicap increases the needs of those who are handicapped.

In an attempt to understand how these associations of handicaps are
made up, three factorial analyses were made and all the combinations
achieved identified. The conclusions drawn may be formulated as follows:

• There is a definite link between the severity of mental deficiency and
the number of associated handicaps; the majority of vegetative and severely
retarded children have two or three extra handicaps, whereas 80 percent of
the children who were "not susceptible to testing" suffered from one
handicap only: a psychotic personality.

• The high frequency of behavior disorders of a psychopathic nature—

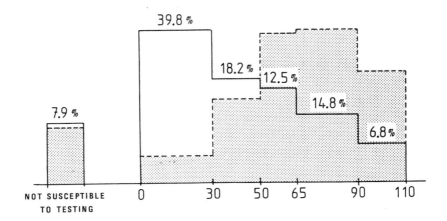

―――― 100 % = 88 CHILDREN WITH SEVERE EPILEPSY
(MORE THAN 12 FITS EACH YEAR).

―――― 100 % = 3,934 CHILDREN IN THE SURVEY (IQ KNOWN)

Figure 6. Gravity of epilepsy according to IQ.
SOURCE: R. Salbreux, J.M. Deniaud, and B. Rougier, "Étude de la Déficience Mentale dans la Région Parisienne. Á Partir des Premiers Résultats d'une Enquête Épidémiologique," *Revue de Pédiatrie* (Paris) 14 (1978): 389-400.

53.6 percent in the epidemiological survey—conditions the number of associations, which, on the one hand, are twice as frequent when these types of manifestations are taken into consideration, and, on the other, are not independent of the level of intelligence, as shown in Figure 1. As can be seen, there is a distinctly high proportion of slight subnormality, that is, IQs of 66-90.

• Above all, the existence of a behavior disorder in a child with an IQ of ≤50, who already has several organic handicaps, will in no way change her/his status as a case of multiple handicaps, whereas the existence of such a disorder in a child with an IQ of between 66 and 90 will be sufficient to give rise immediately to the idea of multiple handicaps.

These findings have led to the formulation of two proposals for exclusive categorization:[17]

• The first is aimed at detecting and isolating the most frequent associations of handicaps, and summarizing the descriptions of them in a single variable that can be applied to a study of the means to deal with severe handicaps. Subjects with multiple handicaps are separated into several groups, determined more by the nature of their handicaps or associations than by their number.

• The second, on the contrary, is based on respecting the accepted classifications; it avoids superimposition by setting up a priority ranking of the handicaps when one obviously dominates the others, as, for example, in severe mental deficiency. At the same time, this allows for a class of multiple handicaps in cases where the association is not limited to one or another of the handicaps present. An attempt has been made in Figure 7 to depict a model for such categorization. In this diagram only the rectangles in unbroken lines correspond to a classification that does not overlap with another. The small rectangles in broken lines concern 541 of the 713 children with a level of intelligence of ≤50. The diagram demonstrates three types of subjects with multiple handicaps whose circumstances are entirely different.

Group A contains associations of organic handicaps in the absence of severe mental deficiency or behavior disorders. These children present original and complex problems of rehabilitation, deaf-blind, for example, and are comparatively few in number.

Group B consists of children with severe mental deficiency (IQ ≤50) who have manifestations of a psychopathic nature, especially so-called psychotic behavior; 76 percent of them have numerous additional problems, however, such as physical impairments, usually malformations, motor disorders, epilepsy, and sensorial—especially visual—deficiencies.[18] Severely retarded children (IQ ≤30) in particular often suffer from a number of impairments, and have two or three handicaps associated with their condition. But mental retardation is always at the center of the clinical picture, and the presence of additional problems simply calls for improvements in their care, especially closer medical supervision.

Group C covers children with medium and, most especially, slight mental subnormality, who suffer from behavior disorders of a psychopathic nature. Although by definition the epidemiological survey is not concerned with children in school, those with psychopathic disorders comprise nearly a quarter of the population analyzed. The number can be calculated from what has been said earlier about slight and medium subnormality; they tend to fail in tests and also to fail in their school work; some are excluded from the normal school system, while others are kept in regular classes or put in special schools. These children represent one of the great social problems of our time, for although their "behavior disorders" expose the turmoil caused by emotional and sociocultural factors, they also reflect intolerance of the environment; but here again we do not consider their

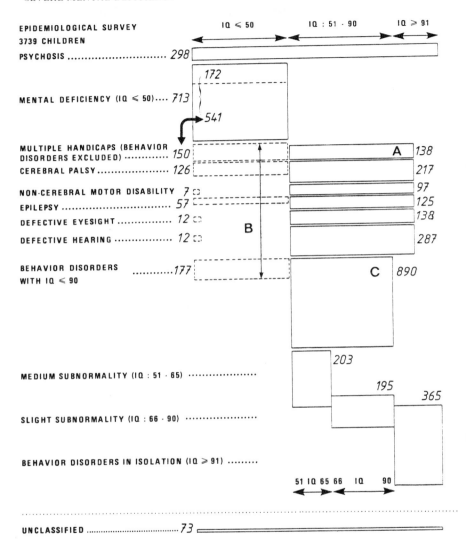

Figure 7. Classification of handicaps into twelve groups.

Source: R. Salbreux, J.M. Deniaud, S. Tomkiewicz, et al., "Typologie et Prévalence des Handicaps Sévères et Multiples dans une Population d'Enfants. Premiers
Résultats de l'Enquête Épidémiologique sur les Inadaptations Sévères dans la
Population Juvénile de la Région Parisienne," *Revue de Neuropsychiatrie de l'Enfance et
de l'Adolescence* (Paris) 27 (1979): 5-28.

association with slight mental subnormality as constituting a multiple handicap.

Mental Deficiency and Social Factors

Whatever the degree of mental deficiency, the environment appears to be a determining factor.

The study in Meurthe et Moselle showed the correlations that exist in school life between intellectual level, on the one hand, and, on the other, sex; the father's professional status; nationality of the parents; family life; birth rank; residence in urban or rural areas; number of people living in the home; and whether or not the child had space for her/himself, and, if so, how much.[19] Inhibition in speech or lateness in speaking and enuresis, which often reflect emotional difficulties in early childhood, seem to be important indicators.[20]

The study in the Paris area also confirmed the inequality of risk according to the social group to which a child belongs, even for the severely handicapped (Figure 8). According to the social and professional categories of the INSEE, a significant difference is apparent in the distribution of the population covered by the study. It will be noted that the more privileged social classes—managerial staff, schoolteachers, and middle-level professional personnel—are poorly represented, whereas there is a high proportion of the less-privileged social classes such as employees, skilled workers, and laborers; semiskilled workers constitute an exception that has not been explained.

Handicaps of "organic" origin appear to be equally distributed among the various social and professional categories. Defective intelligence and personality disorders are unequally distributed, however, and significant differences are apparent among various social groups. The most striking divergence is the high proportion of slight subnormality among children of the managerial class; a similarly high proportion manifest psychotic behavior. Behavior disorders of a psychopathic nature seem to be more frequent at the other end of the social scale, among children of domestic staff, a category in which the highest proportion of slight subnormality is found.

What the study in the Paris area showed up most is the inequality of access to existing facilities, not only according to the nature or degree of the handicap, which is normal, but according to the social and economic status of the family, which is less acceptable.[21]

A few facts are worthy of special note:

 • Requests for simple solutions, such as individual rehabilitation

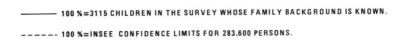

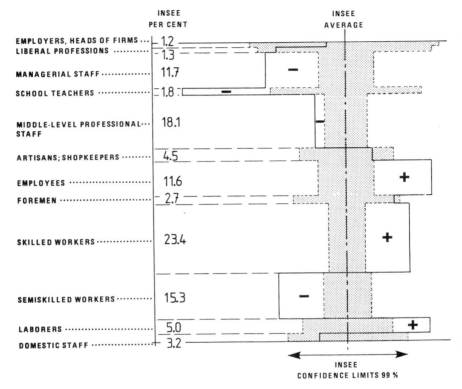

Figure 8. Comparison of the epidemiological survey and the general population of the Paris area: distribution by social and professional categories.
SOURCE: R. Salbreux, J.M. Deniaud, and B. Rougier, "Étude de la Déficience Mentale dans la Région Parisienne. Á Partir des Premiers Résultats d'une Enquête Épidémiologique," *Revue de Pédiatrie* (Paris) 14 (1978): 389-400.

therapy by a professional, ambulatory care through a "centre médico-psycho-pédagogique" (CMPP), or admission to special classes, are *partial* solutions geared to the specific disorders and/or needs of the child—for example, psychotherapy or special instruction for those with defective eyesight or hearing. Such requests are made chiefly on behalf of children with a normal or slightly subnormal level who suffer from physical handicaps or psychological difficulties (Figure 9).

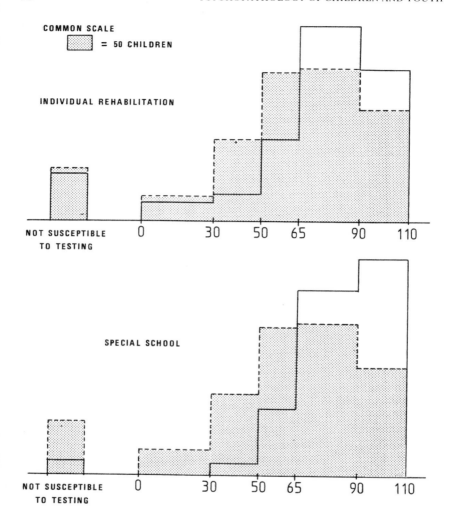

Figure 9. Organization of care and level of intelligence.
Source: R. Salbreux, J.M. Deniaud, S. Tomkiewicz, et al., "Typologie et Préva-
lence des Handicaps Sévères et Multiples dans une Population d'Enfants. Premiers
Résultats de l'Enquête Épidémiologique sur les Inadaptations Sévères dans la
Population Juvénile de la Région Parisienne," *Revue de Neuropsychiatrie de l'Enfance et
de l'Adolescence* (Paris) 27 (1979): 5-28.

• Requests for day care, which entails *global* care without separation from the family group, are for the most part made on behalf of medium or severely subnormal children who may attend medical day care educational institutions; psychopathic children are assigned to day hospitals (Figure 10).

• Requests for residential facilities are made for severely retarded and vegetative children (Figure 10), but they may also be made because of certain multiple handicaps that are difficult to cope with, such as serious psychomotor impairment, severe epilepsy, blindness, or certain psychoses.

An important fact becomes apparent with regard to cases of medium and severe subnormality: it is the number of associated handicaps rather than their severity that determines requests for residential care; this is demonstrated in Figure 11.

For children from the privileged social sector, the parents' request, the team's recommendation, and the implementation of the solution coincide perfectly and result in simple care in specialized classes.

Children from less-privileged social classes appear to be penalized by the fact that their parents are not well-informed and often do not make a request. In such cases the team usually recommends residential care, sometimes against the wishes of the parents.

The number of places available seems for the most part to be satisfactory, except for certain special schools and residential establishments fairly close to the family home. Some switching among categories is observed, however, which leads to unsatisfactory utilization of facilities; furthermore these are poorly distributed geographically. This "perversion" of institutions from their original purposes tends to raise difficult financial problems and to create, artificially, a permanent shortage of facilities to care for the most serious cases of mental deficiency.[22]

Our research on adolescents and adults, which consists of an epidemiological portion and a medical-social portion, had made it possible to clarify the characteristic "path" followed by mentally handicapped persons toward their fate: it traverses a *hermetically closed institutional system*—family, specialized establishment, asylum—in which there is considerable variation in the quality of care and of education. Such "channels" are almost completely watertight, and only in 17.5 percent of cases does the path not follow the usual pattern; indeed some of them describe themselves as going "from birth to death." In particular, the decisive role of the first orientation appears extremely important, and, here again, the type and severity of the handicap obviously are considered, but the subject's social background influences social patterns that determine the future of the mentally deficient.

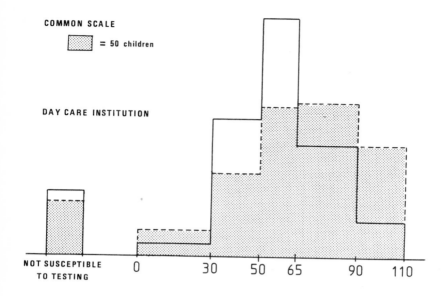

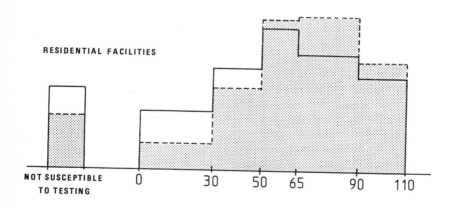

Figure 10. Type of care given and level of intelligence.
SOURCE: R. Salbreux, J.M. Deniaud, S. Tomkiewicz, et al., "Typologie et Préva-
lence des Handicaps Sévères et Multiples dans une Population d'Enfants. Premiers
Résultats de l'Enquête Épidémiologique sur les Inadaptations Sévères dans la
Population Juvénile de la Région Parisienne," *Revue de Neuropsychiatrie de l'Enfance et
de l'Adolescence* (Paris) 27 (1979): 5-28.

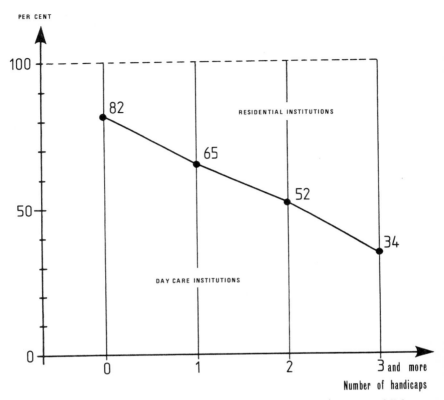

Figure 11. Percentage of placements in residential and day care establishments according to the number of supplementary handicaps.

Source: R. Salbreux, J.M. Deniaud, and B. Rougier, "Étude de la Déficience Mentale dans la Région Parisienne. Á Partir des Premiers Résultats d'une Enquête Épidémiologique," *Revue de Pédiatrie* (Paris) 14 (1978): 389-400.

DISCUSSION

An epidemiological approach tends to confirm that the mentally deficient are divided into two main groups:

• *Cases of slight and medium mental deficiency*, undoubtedly including a number of false mental deficiencies, where the sociocultural and emotional implications are clearly predominant. The association, in many cases due to circumstances, between behavior disorders and this clinical framework of difficulties, mainly connected with school and with no obvious organic origin, should be considered as a manifestation of *unrest* in a child, and a reflection of the degree of *tolerance* of the environment, rather than as a second handicap over and above mental deficiency, thus creating a so-called multiple handicap.

• *Cases of severe mental deficiency*, in which the many additional organic impairments fit into a many-faceted clinical picture, but with mental deficiency predominant; these manifestations make it difficult to give a prognosis of practical autonomy, and sometimes make social integration quite impossible. Nevertheless, in practice it seems feasible to give these mentally deficient subjects a single form of care, whatever the clinical complexity of their encephalopathy.

This distinction is of course oversimplified, but, based as it is on the most recent epidemiological data, it avoids the confusion between serious and slight forms,[23,24] which psychometry helped to foster by showing all mentally deficient children as lacking to differing degrees one particular faculty: intelligence.[25] It dispels the illusion of proportionality attached to the model of linear development suggested by the false concept of constancy in the intelligence quotient, which studies by genetic psychologists, on the one hand, and psychoanalysts, on the other, had already largely brought into disrepute.

These studies highlight the effect of psychosocial factors working at all stages of development, and, in so doing, link up with the considerable contribution made to the understanding of mental deficiency by a psychodynamic approach,[26,27] and even outstrip it on certain points. The formation of a child's personality stands out as decisive, whatever the basic neurobiological data may be, throughout her/his history and in continuous interaction with the family background and the environment.[28] Even in the most serious cases of mental deficiency, with the most obvious organic etiology, however, we find the influence of purely social factors playing their part in guiding handicapped persons into very specific channels of education and care, especially residential establishments,[29] and in maintaining them there.

CONCLUSION

In light of these epidemiological and medicosocial studies, any viewpoint that diminishes the subject strikes us as inconsistent with what we ourselves observe in our daily work. The only conceivable approach seems to be a multidimensional one to a process that is basically multifactorial, complex, and heterogeneous. This should enable mentally deficient persons to exist in other ways than through their disability, deficiency, conflicts and obstructions, social background, or the way they are regarded by society.

NOTES

1. Z.A. Stein and M. Susser, "The Epidemiology of Mental Retardation," in *American Handbook of Psychiatry*, 2nd ed., vol. 2, ed. G. Caplan (New York: Basic Books, 1974): 464-91.

2. C. Lévy, "Les Jeunes Handicapés Mentaux. Résultats d'une Enquête Statistique sur Leurs Caractéristiques et Leurs Besoins," Institut National d'Etudes Demographiques, Travaux et Documentation, Cahier no. 57 (Paris: Presses Universitaires de France, 1970).

3. F. Hatton, L. Tiret, P. Maguin, et al., "La Fausse Insuffisance Mentale. Ses Caractéristiques, son Évolution," *Revue de Pédiatrie* (Paris) 14 (1978): 415-22.

4. R. Salbreux, J.M. Deniaud, S. Tomkiewicz, et al., "Typologie et Prévalence des Handicaps Sévères et Multiples dans une Population d'Enfants. Premiers Résultats de l'Enquête Épidémiologique sur les Inadaptations Sévères dans la Population Juvénile de la Région Parisienne," *Revue de Neuropsychiatrie de l'Enfance et de l'Adolescence* (Paris) 27 (1979): 5-28.

5. C. Col and X. Bied-Charreton, "Étude Épidémiologique de la Déficience Mentale en Auvergne," *Revue de Pédiatrie* (Paris) 14 (1978): 401-06.

6. M. Manciaux, J.P. Deschamps, and J. Martin, "Répartition des Niveaux Intellectuels Mesurés par un Test Collectif dans une Population Scolaire. Une Étude Épidémiologique en Meurthe et Moselle," *Revue de Pédiatrie* (Paris) 14 (1978): 407-14.

7. Ibid.

8. Hatton, Tiret, Maguin, et al., "Fausse Insuffisance Mentale" (See note 3).

9. J.P. Deschamps, G. Valantin, and D. Bardin, "Fausses Insuffisance Mentales, ou Inadaptation Scolaire chez les Enfants de Q.I. Normal," *Revue de Pédiatrie* (Paris) 14 (1978): 423-28.

10. Ibid.

11. R. Salbreux, "Du Concept de la Psychométrie à la Nosographie de la Déficience Mentale," *Quintessence* (Paris) 23 (1979): 9-13.

12. B. Perron, "Á Propos de l'Illusion Nosographique liée au Concept Classique de Débilité Mentale," *Archives Françaises de Pédiatrie* (Paris) suppl. 35 (1978): 62-65.

13. R. Salbreux, *Cursus Scolaire et Institutionnel des Déficients Mentaux Légers et Moyens* (Mimeographed) (Lunéville, France: Office d'Hygiène Sociale de Meurthe et Moselle, 4 November 1978).

14. M. Manciaux, R. Salbreux, and S. Tomkiewicz, "Les Handicapés des Propositions Concrètes," *Preuves* (Paris) 19 (1974): 73-92.

15. M. d'Anthenaise and R. Salbreux, "Prévalence de la Déficience Mentale Profonde chez l'Enfant. Revue de la Littérature. Étude Comparative," *Revue de Neuropsychiatrie de l'Enfance et de l'Adolescence* (Paris) 27 (1979): 45-58.

16. Salbreux, Deniaud, Tomkiewicz, et al., "Prévalence des Handicaps Sévères" (See note 4).

17. Ibid.

18. R. Salbreux, J.M. Deniaud, and B. Rougier, "Étude de la Déficience Mentale dans la Région Parisienne. Á Partir des Premiers Résultats d'une Enquête Épidémiologique," *Revue de Pédiatrie* (Paris) 14 (1978): 389-400.

19. Manciaux, Deschamps, and Martin, "Niveaux Intellectuels Mesurés" (See note 6).

20. Deschamps, Valantin, and Bardin, "Fausses Insuffisances Mentales" (See note 9).

21. B. Rougier, R. Salbreux, J.M. Deniaud, et al., "Prise en Charge des Handicapés en Fonction de Leur Handicap et de la Catégorie Socio-Professionnelle de Leurs Parents," *Revue de Neuropsychiatrie de l'Enfance et de l'Adolescence* (Paris) 27 (1979): 29-44.

22. Manciaux, Salbreux, and Tomkiewicz, "Les Handicapés" (See note 14).

23. S. Tomkiewicz and R. Salbreux, "La Déficience Mentale Existe-t-Elle?", in *Journées de Pédo-Psychiatrie Entretiens de Bichat—Pitié-Salpétrière* (Paris: Expansion Scientifique, 1976): 21-27.

24. S. Tomkiewicz, "Un Regard Social sur la Déficience Mentale," *Journées Parisiennes de Pédiatrie* (Paris: Flammarion, 1978): 399-408.

25. Salbreux, "Concept de la Psychométrie" (See note 11).

26. R. Mises, "Nouvelles Orientations dans l'Approche Psychopathologique des Déficiences Intellectuelles," *Archives Françaises de Pédiatrie* (Paris) 35, suppl (1978): 4-9.

27. R. Mises, "Eléments pour une Approche Psychopathologique des Enfants Déficients Mentaux," in *Journées Parisiennes de Pédiatrie* (Paris: Flammarion, 1978): 384-89.

28. Salbreux, "Concept de la Psychométrie" (See note 11).

29. M. Zafiropoulos, J.M. Deniaud, and R. Salbreux, "Trajet et Destin des Adolescents et Adultes Déficients Mentaux Profonds," *Revue de Neuropsychiatrie de l'Enfance et de l'Adolescence* (Paris) 27 (1979): 91-110.

THE EPIDEMIOLOGY OF MENTAL RETARDATION IN THE UNITED STATES

Margaret E. Hertzig

In recent years in the United States the attention and concern of both professionals and the public is being directed toward consideration of a number of issues of importance in the identification, care, and treatment of mentally retarded persons. The practice of labeling, for example, in and of itself, has become a major social issue, and the consequences of classifying children whose current behavior and/or developmental course does not conform to usual expectations are beginning to be systematically explored. These efforts are resulting in a general reaffirmation of the central importance of classification in providing a basis for diagnoses, treatment, and prevention of disease and disability.

The establishment of a system of classification and the implementation of its use, however, can no longer be regarded as wholly benign. The negative consequences of labels, particularly if indiscriminately or inappropriately applied, have begun to be delineated with increasing precision. In the area of mental retardation, special attention is being directed toward the possible discriminatory and stigmatizing features of the labeling process, particularly as it affects persons who are mildly impaired.[1] Moreover, both the nature and the quality of opportunities available to an individual once a label of retardation has been applied are also coming under scrutiny. Expectations with respect to what constitutes appropriate care, treatment, education, and training for mentally retarded persons of all ages and at all levels of competence are undergoing rapid change.

Thus deinstitutionalization and institutional reforms are matters of national concern.[2] Furthermore, federal legislative action (Public Law 94–142) mandates that all handicapped children, regardless of the severity of their impairment, are to be educated in the least restrictive environment to the maximum extent possible.[3]

DEFINITION

The current social climate is clearly reflected in the 1977 revised edition of the *Manual on Terminology and Classification in Mental Retardation* of the American Association of Mental Deficiency (AAMD).[4] The introduction to this handbook specifies that the association considers mental retardation to be a cultural concept. The development of the proposed schema occurred within the context of an awareness that the definition and the consequences attaching to its application are therefore dependent on social norms, philosophical expectations, and the provisions made for deviant members by various social groups. These are not static, but vary from place to place and from time to time.

How then is mental retardation defined by the AAMD? According to its definition, which has been incorporated essentially without change into the new *Diagnostic and Statistical Manual of Mental Disorders* of the American Psychiatric Association,[5] mental retardation refers to "significantly sub-average general intellectual functioning existing concurrently with defects in adaptive behavior, and manifested during the developmental period." Both manuals specify that onset must occur prior to age eighteen. "General intellectual functioning" is further defined as the results obtained by assessment with one or more of the individually administered intelligence tests; "significant subaverage" refers to an IQ of more than 2 standard deviations (SDs) below the mean; while "adaptive behavior" is considered to reflect the effectiveness or degree with which an individual meets the standards of personal independence and social responsibility expected of her/his age and cultural group. By establishing the IQ cutoff at 2 SDs below the mean of the testing instrument, this current revision continues to apply the narrower standard first introduced by the AAMD in 1973; prior to that date the IQ limit had been set at 1 SD.

Thus the definition stresses the developmental origin and bidimensional character of mental retardation, and describes a level of behavioral performance without reference to etiology. No distinction is made between retardation associated with psychosocial or polygenic influences and that associated with biological deficits. Nor does a description of current behavior imply prognosis. Within the framework of the definition, an individual may meet the criteria of mental retardation at one time in life, but not at some other time.

INCIDENCE AND PREVALENCE

What do we know about the frequency of the occurrence of retardation? The subject of incidence and prevalence has generated considerable discussion and controversy in recent years. Despite the obvious importance, in terms of developing rational plans for service and preventive interventions, of firm knowledge with respect to the prevalence and differential distribution of mental retardation in the population, the picture is still not entirely clear.[6-8]

Rates of retardation determined in the course of epidemiologically based field studies in the United States vary widely; from less than 1 percent in the state of Delaware[9] to over 7 percent in North Carolina.[10] Differences in reported rates may well reflect actual differences in the proportion of mentally retarded persons in various communities, but it is also possible that they may derive, either in part or in whole, from differences in methodology. This problem is illustrated in the following brief summaries of selected epidemiological studies of mental retardation in the United States.

• In the late 1930s P.V. Lemkau and coworkers studied the prevalence of all types of mental disorders, including retardation, in the Eastern Health District of Baltimore, Maryland.[11] The population consisted of 55,000 white and nonwhite persons. The case-finding method involved examining records of community and state agencies, schools, courts, and prisons. Identified mentally retarded persons were classified according to the following IQ ranges: 50-69, 25-49, 24 and under, and untested. The investigators did not examine the subjects directly, and the untested category referred primarily to adults who were classified on the basis of social history. The study found an overall rate of mental retardation of 12.2 per 1,000 population.

• In 1953 the total population of 342,000 residents in Onondaga County, New York, was conducted under the auspices of the state Department of Mental Hygiene.[12] Community agencies were contacted and asked to refer children under age eighteen. Criteria included the request to report all children identified as or suspected of being mentally retarded on the basis of developmental history, poor academic performance, IQ score, or social adaptation when contrasted with their age peers. No direct examination was made of referrals. It is important to note that of the children with known IQ scores included in the survey about 25 percent had scores above 90, and 60 percent above 74. The Onondaga County study found a prevalence rate of 35.2 per 1,000 population.

• The California Test of Mental Maturity was used as a screening instrument in a study conducted in the state of Wyoming in 1957−58.[13] Of the 70,000 children enrolled in school, approximately 65,000 were tested; it was estimated that they comprised about 92 percent of children in public school and 87 percent of private and parochial school enrollments. Children with IQs of 80 or less were classified as mentally retarded. Many, but by no means all, were individually reexamined with the Stanford-Binet Test. Both group and individual measures were combined in calculating a prevalence rate of 50.2 per 1,000 children between the ages of six and twenty-one.

• In 1964 S.H. Wishik studied the prevalence of all handicapped children in two Georgia counties, who were selected as representative of the state's urban-rural and racial distribution.[14] The method of case finding included a communitywide campaign to solicit voluntary referrals, followed by a 10 percent canvass of households. All reports, both voluntary and canvass, were evaluated by pediatricians who made a tentative diagnosis. A sample of children was then invited to undergo individual clinical assessment. The household canvass found twice as many handicapped children as was indicated from voluntary reporting alone. The criteria of retardation was a combination of IQ score and clinical judgment. For IQs below 80 a rate of 36.6 per 1,000 was reported for young people under age twenty-one.

• J.F. Jastak, in a study conducted in Delaware in 1953 and 1954, constructed four indices to provide the basis for defining mental retardation: 1) the average of fifteen separate, subtest standard intelligence scores; 2) the highest subtest standard score or altitude; 3) a scholastic achievement index; and 4) an occupational achievement index.[15] A group of 2,117 persons between age ten and sixty-four, selected by a survey of sample households, were individually examined using three alternative definitions of retardation. In one, persons were considered retarded if they fell in the lowest 25 percent of the population in all indices; corresponding definitions were used for the 9 percent and 2 percent levels. Cutoff points were determined separately for American-born whites, foreign-born whites, and blacks to avoid bias due to foreign language background or lack of educational opportunities. Rates were 88.3, 20.3, and 3.8 per 1,000 at the 25, 9, and 2 percent cutoffs, respectively.

• In 1957 E.J. Levinson used a questionnaire to survey all known schools and residential institutions serving children in the state of Maine.[16] Reports were requested on all children known or believed to be retarded, whether in or out of school. The criterion used was an IQ below 75, either as determined by testing or estimated by the institutional informant. Individuals between the ages of five and twenty were included in the study, and a prevalence rate of 25 per 1,000 population was reported.

• In 1965 W.D. Richardson surveyed the mentally retarded under age twenty-one in an urban and a rural county in North Carolina[17] with a total population of some 150,000. The survey was carried out in three stages: the first consisted of a review of agency records to ascertain the number of handicapped children; in the second, a 5 percent sample of households was surveyed in order to identify handicapped children not otherwise reported; in the third, subsamples of both normal and presumptively handicapped children from the households surveyed were given diagnostic clinical examinations. Using a criterion for mental retardation of an IQ below 70, a prevalence rate of 77 per 1,000 population was found.

• In 1968 Lemkau and P.D. Imre reported the results of a field study conducted in a rural county in the southeastern United States with a population under 20,000; every family in the county was interviewed.[18] The study focused on young people between age one and nineteen. Preschool-children who scored less than a Social Quotient of 81 on a modification of the Vineland Social Maturity Scale were individually examined, as were school-agers who scored below 79 on a group IQ test or were nominated by their teachers. Children were considered retarded if their individual test score was below 70. Overall prevalence was reported as 74.4 per 1,000 population.

DIFFERENCES IN STUDIES

As this brief survey indicates, these field studies differ markedly with respect to the sociodemographic characteristics of the population studied; moreover, differing survey methods were employed. Some studies relied exclusively on nominations by social agencies; others conducted household surveys; still others employed both methods. While some surveys relied on agency reports to identify persons as retarded, others used independent clinical assessment. Finally, the definitions of mental retardation differed. In most studies, IQ was the only criterion for diagnosis; levels required for inclusion ranged from 69 to 90. In other investigations, however, some effort was made to include a measure of adaptive function, although in most cases this was inferred from agency reports. Only in the investigation reported by Jastak was a systematic effort undertaken to measure aspects of adaptive behavior.

Despite the variability in overall prevalence rates as determined in these field studies, certain trends are consistently identified. The more severe forms of retardation constitute a relatively small proportion of the total burden of the disorder. In almost all studies an IQ of less than 50 is found to occur in approximately 4 per 1,000 population;[19] the prevalence of this degree of retardation is greatest in younger age groups, decreasing with maturity. Severely impaired individuals frequently show associated clinical and laboratory pathology, which is most often diagnosed during infancy or early childhood. It has been reported that genetic disorders are found in nearly 50 percent of this group, whose members come from all socioeconomic levels.[20] The impairment is chronic, and, essentially, decrements in age-specific prevalence are the consequences of a higher than average mortality rate.

MILD MENTAL RETARDATION

In contrast, mild mental retardation has a very low prevalence during the preschool years; a very high frequency of occurrence during the period of school attendance; and a precipitous drop thereafter. The preschool-age group includes a number of children with Down's syndrome, who usually gain higher scores in psychometric tests administered early in life. The group of mildly retarded children identified prior to school entrance also includes some individuals with other types of organic impairment in whom intellectual functioning is only slightly depressed.[21]

The mildly retarded individuals diagnosed during their school years are quite different from those identified prior to school entrance. In the vast majority of these children retardation is not accompanied by somatic signs, and their families are economically, socially, and educationally underprivileged. Beyond late adolescence many of these individuals become reabsorbed in the general population and their retardation is no longer suspected, let alone diagnosed. As a consequence, the prevalence of mild retardation again approximates that found before school age. Causation has been attributed to genetic factors; the impact of early childhood experiences; and exposure to noninheritable conditions of risk such as low birth weight or postnatal malnutrition. Most likely the emergent clinical picture is defined by the nature of the interaction among all three sets of conditions.[22]

SUBTYPES OF RETARDATION

The analysis of trends has contributed greatly to our increased understanding of the distribution and natural history of various subtypes of retardation. Nevertheless, efforts to estimate overall prevalence have continued to concern many authorities, particularly as global estimates frequently provide the basis for the drawing up of budgets in many state and local jurisdictions.[23]

It has been frequently stated that some 6 million Americans—about 3 percent of the population—are retarded. G. Tarjan has critically examined this assertion and has pointed out the assumptions upon which it is based.[24] Those who posit a 3 percent prevalence rate are operating from the premise that the criterion for retardation is confined exclusively to that of an IQ below 70; moreover, the 3 percent model implies that incidence and prevalence are equivalent.

Although the incidence of some specific types of retardation associated with inborn errors of metabolism, chromosomal aberrations, congenital abnormalities, trauma, or toxic agents is fairly well established, people with these conditions represent only a small segment of the total retarded population. The incidence of overall mental retardation is much more difficult to determine, for an accurate count is greatly complicated by the gradual clinical onset. Latent retardation can be present for a long period, and overt recognition depends more on the diagnostic process than on the presence of symptoms. Some estimate of incidence can be made, however, if onset is arbitrarily equated with the time of first diagnosis. Analysis of data depicting the age-specific IQ distribution among individuals institutionalized in state facilities for the retarded suggests it is not unreasonable to estimate that, at some point in their lives, about 3 percent of newborns will be suspected or even classified as retarded.

It would be possible and appropriate to equate incidence and prevalence if the diagnosis remained constant over the entire lifespan of an individual, and if the mortality rate of retarded persons were similar to that of the general population. The discrepancy between these requirements, as well as both clinical experience and epidemiological trends, led Tarjan and his colleagues to suggest a downward revision in the estimate of overall prevalence to 1 percent of the population.[25] According to this view, an estimated 2 million individuals exist in whom mental retardation is clinically diagnosed or in whom the diagnosis is ascertained upon examination.

REVISED ESTIMATES

J.R. Mercer's epidemiological studies of mental retardation in the community of Riverside, California, provide considerable empirical support for this revised estimate.[26,27] In the clinical phases of these investigations, attention was directed toward evaluation of intellectual adequacy and adaptive behavior. The former was determined in the course of individualized administration of standardized measures of intelligence; primarily the Stanford-Binet or Kuhlman-Binet tests; adaptive behavior was conceptualized as the individual's ability to play even more complex roles in a progressively widening circle of social systems; it was assessed in terms of the responses made by relatives to a series of twenty-eight, age-grade scales specifically developed for this purpose. The construction of the scales relied heavily on the Vineland Social Maturity Scale and the Gesell Developmental Scale. Items used in the evaluation of older children and adults were augmented to include a substantial focus on the nature and quality of participation in home, neighborhood, educational, occupational, and community activities.

Mercer's research design called for a first-stage screening of a large sample of the population, using the adaptive behavior scales, and a second stage of individualized testing. The screened sample was a stratified-area probability sample of housing units in Riverside, selected so that all geographic areas and socioeconomic levels were represented. The data permitted analysis of the impact of various definitions of mental retardation on prevalence.

THE IQ FACTOR

When the diagnosis of mental retardation was based on the single criterion of measured intelligence, setting the IQ cutoff at 80—the usual level employed by educational authorities in this community—it resulted in an overall prevalence of 3.7 per 1,000 population. When the IQ cutoff was reduced to 70 (approximately 2 SDs below the mean of the testing instruments) prevalence declined to 2.1. The imposition of a two-dimensional definition caused the prevalence rate to fall still further. A prevalence rate of 18.9 per 1,000 resulted when educational criteria were used to set the limits of both intellectual level and adaptive behavior. If the definition of mental retardation was formulated to include only those individuals functioning 2 SDs below the mean of both measures, the rate was reduced to .97 per 1,000 population.

As anticipated, variation in definition had the greatest impact on the prevalence of mild retardation. Most individuals whose IQs were under 50 also failed the adaptive behavior measure. On the other hand, many persons with IQs between 50 and 69 and between 70 and 79 were performing their social roles in the family, neighborhood, and broader community in a manner comparable to the performance of their age peers. In accordance with the requirements of a two-dimensional definition, they were not considered mentally retarded, even though their IQs fell below established cutoff scores. The number of individuals so affected was not inconsiderable. The percentage shrinkage in prevalence, as a consequence of the introduction of dual criteria, was approximately 50 at each IQ level examined.

Mercer has emphasized that these data derive from the examination of mental retardation from a clinical perspective.[28] From that vantage point mental retardation is a designation that, in providing a summary description of intelligence and behavior, presumably transcends cultures and social settings. It is also possible to examine both the definition and the frequency of occurrence of retardation from a social system perspective. According to this view, mental retardation is considered an achieved status in a social system, reflecting the role played by people holding that status. Thus a person is retarded only by virtue of having been labeled as such, with the social structure in a particular area being the primary determination of who is so designated.

As an extension of this line of thinking, Mercer attempted to determine who had been labeled as retarded by whom in the Riverside community.[29] Reports were obtained from formal organizations that might number the retarded among their clientele and from an appropriately selected sample of community residents. The overall prevalence rate for individuals nominated by one or more social system in the community was found to be 1.2 per 1,000; this rate closely approximated that found when mental retardation was clinically defined in terms of IQ and adaptive behavior, with levels set at 2 SDs below the mean.

Severity of retardation can be defined within the framework provided by a social system perspective, in terms of the number of different systems that so label an individual. Thus if a person holds the status of retardate in all the social systems in which she/he participates, that person is comprehensively retarded. Individuals living in institutions for the retarded provide examples of such labeling; those living in the community may also be comprehensively retarded, or they may be considered retarded in some systems or situations and not in others. A scale defining the comprehensively retarded at one pole and the most situationally retarded at the other was developed and applied to persons designated as retarded by organizations and individuals in Riverside.[30]

The comprehensively retarded were found to have significantly lower IQs and displayed much more evidence of physical disability than the situationally retarded. Minority ethnic groups and low socioeconomic levels were *not* overrepresented among the comprehensively retarded. In contrast, however, the situationally retarded were more likely to be members of minority ethnic groups of lower socioeconomic status than were the comprehensively retarded. The public schools, more than any other social system in the community, designated individuals who were the most situationally retarded.

TWO DISSIMILAR POPULATIONS

Thus findings of epidemiological investigations, both those employing the more usual and familiar clinical approach and those designed to encompass a social system perspective, have made explicit what is only implied in the current definition of mental retardation.

As now formulated, two quite dissimilar populations are subsumed into a single diagnostic entity. The smaller group of moderately to profoundly handicapped individuals, often referred to as the "clinically" retarded, are consistently identified by both the clinical and social system approaches. The two systems begin to diverge in relation to what is currently classified as "mental" retardation due to psychosocial disadvantage. Clinical diagnostic procedures, even when measures of IQ and adaptive behavior are both employed, consistently identify as retarded a higher proportion of individuals, particularly among those from minority groups, than do their families or neighbors in the community. Mercer has suggested that this difference is a consequence of the fact that the category of psychosocial retardation is not, in and of itself, homogeneous; rather, it may be composed of both socioculturally modal and nonmodal individuals.[31]

The socioculturally modal are conceptualized as a group of relatively nondisabled persons from homes that conform to the sociocultural configuration of the larger community. Presumably they fail the IQ and adaptive behavior measures, not because of a lack of opportunities to acquire the necessary knowledge and skills, but because they are unable to take advantage of them. By way of contrast, the socioculturally nonmodal come from homes that do not conform to the sociocultural mode of the community. Presumably many of these individuals have not been exposed to the cultural materials and have not acquired the knowledge needed to perform acceptably on intelligence tests and measures of adaptive behavior.

In order to more clearly distinguish between these two groups, Mercer has urged the option of a pluralistic evaluation procedure that would interpret the scores attained by an individual child against the norms of her/his particular sociocultural grouping, rather than those of the standard population.[32,33] Such a procedure, it is argued, would more accurately identify people who require special services without unnecessarily stigmatizing those who are likely to adequately fulfill adult role expectations.

LABEL OF RETARDATION

How to define and how to ascertain retardation, particularly mild retardation, once so designated, are not merely matters of academic interest: they are issues of major social and practical import to the retarded, their families, and relevant social institutions. Although many educators and child psychiatrists, sensitive to the high frequency of occurrence of specific learning problems and behavioral disturbances among individuals in the borderline category, believe the elimination of this designation may well result in a denial of service to large numbers of persons with special needs, others view the label of retardation as inevitably harmful, and one to be avoided at all costs. Members of minority groups, in particular, consider the labeling process to be but another manifestation of discrimination.

Concern about stigmatization is of course by no means new. As early as 1905 A. Binet stated that "it will never be to one's credit to have attended a special school. We should at least spare from this mark those who do not deserve it."[34] In recent years, however, this concern has been translated into actions that have had and are having a major impact on the provision of services to the mildly retarded. In many states the imposition of new criteria has resulted in the decertification of some retarded children for special educational programs. In accordance with federal legislative requirements, this de facto "mainstreaming" has been accompanied by the active movement of many special-class children into regular grades. The impact of these trends has yet to be satisfactorily evaluated. Comparisons of children from special versus regular classes offer little conclusive evidence as to the relative merits of each setting.[35,36]

METHODOLOGICAL PROBLEMS

The interpretation of findings is complicated by significant methodological problems. Special classes differ from regular classes in many ways, including curriculum; teacher-pupil ratios; level of teacher training; degree of segregation; and the imposition of labels. Any or all of these factors may influence outcome. Nevertheless, additional empirical data is badly needed if professionals, as well as regulatory and funding agencies, are to be appropriately guided in their efforts to best meet the needs of mildly retarded persons.

Similar concerns may be raised about trends toward deinstitutionalization and normalization as they relate to the care and treatment of the more severely handicapped. While the need to remove retarded persons from the inhumane living conditions and stultifying atmosphere that characterizes some institutions is undeniable, the form in which alternative care should be provided is not as readily apparent. The impact of massive programs to relocate retarded persons is only beginning to be systematically evaluated. Yet is is becoming increasingly clear that not all institutions are bad; that deterioration is not an inevitable consequence of institutional placement; and that not all community-based programs offer opportunities for the maximization of function that was anticipated or hoped for.[37] Our understanding of which factors in these various settings facilitate or impede the adjustment and progress of which individuals being served is, however, still rudimentary.

In summary, the present period in the United States is one in which new theories about mental retardation have developed in response to and, in turn, have influenced the emergence of changing concepts of how affected persons should be educated and cared for. Our coming needs therefore lie not only in the direction of more precise enumeration, but in the systematic evaluation of the impact of different models of service delivery on the lives of the retarded and their families.

NOTES

1. N. Hobbs, ed., *Issues in the Classification of Children,* vol. 1 (San Francisco: Jossey-Bass, 1975).

2. R.C. Scheerenberger, "Public Residential Services for the Mentally Retarded," in *International Review of Research in Mental Retardation,* vol. 9, ed. N.R. Ellis (1975): 187-208

3. L. Corman and J. Gottlieb, "Mainstreaming Mentally Retarded Children: A Review of Research," in ibid.: 251-73.

4. H.J. Grossman, ed., *Manual on Terminology and Classification in Mental Retardation,* rev. ed. (Washington: American Association of Mental Deficiency, 1977).

5. Task Force on Nomenclature and Statistics, *Diagnostic and Statistical Manual of Mental Disorders,* 3rd ed. (Washington: American Psychiatric Association, 1978).

6. R.W. Conley, *The Economics of Mental Retardation* (Baltimore: Johns Hopkins University Press, 1973).

7. E. Gruenberg, "Epidemiology," in *Mental Retardation: A Review of Research,* ed. H.A. Stevens and R. Heber (Chicago: University of Chicago Press, 1964).

8. R. Lapouse and M. Weitzner, "Epidemiology," in *Mental Retardation: An Annual Review*, ed. J. Wortis (New York: Grune and Stratton, 1970).

9. J.F. Jastak, M.Mc. Halsey, and M. Whiteman, *Mental Retardation—Its Nature and Incidence* (Newark, Delaware: University of Delaware Press, 1963).

10. W.D. Richardson and A.C. Higgins, *The Handicapped Children of Alamance County, North Carolina: A Medical and Sociological Study* (Wilmington, Delaware: Nemours Foundation, 1965).

11. P.V. Lemkau, C. Tietze, and M. Cooper, "Mental Hygiene Problems in an Urban District," *Mental Hygiene* 25 (1941): 642-46; 26 (1942): 100-19; 275-88.

12. New York State Department of Mental Hygiene, Mental Health Research Unit, "A Special Census of Suspected Referred Mental Retardation, Onondaga County, New York," in *Technical Report of the Mental Health Research Unit* (Syracuse: University of Syracuse Press, 1955).

13. *Wyoming Mental Ability Survey, 1957–1958* (Cheyenne: State Department of Education, 10 May 1959).

14. S.H. Wishik, *Georgia Study of Handicapped Children; Report on a Study of Prevalance, Disability, Needs, Resources, and Contributing Factors,* Publications for Program Administration and Community Organization (Atlanta: Georgia Department of Public Health, 1964).

15. Jastak, Halsey, and Whiteman, *Mental Retardation* (See note 9).

16. E.J. Levinson, *Retarded Children in Maine. A Survey and Analysis,* University of Maine Studies, 2nd ser., no. 77 (Orono: University of Maine Press, 1962).

17 Richardson and Higgins, *Handicapped Children* (See note 10).

18. P.V. Lemkau and P.D. Imre, "Results of a Field Epidemiologic Study," *American Journal of Mental Deficiency* 73 (1968): 858-63.

19. H.K. Abramovicz and S.A. Richardson, "Epidemiology of Severe Mental Retardation in Children: Community Studies," *American Journal of Mental Deficiency* 80 (1975): 18-39.

20. B.F. Crandall, "Genetic Disorders and Mental Retardation," *Journal of the American Academy of Child Psychiatry* 16 (1977): 88-108.

21. G. Tarjan, S. Wright, R.K. Eyman, et al., "Natural History of Mental Retardation: Some Aspects of Epidemiology," *American Journal of Mental Deficiency* 77 (1973): 369-79.

22. G. Tarjan, "Mental Retardation and the Organization of Services," *Psychiatric Annals* 6 (1976): 325-29.

23. R.L. Luckey and R. Neman, "Practices in Estimating Mental Retardation Prevalence," *Mental Retardation* 14 (1976): 44-46.

24. Tarjan, Wright, Eyman, et al., "Natural History of Retardation" (See note 21).

25. Ibid.

26. J.R. Mercer, *Labeling the Mentally Retarded* (Berkeley: University of California Press, 1973).

27. ———, "The Myth of 3% Prevalence," in *Sociobehavioral Studies in Mental Retardation,* ed. G. Tarjan, R.K. Eyman, and C.E. Meyers, Monographs of the American Association of Mental Deficiency, 1 (1973): 1-18.

28. ———, *Labeling the Retarded* (See note 25).

29. Ibid.

30. Ibid.

31. Ibid.

32. J.R. Mercer, "A Policy Statement on Assessment Procedures and the Rights of Children," in *Annual Progress in Child Psychiatry and Child Development*, ed. S. Chess and A. Thomas (New York: Brunner Mazel, 1975): 20-35.

33. ———, "Cultural Diversity, Mental Retardation and Assessment. The Case for Nonlabeling," in *Research to Practice in Mental Retardation*, vol. 1, *Care and Intervention*, ed. P. Mittler (Baltimore, Maryland: University Park Press, 1977): 353-62.

34. A. Binet, quoted in Mercer, "Policy Statement on Assessment" (See note 32).

35. D.L. MacMillan, R.L. Jones, and G.F. Aloia, "The Mentally Retarded Label: A Theoretical Analysis and Review of Research," *American Journal of Mental Deficiency* 79 (1974): 241-53.

36. Corman and Gottlieb, "Mainstreaming" (See note 3).

37. M. Begab, "Some Priorities for Research in Mental Retardation," in *Research to Practice in Mental Retardation*, vol. 1, *Care and Intervention*, ed. P. Mittler (Baltimore, Maryland: University Park Press, 1977): A21-30.

DISCUSSION

Methods of Sampling

Epidemiological studies of serious retardation in France are concerned with distribution of various kinds of handicaps in the population, not only mental deficiency.

Salbreux's study dealt with rare handicaps, the appearance of which could not have been ascertained in a smaller sample. For example, in the field of mental deficiency he found cases of encephalopathy through vaccination records; they were but a few of thousands of cases on file.

One participant commented on appropriate methods of sampling for conditions with quite varying levels of incidence and prevalence; it seems important to grapple with this problem. As far as children with mild retardation are concerned, when it is clear that one is going to miss very large numbers of them if one relies on documentary evidence, an attempt should be made to find another method to identify them. Group testing of children in classrooms is a reasonably reliable and valid method for identifying disorders; if that is not done one will find one has overidentified children with multiple handicaps, with behavior problems, and other disorders, sometimes severe, sometimes mild. As far as the rarer disorders are concerned, severe mental retardation, with IQs below 50, falls into this group. It seems perfectly acceptable to identify such children on the basis of documentation because it is known from massive evidence that the vast majority of them are in fact receiving a special education of some sort.

As for very rare disorders—and mention was made of vaccinea encephalopathy—neither documentation or total population screening is likely to be effective; other measures may be necessary.

Collaborative Study in the United Kingdom

In the United Kingdom there are two areas where additional studies have been undertaken because of the ability and willingness of pediatricians to collaborate. The National Phenylketonuria Registry has enabled researchers to pick up about fifty cases a year, and the condition has been studied in a way that would not be possible by even quite a large center depending on its own resources.

Vaccinea, the question of pertussis and encephalopathy from immunization, has been greatly clarified by a collaborative study in which all pediatricians were asked to provide information. Indeed it has been possible to demonstrate that post-whooping-cough immunization does not exist. Unfortunately that theory is out of favor because of alarming reports by epidemiologically unsophisticated people: deaths from whooping-cough are now occurring in the unprotected population.

Sex-Linked Study

The Mannheim study on mental retardation found a sex-linked result for boys having more handicaps and lower IQs than girls. This is something that has been generally found, not only in relation to severe mental retardation where there is a biological component. It seems to go along with the general fact that although more boys are conceived, fewer survive; they appear to be somewhat more biologically inferior. This is also found in relation to mild mental retardation, where the frequency of occurrence is also greater among boys.

One explanation has been that they are more likely to engage in behavior that brings them to the attention of people who are particularly concerned with moving children from one educational track to another. Parents and society pay more attention to boys, and are more demanding of boys than of girls. Perhaps this is one reason they have more trouble adapting.

Chromosomal Anomalies

In recent years people who work with chromosomal anomalies have become interested in what is known as the fragile X syndrome, in which the cells and tissue culture of males with mental retardation exhibit some unusual lysis of the X chromosome. That is an uncommon condition, but perhaps the multiplication of uncommon conditions suffices. Studies of that trait in meningitis in the first year of life show a predominance of males. The impact of hyperbilirubinemia in infants is associated with higher rates of kernicterus, at the same level of elevated bilirubin, in the male than in the female infant.

Mary Lyon, the geneticist, has offered one hypothesis to explain the vulnerability of the male: it is to the effect that female heterozygousness in the X chromosome allows the female, who has a deleterious gene on one, to be protected if the normal allele is present on the other; the male, on the other hand, is stuck with one allele on the X, and if that is defective he is in difficulty. Whether this explains it fully or not, they are the weaker of the sexes; there is no question of that.

Labeling the Retarded

The question was raised about the consequences of labeling mildly retarded, or presumably mildly retarded, children in the United States. When the definition of mental retardation is restricted to the dimensions of intellectual level and adaptive functioning, each set at 2 standard deviations (SDs) from the mean, very few children who fall into the category of me.itally retarded are there by virtue of psychosocial phenomena. If that is the case, what use is there to redefine or create new categories of psychosocial retardation based on the degree to which characterization is socioculturally modal or nonmodal?

The narrower the definition gets, by the imposition of the two dimensions and the establishment of cuts at 2 SDs or more below the mean, the more individuals—primarily those previously categorized as mildly or borderline retarded—in the lowest socioeconomic, ethnic minority groups are eliminated. This is a substantial group; tightening the definition does not completely remove the social class gradient for mild retardation.

Functioning in the School System

People who feel the label is important also raise another question: "What are you going to do with these young people within the school system if you don't call them that?" Perhaps calling them something else will be equally detrimental. They clearly are individuals who need special services.

It is important to make the distinction between those individuals who come from sociocultural, nonmodal groups and those who have grown up in a social system fairly coincident with the society at large. The first group probably will respond more than the second group to different kinds of educational intervention; the second group has been exposed to a greater frequency of the occurrence of the whole host of risk conditions that add CNS impairment to sociocultural factors and contribute to outcome, so it may contain a higher proportion of prematurely born children; as a group they are much more frequently found in lower socioeconomic groups. There is a good deal of evidence that prematurity, if individuals with clear-cut neurological disturbances such as cerebral palsy are excluded, has no effect on the IQ or on school functioning of youngsters from middle- and upper-class groups; but it does have a major impact on the school performance of children in lower socioeconomic groups when they are compared with full-term children.

This is an important issue. One cannot simply change labels and think one has done away with the issue of discrimination. The law provides for special programs, and the schools are wrestling with the problem this creates. Children are no longer in a retarded class or retarded school; they go to the resource room for half the day. But they frequently are just as stigmatized and just as labeled as if they stay there the whole day.

III. BRAIN DAMAGE

BRAIN DAMAGE: EVIDENCE FROM MEASURES OF NEUROLOGICAL FUNCTION IN CHILDREN WITH PSYCHIATRIC DISORDER

Eric Taylor

Two major strategies have guided efforts to understand the contribution of disordered brain function to psychiatric disturbance in childhood. The first of these, reviewed in this volume by Dennis P. Cantwell, is to study the psychiatric status of children with evidence of definite injury to the brain; the second is to examine the neurological status of psychiatrically defined groups. The first strategy has perhaps led to the clearer lessons,[1] which are set out briefly as the background to this paper:

• Definite brain damage can lead to disorders of behavior and cognition without any other neurological impairment; if that is indeed the definition of "minimal brain dysfunction" (MBD), it obviously exists. Possibly, however, it is only found after rather severe injury to the brain; the evidence concerning subtler influences remains unsatisfactory and inconclusive. If such subtle influences are to be identified, it may well be by the study of particular psychiatric diagnoses.

• Alteration of the physiological functioning of the brain is likely to be one important factor in the pathogenesis. This is not to say that dysfunction is necessarily directly expressed in behavior; the links might be much less direct, through, for example, the mediation of cognitive impairment, educational failure, temperament distortion, or altered self-image.

• Brain damage does not lead to a specific psychiatric syndrome, but rather to a general vulnerability to the whole range of psychiatric problems. Since there is no "brain damage syndrome," it follows, a fortiori, that a "MBD syndrome" is implausible.

98

PSYCHOPATHOLOGY OF CHILDREN AND YOUTH

One of the unanswered questions concerns precisely the area of most controversy: the possibility that damage to the functioning of the brain by external insults is a major cause of psychiatric syndromes in children. This paper addresses the question by giving an overview of some recent evidence, obtained in part by workers connected with the Institute of Psychiatry in London, derived from applying a variety of measures to do with brain dysfunction to psychiatric populations. Not only can the question be pursued in this way; for some purposes it must be.

Consider, for example, the clinician who seeks to understand the psychiatric problems of a child whose birth history is abnormal. It is not enough for him to know that perinatal accidents are associated with a higher risk of psychiatric problems, for they are much more commonly not so associated; he needs to know how likely it is that such a psychiatric problem will prove to have an entirely nonneurological basis. Furthermore, most causes of brain damage have multiple, diffuse effects. It is neurologically implausible that all kinds of brain damage should be equivalent. There may be specific relationships between brain and behavior that are quite obscured by considering together all forms of injury to the brain. It is therefore necessary to study different kinds of behavior problems and to continue the effort of diagnostic refinement. A few of the methods open to us are:

• Clinical neurological evaluation, including the appraisal of the history, the conventional examination, gross developmental delay, and radiological investigation.

• The use of specific behaviors or behavioral patterns as indices of brain disorder.

• Neurophysiological measures of function.

• Measures of clumsiness and lack of coordination—one kind of "soft neurological sign."

• Psychometric measures.

• Pharmacological methods: although these may be powerful ways of dissecting the biological basis of behavior, and although they are being used in current research at the Institute of Psychiatry, I shall not refer to them further as they are the subject of a later session of this symposium.

STRUCTURAL NEUROLOGICAL EVALUATION

Structural abnormality can exist in the absence of brain damage, which can cause functional abnormality without structural abnormality. Evidence of structural damage in the nervous system is, however, seldom found. N. Geschwind and his colleagues recently provided the first post-mortem evidence of structural change in the brain of a man with a serious difficulty in language development, and they have focused attention on the anatomical asymmetry of the planum temporale.[2] Computerized axial tomography has wrought a revolution in neurological investigation. D.B. Hier and his coworkers have shown that some patients with developmental dyslexia have a reversal of the normal pattern of cerebral asymmetry, and suggest that in these patients language is lateralized to a hemisphere structurally unsuited to the purpose.[3] Even such structural measures, however, have similar problems to those I shall consider, and show high rates of "abnormality" in the normal population.

In Figure 1 are abstracted some of the data from Hier's study as they would apply to a population of 1,000 children. It is clear that children with reversed asymmetry are very much more likely to be normal readers then

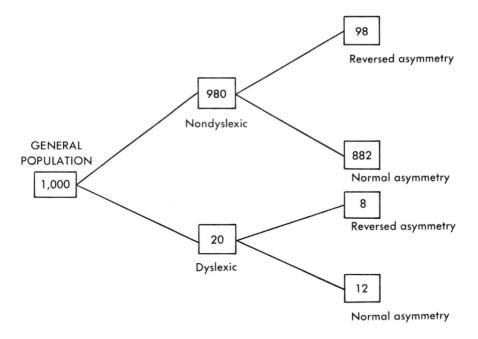

Figure 1. Normal and reversed cerebral asymmetry in normal and dyslexic populations of children.
SOURCE: Based on data in D.B. Hier, M. Lemay, P.B. Rosenberger, et al., "Developmental Dyslexia: Evidence for a Subgroup with a Reversal of Cerebral Asymmetry," *Archives of Neurology* 35 (1978): 90-92.

impaired readers; that prediction on this basis would be seriously inadequate and would not be acceptable as a screening test; and that it can be conceived better as a risk factor than as a cause.

Further, the pattern of reversed cerebral asymmetry and the microscopic structure of the planum temporale are not pointers to brain damage. Genetic determination is a more plausible explanation, given the absence of other indicators of brain damage.

NEUROLOGICAL EVALUATION
OF SPECIFIC PSYCHIATRIC SYMPTOMS

A substantial body of literature exists to argue the proposition that some behaviors—particularly the frequently diagnosed syndrome of hyperactivity—are specifically biologically determined;[4] to argue it, but not to establish it. Indeed there is considerable evidence that the behavioral components of the syndrome—overactivity, impulsiveness, inattention—are not associated with each other or with neurological measures,[5] and that different neurological measures do not associate into a single factor of brain impairment.[6] It is frequently diagnosed in North America, but seldom in England; yet our questionnaire study in South London classrooms has indicated that teachers completing the symptom rating scale of C.K. Conners[7] do so in very similar ways to their counterparts in America and New Zealand, as shown in Table 1.[8]

Furthermore, children diagnosed in London as exhibiting "conduct disorder" are very similar to those diagnosed as "hyperkinetic" in the United States: both are equally deviant on the scale that measures hyperactivity. Presumably the difference lies in the diagnosticians rather than in the children. We therefore doubted the specificity of the syndrome and proceeded to investigate how far the overactivity behaviors of the children attending our clinic could be seen as specific; how far they were associated with biological factors such as abnormal birth history, abnormal neurological examination, minor congenital anomalies, and early onset of symptoms; how far with psychological factors such as IQ, reading retardation, cognitive impulsiveness, and galvanic skin response; and how far with social and family factors.[9]

The results are readily summarized, because we found very few associations. Parent and teacher questionnaire measures of overactivity were not related at all, either to each other or to observational measures taken at the clinic. Neither did these measures relate to biological factors—but there was an association with IQ.

TABLE 1. MEAN SCORES ON HYPERACTIVITY FACTOR[1]
OF C.K. CONNERS'S TEACHER'S QUESTIONNAIRE

Boys in normal school in the United States Midwest	1.56
Boys in normal school in South London	2.07
Boys in normal school in Auckland, New Zealand	1.83
"Hyperkinetic" boys in the United States Midwest	3.17
"Conduct disorder" boys in South London	3.11

NOTE: 1) Range of 1.0 to 4.0.
SOURCES: Data adapted from J. Werry, R. Sprague, and M. Cohen, "Conners' Teacher Rating Scale for Use in Drug Studies with Children," *Journal of Abnormal Child Psychology* 3 (1975): 217-29; S. Sandberg, M. Rutter, and E. Taylor, "Hyperkinetic Disorder in Psychiatric Clinic Attenders," *Developmental Medicine and Child Neurology* 20 (1978): 279-99; and J. Werry and D. Hawthorne, "Conners' Teacher Questionnaire—Norms and Validity," *Australian-New Zealand Journal of Psychiatry* 10 (1976): 257-62.

The observation of this lack of associations with biological factors has since then been replicated by S. Sandberg, M.W. Wieselberg, and D. Shaffer in a sample of children drawn from the general population. We conclude that there is no support for the notion that this rather broadly defined set of symptoms is neurologically based; that conclusion is of course restricted to the measures we used.

Rarer symptoms may, however, have stronger associations. General population studies have to be very large indeed to yield groups of rare conditions, and we therefore turn to studies based on the case records of the children seen at our clinic over the years 1973 to 1978. Of some 2,400 such children, thirty-one were diagnosed as manifesting hyperkinetic syndromes. This is of course enormously less common than in practice in many other countries. Figure 2 indicates, however, that the diagnosis was meaningful in terms of predicting differences from other children attending the clinic who were diagnosed as having conduct disorder.

Normal family relationships, as judged by the clinician responsible, were more frequent in the hyperkinetic children, as were intellectual retardation and an early onset of symptoms. All these can be seen as

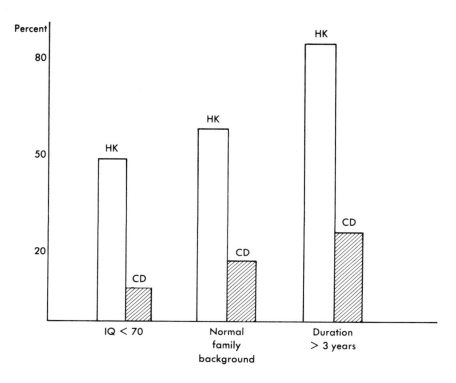

Figure 2. Comparisons of hyperkinetic (HK) and conduct-disordered (CD) children in the frequency of other clinical features (see text).
SOURCE: Data based on the records of Bethlem Royal and Maudsley hospitals in London.

pointers to a biological basis, but might of course represent no more than the grounds on which the clinicians based their diagnoses.

We then turned from the diagnoses of hyperkinetic syndrome to the symptom of "gross overactivity" recorded as present or absent by the clinicians in charge of the 2,400 cases; 106 of them were regarded as showing the definite presence of the symptom. This should be much less contaminated by etiological consideration, yet comparison of these grossly overactive children who definitely did not show the symptom yields a rather similar pattern, as shown in Figure 3.

Intellectual retardation, clumsiness, specific developmental delays, and

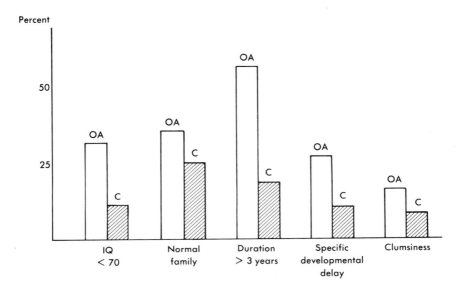

Figure 3. Comparisons of children with the symptoms of gross overactivity (OA) and controls (C) in the frequency of other clinical features (see text).

long duration of symptoms were all present in excess, to a statistically significant degree, in the grossly overactive children. This relationship still held when corrected for age and for diagnostic differences.

The same pattern of associations was found for the symptom of "social disinhibition," and indeed this was strongly associated with gross overactivity. Social disinhibition is of particular interest, as it was one of the very few features of head-injured children specifically associated with the injury.[10] By contrast, this pattern of associations did not hold for individual symptoms of conduct disorders such as "defiance."

While this gives some support to the idea that a rather rare pattern of symptoms may be based in brain function, there is considerable uncertainty about the precise definition of these symptoms.

A clue comes from the clinic study of overactive children referred to earlier.[11] When we selected only those children who showed the *combination* of rated overactivity at home and at school, and observed overactivity in the clinic, they were indeed different from children who did not have those problems. To begin with they were younger and of lower IQ than the children normal in this respect. Even when matched for age, IQ, and diagnosis, they were significantly more impaired on developmental neurological examination; significantly more impulsive cognitively; and significantly more likely to have had an early onset of their symptoms.

The suggestion that emerges is that *pervasive* overactivity, seen in all contexts of a child's life, is a rare problem, but one that is intimately bound up with developmental delay and cognitive difficulties. R. Schachar and M. Rutter have found some confirmation for this in a reanalysis of the data from the Isle of Wight studies.[12] Teacher and parent questionnaires each yield a factor of hyperactivity, but the two are not strongly related. The small number of children rated high for hyperactivity in *both* situations show the same kind of pattern of a higher rate of cognitive impairment, an earlier onset of symptoms, and a worse psychiatric prognosis at follow up. This is not of course to argue that they are necessarily brain damaged, but rather to suggest they are vulnerable to psychiatric difficulties by reason of closely related cognitive and behavioral problems that arise early in life.

NEUROPHYSIOLOGICAL MEASURES

Electrophysiological measures of children with a variety of psychiatric problems have been reviewed elsewhere.[13] Some hypotheses in this area concern rather specific processes, such as the transfer of information from one cerebral hemisphere to the other. The most generally interesting hypotheses, however, are those that suggest that the whole pattern of responsiveness of the brain to stimuli may be systematically altered as the result of neurological injury, and that this is reflected directly in disordered learning and behavior.

E. Kraepelin, for example, regarded "hyperprosexia" as a consequence of brain damage;[14] this is a tendency to excessive responsiveness to stimuli, and is very much akin to some theoretical formulations of the basic problem in hyperactivity.[15] On the whole, the physiological evidence refutes this. Findings are richest in the field of learning disorders where multiple physiological changes have been described. Children with reading problems show smaller autonomic reactions to signal stimuli;[16,17] a deficit in the high frequency 40 Hz component of the EEG;[18] a smaller amplitude of late components of the averaged visual evoked response;[19,20] less attenuation of the alpha rhythm by mental activity;[21] greater coherence between the hemispheres;[22] a smaller contingent negative variation;[23,24] and more power at all frequencies of the EEG.[25] Indeed the findings are so rich that an adequate description may well require the complex statistical techniques employed by E.R. John in the approach he has called "neurometrics."[26] If there is one feature common to all the findings, it is a general under-responsiveness to meaningful stimuli, and generalized evidence of diminished processing of information from the outside world.

One description of this tendency is the general underarousal of the cortex, which has been suggested as a pathology specific to hyperactive children. Table 2, however, indicates that underarousal as indexed by autonomic measures is probably not characteristic of such children. Data gathered on hyperactive children at a North American clinic confirm the lack of any necessary connection between underarousal and overactivity (Figure 4), although low arousal is connected with whatever abnormality is measured by the developmental neurological examination.[27,28]

It may make more sense to consider not the arousal but the arousabil-

TABLE 2. TONIC AUTONOMIC AROUSAL LEVELS IN HYPERACTIVITY

Investigators	Year	Measure Used	Findings in Hyperactive Children
J. Satterfield and D. Dawson (16)	1971	Skin conductance	Reduced
J. Satterfield, G. Atoian, G. Brashears, et al. (49)	1974	Skin conductance	Elevated
R. Dykman, P. Ackerman, S. Clements, et al. (17)	1971	Skin conductance; heart rate	Unchanged
N. Cohen and V. Douglas (32)	1972	Skin conductance	Unchanged
T.P. Zahn, F. Abate, B.C. Little, et al. (50)	1975	Skin conductance; heart rate; skin temperature	Unchanged
C. Spring, L. Greenberg, J. Scott, et al. (51)	1974	Skin conductance in drug responders	Unchanged
R.A. Barkley and T.L. Jackson, Jr. (52)	1977	Skin conductance in drug responders after drug withdrawal	Unchanged

NOTE: Numbers in parentheses after authors' names refer to notes at the end of this chapter.

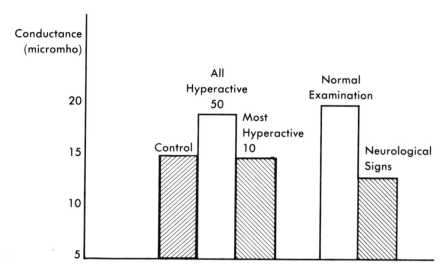

Figure 4. Skin conductance in hyperactive children. (N=50) and normal controls (N=19) (see text).

ity of overactive children. The tendency to diminished reponsiveness has also been suggested for this group.[29] Children with the broad diagnosis of overactivity do appear to be less responsive than normal children to a novel stimulus or a stimulus that acts as the signal to perform a test.[30-32] When they are presented with familiar stimuli that do not carry any signal value, however, they are not less responsive. Figure 5 shows the course of habituation of the skin conductance response to tones that do not act as a signal for any response.[33]

It seems preferable to regard the pattern of response of overactive children as a failure of selectiveness in response. This failure appears to be a nonspecific risk factor rather than a direct cause, for it is associated with a wide range of behavior deviation and not with the symptom of overactivity per se—or indeed with any symptom. It may well be neurologically determined, since even within a group of children diagnosed as overactive it is associated with the presence of signs of sensorimotor incoordination in a neurological examination (Figure 6). At present this is about the only evidence for a neurological cause. It could be that unselectiveness is not directly associated with behavior but with a disturbance of concentration. This awaits further investigation, but it is plausible in that a failure of selectiveness at the physiological level may well be associated with a similar

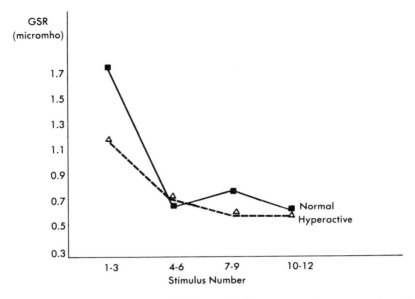

Figure 5. Galvanic skin response (GSR) amplitudes to successive presentations of an auditory tone in hyperactive children and normal controls (see text).

pattern at the psychological level of description. (Central EEG measures in hyperactivity are sufficiently contradictory as to shed no clear light on this.[34])

Not the least of the inadequacies of the concept of "minimal brain dysfunction" is that it systematically confounds behavior problems such as overactivity, and cognitive problems such as inattention and specific learning disability. It is clear that learning disorders are overrepresented in *all* the disorders of conduct by comparison not only with normal children but with emotionally disordered children. We have already seen that neurophysiological abnormalities are indeed associated with learning disorders. It remains to be discovered whether there is any neurophysiological basis for disturbances in behavior that is separate from the cognitive associations of both.

Further, it is important to avoid the "fallacy of physiological primacy," which asserts that a physically measured variable must reflect a physically based process—which of course is not so. EEG changes and autonomic nervous system actions are forms of behavior; they may as well be the effect as the cause of psychological abnormalities. Perhaps the major value of

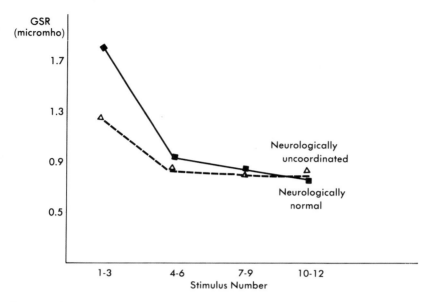

Figure 6. Galvanic skin response (GSR) amplitudes to successive presentations of an auditory tone in hyperactive children with a normal neurological examination and hyperactive children with evidence of lack of coordination on neurological examination.

these measures lies in their taking us away from the idea of "brain damage" as a unitary condition and toward the more precise description of function.

MEASURES OF COORDINATION

At first sight, the measurement of delays in acquiring sensorimotor coordination lacks some of the interest of the measures we have considered. It is not guided by theory, and it does not yet provide any useful description of functions that might take the place of the global idea of brain damage. Such an examination can indeed distinguish between normal and neurologically damaged children,[35] albeit the distinction in that study was not complete; for example, epileptic children were no different from normals. Its validity as a measure of brain damage is compromised by the clear findings that other factors, including age, sex, and IQ, can also influence the results of the examination.[36-38] Even allowing for these factors, there is some evidence that the examination is more likely to be abnormal in children with hyperactive behavior than in those with neurotic symptoms,[39] and in those with learning problems rather than in normal controls.

It may be that, just as with the neurophysiological measures, the major association is between clumsiness and cognitive problems; this could by itself account for the greater frequency of minor degrees of incoordination in children with behavior disorder. Could clumsiness be a direct reflection of an important neuropsychological impairment? First of all, clumsiness is in all probability not a unitary problem. Factor analysis of the items from the neurological examination of minor signs does not suggest a single important factor, but rather a number of loosely related abilities that bear no self-evident relationship to psychological functions.[40] It seems unlikely that an overall score from such an examination will bear much relationship to any particular cognitive skill. Second, an overall measure of coordination is not likely to be of much value in the prediction of children at risk. The very high rate of abnormalities in the general population precludes this, as it did for the radiological sign considered earlier.

Nevertheless the kind of sign that most validly discriminates among psychiatrically defined groups is that in which control functions appear to be most implicated. Dysdiadochokinesia and dysgraphesthesia have been stressed.[41] In a search for the most discriminating items I examined nineteen normal children and fifty children with disorders of conduct, using ninety "soft signs" frequently included in the developmental examination. Those that most clearly tapped a simple motor function, such as unequal reflexes or equivocal plantar responses, did not distinguish between the groups. Similarly, the presence of twitches of the fingers or strength of movements and of pointing; graphesthesia; and skill in balance. They have in common the requirements for a complex processing of information movements and of pointing; graphaesthesia; and skill in balance. They have in common the requirement for a complex processing of information in the guiding of movements. They invite experimental analysis, and indeed further progress in this area will probably come from the closer investigation of the processes required for such skills.

The interest of such an analysis is further suggested by some findings from studies on minor neurological abnormalities in adult psychiatric patients.[42] F. Quitkin and his colleagues, for example, found such signs to be present in excess in medicated psychiatric patients, as well as in unmedicated patients diagnosed as "schizophrenia with premorbid asociality" and "emotionally unstable character disorder."[43] In both groups there were problems going back to childhood; and for the first group, certainly, and for the second group, possibly, cognitive difficulties of long standing were a part of the condition. The implication is that these signs may be acting as a marker for a disturbance of function that has some influence on the form of adult psychiatric disturbance.

PSYCHOMETRIC METHODS

All the sources of evidence considered in the foregoing pages suggest the central importance of cognitive impairment in some behavior disorders, but do not specify the nature of the impairment. Psychometric tests are not of course directly useful in establishing the etiology of the abnormalities they describe. W. Yule has concisely outlined the pitfalls in any such procedure, especially in the use of profiles of test performance.[44] Their value should be a clearer description of abnormalities. Impairment of language and of attention appear to be particularly strongly in need of clearer experimental definition and measurement.

The ability to pay attention has been emphasized as a cognitive skill whose neurological impairment can lead directly to symptoms of "hyper-activity."[45] Unfortunately, there is very little consensus on what attention means or how one measures it;[46] indeed there is little information on what factors influence the development of attention. D. Shaffer and colleagues found inattention and overactivity to be associated with conduct disorder rather than with brain damage.[47] The close link between inattention and behavior problems supports the view presented here. Shaffer's study, however, is often presented as evidence against the view that inattention may be caused by brain damage. It does not in fact support this proposition, since the brain-damaged children in the study were selected for their psychiatric features, not because they represented the whole population of brain-damaged children. There is in fact evidence that both brain damage and psychological understimulation can diminish the capacity to concentrate and to sustain prolonged concentration.[48] The consequences for behavior have still to be elucidated.

CONCLUSIONS

A rather wide, though not extensive, range of measures has been considered. There is no evidence that they cohere into a single factor of brain dysfunction. Even singly, none of them can be regarded as an unequivocal index of brain abnormality. Indeed it would probably be a mistake to seek such an index, since so many lines of evidence now cast doubt on the value of a single psychological construct of brain damage. There is no "MBD syndrome," and hyperactivity is not a syndrome of brain damage.

Such uncommon symptoms, however, notably pervasive overactivity and social disinhibition, seem likely to have a developmental neurological origin that may be mediated through cognitive abnormalities. Furthermore there are signs that we are moving more closely toward useful neurophysiological accounts of important kinds of behavior. This could add an extra level of description to illuminate the pathogenesis of problems in learning and in behavior. It is likely to be applicable to the other strategy of investigation that begins with the study of neurologically defined groups of children.

NOTES

1. M. Rutter, "Brain Damage Syndromes in Childhood: Concepts and Findings," *Journal of Child Psychology and Psychiatry* 18 (1977): 1-22.

2. A.M. Galaburda, "Right-Left Asymmetries in the Brain," *Science* 199 (1978): 852-56.

3. D.B. Hier, M. Lemay, P.B. Rosenberger, et al., "Developmental Dyslexia: Evidence for a Subgroup with a Reversal of Cerebral Asymmetry," *Archives of Neurology* 35 (1978): 90-92.

4. D.P. Cantwell, "Hyperkinetic Syndrome," in *Child Psychiatry: Modern Approaches*, ed. M. Rutter and L. Hersov (Oxford: Blackwell Scientific Publications, 1977): 524-55.

5. J. Schulman, J. Kaspar, and F. Throne, *Brain Damage and Behavior: A Clinical-Experimental Study* (Springfield, Illinois: C. C Thomas, 1965).

6. J. Werry, "Studies on the Hyperactive Child. IV: An Empirical Analysis of the Minimal Brain Dysfunction Syndrome," *Archives of General Psychiatry* 19 (1968): 9-16.

7. C.K. Conners, "A Teacher Rating Scale for Use in Drug Studies with Children," *American Journal of Psychiatry* 126 (1969): 884-88.

8. E. Taylor, "The Drug Treatment of Hyperkinetic States: Clinical Issues," *Neuropharmacology*, in press.

9. S. Sandberg, M. Rutter, and E. Taylor, "Hyperkinetic Disorder in Psychiatric Clinic Attenders," *Developmental Medicine and Child Neurology* 20 (1978); 279-99.

10. D. Shaffer, O. Chadwick, and M. Rutter, "Psychiatric Outcome of Localised Head Injury in Children," in *Outcome of Severe Damage to the Central Nervous System*, ed. R. Porter and D. FitzSimons (Amsterdam: Elsevier, Excerpta Medica, North Holland, 1975).

11. Sandberg, Rutter, and Taylor, "Hyperkinetic Disorder" (See note 9).

12. R. Schacher, M. Rutter, and A. Smith, "The Characteristics of Situationally and Pervasively Hyperactive Children: Implications for Syndrome Definition," *Journal of Child Psychology and Psychiatry*, in press.

13. E. Taylor, "Psychophysiology of Childhood Disorders," in *Handbook of Biological Psychiatry*, eds. H.M. van Praag, M.H. Lader, O.J. Rafaelsen, et al. (New York: Marcel Dekker, 1980).

14. E. Kraepelin, *Psychiatrie. Ein Lehrbuch für Studierende und Aerzte*, 5th ed (Leipzig: Barth, 1896).

15. P. Wender, "Minimal Brain Dysfunction in Children" (New York: John Wiley, 1971).

16. J. Satterfield and D. Dawson "Electrodermal Correlates of Hyperactivity in Children," *Psychophysiology* 8 (1971): 191-97.

17. R. Dykman, P. Ackerman, S. Clements, et al., "Specific Learning Disabilities: An Attentional Deficit Syndrome," in *Progress in Learning Abilities*, vol. 2, ed. H. Mykelbust (New York: Grune and Stratton, 1971).

18. D.E. Sheer, "Focused Arousal and 40 Hz EEG," in *The Neuropsychology of Learning Disabilities*, ed. R. Knights and D. Bakker (Baltimore, Maryland: University Park Press, 1976).

19. C.K. Conners, "Cortical Visual Evoked Response in Children with Learning Disorders," *Psychophysiology* 7 (1970): 418-28.

20. A. Preston, J.T. Guthries, and B. Childs, "Visual Evoked Responses in Normal and Disabled Readers." *Psychophysiology* 11 (1974): 452-57.

21. P.W. Fuller, "Computer-Estimated Alpha Attenuation during Problem Solving in Children with Learning Disabilities," *Electroencephalography and Clinical Neurophysiology* 42 (1977): 149.

22. B. Sklar, J. Hanley, and W.W. Simmons, "An EEG Experiment Aimed towards Identifying Dyslexic Children" *Nature* 240 (1972): 414.

23. Dykman, Ackerman, Clements, et al., "Specific Learning Disabilities" (See note 17).

24. J. Cohen, "A New Psychophysiological Approach to the Diagnostic Evaluation of Children," quoted in ibid.

25. A.E. Maxwell, P. Fenwick, G.W. Fenton, et al., "Reading Ability and Brain Function: A Simple Statistical Model," *Psychological Medicine* 4 (1974): 274-80.

26. E.R. John, B.Z. Karmel, W.C. Corning, et al., "Neurometrics," *Science* 196 (1977): 1393-1410.

27. C.K. Conners, "Minimal Brain Dysfunction and Psychopathology in Children," in *Child Personality and Psychopathology: Current Tapes*, vol. 2, ed. A. Davis (New York: John Wiley, 1975).

28. E. Taylor, "Physiological and Clinical Features in the Hyperkinetic Syndrome" (Paper presented at a meeting of the Royal College of Psychiatrists, Child Psychiatry Section, 1976).

29. J.E. Hastings and R.A. Barkley, "A Review of Psychophysiological Research with Hyperkinetic Children," *Journal of Abnormal Child Psychology* 6 (1978): 413-47.

30. Dykman, Ackerman, Clements, et al., "Specific Learning Disabilities" (See note 17).

31. Satterfield and Dawson, "Electrodermal Correlates" (See note 16).

32. N. Cohen and V. Douglas, "Characteristics of the Orienting Response in Hyperactive and Normal Children," *Psychophysiology* 9 (1972): 238-46.

33. Taylor, "Hyperkinetic Syndrome" (See note 28).

34. _____, "Childhood Disorders" (See note 13).

35. M. Rutter, P. Graham, and W. Yule, *A Neuropsychiatric Study in Childhood* (London: SIMP/Heinemann, 1970).

36. J.E. Peters, J.S. Roming, and R.A. Dykman, "A Special Neurological Examination of Children with Learning Disabilities," *Developmental Medicine and Child Neurology* 17 (1975): 63-78.

37. R.M. Adams, J.J. Kocsis, and R.E. Estes, "Soft Neurological Signs in Learning—Disabled Children and Controls," *American Journal of Diseases of Children* 128 (1974): 614-18.

38. H.R. Myklebust, "Identification and Diagnosis of Children with Learning Disabilities: An Interdisciplinary Study of Criteria," *Seminars in Psychiatry* 5 (1973): 55-77.

39. J. Werry, K. Minde, W. Guzman, et al., "Studies on the Hyperactive Child. VII: Neurological Status Compared with Neurotic and Normal Children," *American Journal of Orthopsychiatry* 42 (1972): 441-50.

40. Peters, Roming, and Dykman, "Neurological Examination" (See note 36).

41. D. Shaffer, "Brain Injury," in *Child Psychiatry: Modern Approaches*, ed. M. Rutter and L. Hersov (Oxford: Blackwell Scientific Publications, 1977): 185-215.

42. _____, "Longitudinal Research and the Minimal Brain Damage Syndrome," in

Minimal Brain Dysfunction: Fact or Fiction, ed. A.F. Kalverboer, H.M. van Praag, and J. Mendlewicz (Basel: S. Karger, 1978): 18-34.

43. F. Quitkin, A. Rifkin, and D.F. Klein, "Neurological Soft Signs in Schizophrenia and Character Disorders," *Archives of General Psychiatry* 33 (1976): 845-53.

44. W. Yule, "Diagnosis: Developmental Psychological Assessment," in *Minimal Brain Dysfunction: Fact or Fiction*, ed. A.F. Kalverboer, H.M. van Praag, and J. Mendlewicz (Basel: S. Karger, 1978): 35-54.

45. V. Douglas, "Stop, Look and Listen: The Problem of Sustained Attention and Impulse Control in Hyperactive and Normal Children," *Canadian Journal of Behavioural Science* 4 (1972): 259-82.

46. E: Taylor, "Development of Attention," in *Scientific Foundations of Developmental Psychiatry*, ed. M. Rutter (London: Heinemann, forthcoming).

47. D. Shaffer, N. McNamara, and J.H. Pincus, "Controlled Observations on Patterns of Activity, Attention and Impulsivity in Brain-Damaged and Psychiatrically Disturbed Boys," *Psychological Medicine* 4 (1974): 4-18.

48. Taylor, "Development of Attention" (See note 46).

49. J. Satterfield, G. Atoian, G. Brashears, et al., "Electrodermal Studies in Minimal Brain Dysfunction Children," in *Clinical Use of Stimulant Drugs in Children*, ed. C.K. Conners (Amsterdam: Excerpta Medica, 1974).

50. T.P. Zahn, F. Abate, B.C. Little, et al., "Minimal Brain Dysfunction, Stimulant Drugs and Autonomic Nervous System Activity," *Archives of General Psychiatry* 32 (1975): 381-87.

51. C. Spring, L. Greenberg, J. Scott, et al., "Electrodermal Activity in Hyperactive Boys Who Are Methylphenidate Responders," *Psychophysiology* 11 (1974): 436-42.

52. R.A. Barkley and T.L. Jackson, Jr., "Hyperkinesis, Autonomic Nervous System Activity and Stimulant Drug Effects," *Journal of Child Psychology and Psychiatry* 18 (1977): 347-57.

BRAIN DAMAGE AND PSYCHIATRIC DISORDER IN CHILDHOOD

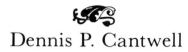

Dennis P. Cantwell

The idea that brain damage may lead to psychiatric disorder in childhood has been prevalent for well over a century.[1] This paper will discuss current knowledge about the relationship between brain damage and psychiatric disorder in childhood in terms of: 1) problems in terminology, in nosology, and in diagnosis of both brain damage and psychiatric disorder; and 2) the epidemiological evidence regarding the relationship of brain damage to the development of psychiatric disorder in children.

TERMINOLOGY

"Brain damage" in its literal sense should be used to describe a condition in which there is a definite structural change in the brain. "Brain dysfunction" should be used when there is an abnormal functioning of the brain, such as an abnormal electrical discharge. Abnormal functioning of the central nervous system (CNS) may occur with or without evidence of an abnormality in the anatomical brain structure; the terms are often used interchangeably, however.[2] Adding the word "minimal" to terms such as brain damage and brain dysfunction serves to complicate the picture even more. The concept of minimal is a quantitative one, which implies we can quantitate something—brain damage or brain dysfunction—that we have a hard time even measuring in children. In addition, at least on the American side of the Atlantic, the diagnosis of minimal brain damage and brain dysfunction is often made *solely* on the basis of the presence of psychiatric

114

and behavioral abnormalities, especially the syndrome of hyperactivity, inattentiveness, and impulsive behavior. Thus, in such cases, brain damage is always associated with psychiatric disorder.

Workers on the European side of the Atlantic, particularly in Britain, have rightly criticized this broad concept of minimal brain damage and minimal brain dysfunction. The European view, generally, is that if a psychiatric disorder develops as a result of brain damage it does so primarily because of the locus of the lesion in the brain, the patient's age at the time the lesion occurred, and the severity of the lesion. Moreover brain damage does not lead to a specific form of psychiatric disorder characterized by a particular symptom pattern.

PROBLEMS IN THE DIAGNOSIS OF PSYCHIATRIC DISORDER

If one is to infer a causal relationship between brain damage or dysfunction and psychiatric disorder, one is faced with the problem of reliably and validly measuring both the damage or dysfunction and the disorder. The voluminous literature on this topic gives negligible recognition to the methodological difficulties of such measurements.

From the standpoint of psychiatric disorder, the official nomenclatures that have been used in the United States—those in the first and second editions of the *Diagnostic and Statistical Manual of Mental Disorders* (DSM)—provide little in the way of psychiatric diagnoses in childhood. DSM I provides no section specifically related to psychiatric disorders of childhood; DSM II has one section with six possible diagnoses, the reliability of which have never been determined in a systematic study. Moreover the validity of some of the categories, such as "runaway reaction of childhood," has never been demonstrated.

The classification system in the third and most recent edition of the DSM,[3] which will become the official system in July 1980, is a vast improvement in this area. There is a much more inclusive childhood and adolescence section. Each disorder is described in a systematic and comprehensive fashion, with essential features; associated features; complications; natural history; familial pattern of illness; predisposing factors; severity; and prevalence. In addition, operational diagnostic criteria are specified for the diagnosis of each psychiatric disorder of childhood and adolescence.

This comprehensive description and the specified diagnostic criteria increase reliability and increase the likelihood of both face validity and descriptive validity for these categories. Whether all the categories will be determined to have predictive validity must await further study. But this edition promises to be a considerable improvement over its predecessors.

The system is a multiaxial one: psychiatric syndromes are coded on either Axis I or Axis II. Axis III allows the clinician to code all biological features outside the mental disorders section of the *Manual of International Statistical Classification of Diseases*[4] that are thought to play a role in the genesis or management of the disorder. This will allow data to be collected in a systematic fashion in order that we may determine how often specific biological factors are related to the presence of specific psychiatric syndromes in childhood and adolescence.

PROBLEMS IN THE DIAGNOSIS OF BRAIN DAMAGE

However great the problems of diagnosis of psychiatric disorder are in childhood, they do not appear to be as great as the problem of diagnosing brain damage and dysfunction. Major techniques used for the diagnosis of brain damage include the following: history from the parents; medical records; physical and neurological examination; laboratory studies, including psychological tests; highly specialized neurological investigative techniques; and autopsy and biopsy.[5]

The *history from the parents* is probably the most frequently used, and definitely the least useful and most inaccurate technique. A number of studies have shown that developmental histories are extremely unreliable.[6] Many important details of pregnancy, delivery, and neonatal status are not recalled by parents, who may have selective recall of potentially traumatic events only for children who later turn out to have psychiatric disturbance. This suggests that the use of medical records may be a more fruitful approach.

When *medical records* are examined, however, it becomes apparent that the information they contain is seldom recorded systematically. When an item is not mentioned one has no way of knowing whether it was not observed or whether it was not inquired about. Thus critical data necessary to make a positive diagnosis of potentially traumatic events are often missing. Even if evidence of potentially traumatic events is available in the records, one cannot make a one-to-one relationship between a history of pre- and perinatal complications and actual damage to the brain. Events that are *potentially* traumatic actually lead to some type of brain damage only in some cases; D. Shaffer's review of the sequelae of perinatal difficulties aptly points this out.[7] Finally, potentially traumatic events that *do* eventually result in brain damage may lead to behavioral abnormality only in certain cases. Perinatal abnormalities are not independent of disadvantageous social and family conditions, which may themselves lead to psychiatric disorder. Thus, even if a relationship is discovered between possible brain damage in early life and later psychiatric disorder, the disorder may be due to some antecedent factor that causes both the damage and the disorder.

A properly conducted and systematically recorded *physical and neurological examination* is of value in detecting major degrees of brain damage. In these cases the brain lesion impinges on a nonsilent area of the brain, giving rise to specific signs such as the Babinski reflex.[8] These "hard" signs, however, are prevalent only in a minority of children with psychiatric disorder. In the United States, particularly, the concept of equivocal or "soft" neurological signs has been advocated as evidence of "minimal brain damage," especially in psychiatrically disordered children.

Unfortunately, until recently most of the relevant literature presented data collected by examinations that were not standardized and for which there are no known normative values.[9] As J.S. Werry has pointed out, what is needed is a wide-ranging system of pediatric-neurological examinations with demonstrated reliability that have been standardized for the general population.[10] This would enable one to establish validity by comparing the results of the examinations of brain-damaged and normal groups. Four such examinations have been developed in recent years: the physical and neurological examination for soft signs (PANESS); the developmental-neurological examination designed by J. Peters; a similar one by Werry and his colleagues; and one by M. Rutter on the Isle of Wight.[11]

In his review of these examinations, Werry concludes that the best, especially in terms of reliability and validity, is that developed by Rutter, who distinguished three types of signs:

• The traditional hard neurological signs such as the Babinski, which almost always indicate neurological abnormality.

• Signs such as ataxia and nystagmus, which sometimes indicate brain damage.

• Signs that represent isolated deficits of function, which are normal for young children; these might include mirror movements, enuresis, and coordination difficulties.

Shaffer's review of soft neurological signs and their relationship to psychiatric disorder in adolescence and later life suggests they are found in older patients suffering from particular types of psychiatric disorder.[12] The studies made to date, however, have been on adult patients who have not been followed from childhood on.[13] Thus we are unable to tell whether the soft signs present in adult life have indeed been present since childhood; nor is it possible to ascertain if any psychiatric disorder was diagnosed in childhood, and if so what type. These studies suggest it might be a fruitful research exercise to examine psychiatric correlates of soft signs in unselected adult populations, and to follow up populations of children with the same type of psychiatric disorder, whether or not there are neurological soft signs.

Certain *laboratory studies* such as the EEG have long been performed on populations of psychiatrically disordered children with the intent of suggesting they indicate brain damage or dysfunction. These interpretations are made despite the fact that there is often lack of agreement among readers of the EEG on both the criteria of the abnormality and its neurological significance.[14] More sophisticated techniques, such as power-spectral analysis of the EEG and evoked potential studies, may give greater promise. Some studies have suggested very specific types of abnormalities associated with certain disorders, such as attention-deficit disorder with hyperactivity.[15] These techniques, however, and the results obtained from them must still be considered in the exploratory stage. In general, comparative studies have not been made using the same techniques with different types of psychiatric disorders in childhood. Investigators have usually concentrated on studying one type of disorder; and different investigators studying the same type of disorder have often come up with contradictory results.

Studies of blood levels and urinary metabolites of biogenic amines have indicated certain types of brain dysfunction in adult patients with various types of psychiatric disorders, such as affective disorders. Similar types of studies of psychiatric disorders of childhood are in their first stages, but some of them do show promise. Biogenic amine studies have been conducted in infantile autism, affective disorder, and attention-deficit disorder with hyperactivity.[16] Again, they must be regarded as exploratory, but they may point the way for more careful delineation of subgroups of these disorders, which do in fact have as their basis some disturbances in biogenic amine metabolism.

Certain psychological tests have been evaluated for their ability to diagnose brain damage, and even to localize it in children. The evidence for such a view is questionable. R. Gittelman-Klein's recent review of psychodiagnosis in childhood[17] suggests there is very little evidence for the notion. Reviews by F.K. Graham and P.W. Burman,[18] M. Herbert,[19] V. Meyer,[20] and A.J. Yates[21] have clearly shown that the validity of using any psychological tests or combination of tests to make a diagnosis of brain damage in children is not established. A number of individuals such as R. Reitan and his associates[22] have attempted to develop neuropsychological test batteries for detecting and localizing brain damage in children. While these may be promising, as are the newer methods developed by workers such as P.E. Tanguay,[23] who follow the neuropsychological model of A.R. Luria, they remain unproven as agents for making a definite diagnosis.

Specialized medical and neurological evaluations, including older techniques such as skull X-rays, angiograms, pneumoencephalograms, and brain scans are rarely done in psychiatrically disordered children unless major cerebral pathology is suspected clinically. Generally these techniques need major degrees of cerebral pathology before they detect any abnormality. More promising results may be obtained with the Emi-Scan, which is not an invasive procedure and which may be more likely to turn up pathology— but also only of a fairly substantial nature.

Biopsy and autopsy are obviously relevant in a minority of cases. Autopsy of course provides the most thorough way to make a diagnosis of brain damage, but it is usually helpful only in cases where the diagnosis is already clear.

A negative brain biopsy does not rule out the possibility that the area sampled is not damaged. Ethical considerations make brain biopsy a feasible procedure in a very small minority of children with psychiatric disorder.

Thus, in reviewing the state of the art in 1979, Werry has summarized the accuracy of the diagnosis of brain damage or dysfunction in children with psychiatric disorders as being "no more than an enlightened guess."

BRAIN DAMAGE AND THE GENESIS OF PSYCHIATRIC DISORDER IN CHILDREN

There is a rather voluminous literature on children with various types of psychiatric disorder who have been studied from a number of standpoints to determine the relative frequency of brain damage and dysfunction. Children studied include inpatients and outpatients of all ages, from infancy through adolescence. The foregoing methods of diagnosis for damage and dysfunction have been used in a variety of combinations in these studies.

Werry has reviewed this literature and has come to the conclusion that when *groups* of psychiatrically disturbed children are studied they do show an increased incidence of signs and symptoms *suggestive* of damage or dysfunction. These include such factors as minor physical anomalies; soft neurological signs; abnormalities in the EEG; and possible pre- and perinatal complications. These studies are far from conclusive, however. As pointed out earlier, the relationship between pre- and perinatal complications and actual damage to the brain is a very tenuous one; that between soft neurological signs or EEG abnormalities and brain damage and dysfunction is even more tenuous. Even if the diagnosis of brain damage can be firmly established in groups of children with a psychiatric disorder, there is usually no way of proving conclusively in individual cases that it is a cause rather than a correlate of the disorder. Alternatively, it may be that certain "X factors," such as adverse environmental and social circumstances, lead to both the brain damage and the disorder.

One of the best of these studies was done on the Isle of Wight.[24] Rutter and his colleagues found that less than 5 percent of children age ten and eleven who had clinically significant psychiatric disorders also had detectable pathological disorders of the brain. That compares with a prevalence rate of 6.4 per 1,000 for pathological disorders of the brain in the total child population of the island. This is a minimal figure, since it does not include children with uncomplicated epilepsy, language delay, coordination problems, and other conditions that may in fact be due to an anatomical brain lesion, but that cannot be detected by current neurological techniques. The figures from this large scale, carefully conducted and controlled epidemiological study indicate that only a minority of children with clinically significant psychiatric disorder have demonstrable evidence of damage to the brain. They also indicate, however, that, compared to the general population of children, those with psychiatric disorder do have an increased prevalance rate of abnormality of the brain.

Another way of looking at the same question would be to observe specific populations of children with various types of psychiatric disorder, rather than large groups of children with heterogeneous disorders. The classes of disorders described in the childhood and adolescence section of DSM III can be separated into five major groupings on the basis of the predominant area of disturbance:

1. Intellectual
   Mental retardation
2. Overt Behavior
   Attention-deficit disorder; conduct disorder
3. Emotional
   Anxiety and other disorders of infancy, childhood, and adolescence
4. Physical
   Eating disorders; stereotyped-movement disorders; and other disorders with physical manifestations
5. Developmental
   Pervasive and specific developmental disorders

If we begin with *mental retardation*, etiological factors may be primarily biological or psychosocial, or an interaction of both. In 25 percent of the cases the etiological factors are known biological abnormalities. Mentally retarded individuals with IQs below 50 almost always have a biological disorder as the basis for their retardation.

Moving on to *overt behavioral disorders*—attention-deficit disorder with hyperactivity; attention-deficit disorder with no hyperactivity; and conduct disorder—the following general statements seem warranted. Attention-deficit disorder with no hyperactivity is a syndrome described for the first time in DSM III, and no systematic studies have been done to either confirm or deny the presence of organic etiology. Attention-deficit disorder with hyperactivity is the new term for what in DSM II was called hyperkinetic reaction; it is also referred to by many other terms, such as the minimal brain dysfunction syndrome. The condition is diagnosed much more frequently in the United States than in Great Britain, probably due to the British requirement of severe persistent hyperactivity as a diagnostic criterion. The British view is that this disorder may not be distinct from the more general group of conduct disorders; the American view is that conduct disorder may coexist with attention-deficit disorder with hyperactivity, which is in itself a distinct syndrome.

An overall review of the literature on the latter syndrome suggests that children with this disorder are more likely than normal children of the same age and intellectual level to have neurological, perceptual, cognitive, and EEG indices *suggestive* of brain damage or dysfunction.[25,26] Psychophysiological studies indicate that, as a group, these children may have a defect in arousability—that is, they may be unable to respond to stimulation.[27] Biochemical studies, although in their infancy, suggest that, as a group, these children may also have a disorder of the central neurotransmitter system.[28] It is clear, however, that many children with this disorder show no evidence of brain damage or dysfunction by whatever indices used. Thus the clinical syndrome alone cannot be taken in and of itself as diagnosis of CNS organicity. Likewise, as will be reviewed later, when brain damage does lead to a psychiatric disorder it certainly does not result uniformly in this symptom pattern of hyperactivity, short attention span, and impulsive behavior.

Many of the foregoing statements about attention-deficit disorder with hyperactivity may also be made about conduct disorder. A number of studies do suggest that children with this disorder are more likely than normal children to have certain indices suggestive of brain damage or brain dysfunction. Indeed the psychophysiological findings for children with attention-deficit disorder with hyperactivity are similar to those presented by H. Quay for both adults and children with conduct disorders.[29]

Since many of these studies probably contain overlapping groups of children with conduct disorders, attention-deficit disorder with hyperactivity, and both disorders, it is difficult to make statements about conduct disorder that may not be attributable to the fact children with attention-deficit disorder with hyperactivity were included in the population studied. Indeed in the British view they may not be separate disorders.

The large category of *emotional disorders* in DSM III includes *anxiety disorders*; separation anxiety disorder; avoidant disorder; and overanxious disorder. Although they have not been studied as extensively as conduct disorders or attention-deficit disorders, what little evidence there is suggests that CNS organic factors are much less important in the genesis of anxiety disorders than they are in the others that have been studied.[30]

Other disorders of infancy, childhood, or adolescence grouped under the emotional disorder category in DSM III include reactive-attachment disorder of infancy; schizoid disorder; elective mutism; oppositional disorder; and identity disorder. Reactive-attachment disorder of infancy is characterized by lack of physical development (failure to thrive); apathy; and lack of age-appropriate signs of social responsiveness due to a physical disorder. When care of these children is grossly inadequate, severe malnutrition can cause permanent brain damage. The evidence for organic factors playing a role in schizoid disorder, oppositional disorder, and identity disorder is essentially nonexistent, primarily due to a lack of studies. In elective mutism, mental retardation is a predisposing factor, and some children have delayed language development suggestive of possible CNS dysfunction.

The large group of *physical disorders* in DSM III include three subgroups: *eating disorders, stereotyped-movement disorders*, and *other disorders with physical manifestations*.

Eating disorders include anorexia nervosa, bulimia, pica, and rumination disorder of infancy. Mental retardation is a predisposing factor to pica, but the evidence for brain damage or dysfunction in the other eating disorders is lacking.

Stereotyped-movement disorders include transient-tic disorder, chronic motor-tic disorder, and Tourette's syndrome. It is not known whether these three tic disorders represent distinct conditions or a continuum of severity. About half the individuals with Tourette's syndrome exhibit nonspecific EEG abnormalities, soft neurological signs, and minor physical anomalies.

The subclass, *other disorders with physical manifestations*, includes categories in which the predominant disturbance is a physical function, such as stuttering, functional enuresis, functional encopresis, sleepwalking, and sleep terrors. Seizure disorders, infections of the CNS, and CNS trauma are all predisposing factors in the development of sleepwalking. Episodes usually occur between a half-hour and three hours after the onset of sleep, in the period of nonrapid eye movement sleep. Sleep terror disorder also occurs in roughly the same time period; there is no solid evidence for organic factors playing a role in its etiology.

Functional enuresis and functional encopresis by definition exclude cases due to organic etiology. Likewise there is no solid evidence that brain damage or brain dysfunction play an etiological role in stuttering.

Pervasive developmental disorders in DSM III include infantile autism and pervasive developmental disorder, childhood onset. These are children whose disorder has formerly been described by such terms as childhood schizophrenia, symbiotic psychosis, and atypical. These disorders are characterized by distortions in the development of multiple basic psychological functions involved in the development of social skills and language. Studies suggest that the great majority of these children probably have some form of CNS dysfunction as at least one etiological factor. Even careful testing of autistic children, however, indicates that about 25 percent have no definite evidence of brain damage or dysfunction.[31]

In summary, certain types of psychiatric disorders in childhood are much more likely to be associated with brain damage and brain dysfunction. Pervasive developmental disorder and mental retardation of at least a moderate degree are most likely to be associated with brain damage. Anxiety disorders are probably least likely to have an organic basis, with other disorders falling somewhere in between.

DOES BRAIN DAMAGE INCREASE THE RISK OF PSYCHIATRIC DISORDER?

The prevalence rates for psychiatric disorder have been studied in children selected because they have either definite or suspected brain damage of a variety of types. Most of the studies have been retrospective; a few have been prospective. The types of proven and suspected brain damage in these studies include pre- and perinatal abnormalities; prematurity; encephalitis; epilepsy; cerebral palsy; head injury; and lead poisoning. Werry concludes that there probably is an increased risk of psychiatric disorder in children with suspected and proven brain damage.[32] A. Sameroff and M. Chandler have pointed out the strong influence of the psychosocial environment, however, which they labeled the "continuum of caretaking casualty," on the subsequent development of psychiatric disorder in children with definite and suspected brain damage.[33]

Rutter and his colleagues on the Isle of Wight used assessment techniques of known reliability to examine a total population of children unbiased by selective referral practices.[34] They chose for their study all children born between 1 March 1950 and 31 August 1960 who suffered from any type of chronic neuroepileptic disorder present at the time of the assessment and associated with a current or persistent handicap. Children were excluded in whom the diagnosis of brain damage had to be made *solely* on the basis of soft signs, or in the presence of some type of behavioral or cognitive abnormality that may or may not have been due to actual damage to the brain. Thus this was a study of truly brain-damaged children.

There were 186 children with a definite neuroepileptic disorder, and the diagnostic breakdown was as follows: sixty-four, uncomplicated epilepsy; forty, severe intellectual retardation; thirty-five, cerebral palsy; twenty, some other brain disorder; nineteen, a lesion below the brain stem; fifteen, blind; fourteen, deaf; nine, a developmental language disorder; and two, a spinal defect but no other associated neurological problem. There was some overlap among these diagnostic groups. A comparison of the prevalence rate of psychiatric disorder was made of the various groups of Isle of Wight children.

About 7 percent of the ten- and eleven-year-olds were found to have a clinically significant psychiatric disorder. Those with chronic physical disorders *not* involving the brain, such as asthma and diabetes, had a rate of psychiatric disorder of about 12 percent—almost twice as high as that of the general population. Psychiatric disorder was found in approximately 17 percent of the blind children; 16 percent of the deaf children; and 13 percent of children with lesions at or below the level of the brain stem. The evidence suggests that the disorder was significantly higher in children with a variety of physical disabilities not directly involving the brain than in children in the general population.

The most striking finding of the study was the very high psychiatric rate—35 percent—among children with definite brain disorders. This is five times higher than the rate for the general population, and three times higher than that for children with chronic disorders that did not involve anatomical abnormality in brain structure. Children with uncomplicated epilepsy had a psychiatric disorder rate of about 28 percent; children with epilepsy who *also* had definite abnormalities above the level of the brain stem had a rate of about 58 percent. Children who had lesions above the brain stem without epilepsy had a rate of about 37.5 percent.

This carefully designed study indicates very definitely an increased prevalence rate of psychiatric disorder in children with demonstrable brain damage, and, likewise, a comparable prevalence rate in children with at least one form of abnormal brain function but with no demonstrable physical abnormality of the brain: uncomplicated epilepsy. Those who have both an abnormality in brain structure and in brain function have an even higher rate of psychiatric disorder.

Another major finding of the Isle of Wight study is that no specific behavior syndrome occurs in children with known brain damage. Neurotic and antisocial disorders were the most common psychiatric disorders seen in children in the general population; they were also the most common in children with uncomplicated epilepsy and in those with lesions above the brain stem.

WHICH BRAIN-DAMAGED CHILDREN DEVELOP A PSYCHIATRIC DISORDER?

As not all children who have brain damage develop a psychiatric disorder, the next important question is: What are the factors associated with psychiatric disorder in children with brain damage? Some factors that have been considered include sex of the child; locus of the lesion in the brain; age of the child at the time of the brain injury; severity of the injury; etiological type of injury; and presence of associated factors such as intellectual retardation, abnormal physiological brain functioning, and certain environmental variables.

Although psychiatric disorder in childhood is more common in males than in females, the evidence from some studies suggests that psychiatric disorder in brain-damaged children is just as common in girls as it is in boys.[35]

A study by Shaffer and his colleagues on the psychiatric outcome of localized head injury in children provides some answers to the question of whether age at the time of the injury and severity and locus of the injury play an important role in the onset of psychiatric disorder.[36] They studied children with unilateral, compound, depressed fractures of the skull, with an associated tear of the dura; associated gross damage to the underlying brain substance had been confirmed at the time of surgery. Locus, age, and severity could thus be well determined. The rate of psychiatric disorder in this group was 62 percent.

No significant difference was observed in the rate of psychiatric disorder among children who had right or left hemisphere injuries, or injuries to the frontal, temporal, or parieto-occipital areas; the rate among those with right parieto-occipital injuries, however, was significantly lower than in the others—39 percent compared to 67 percent. No significant difference in the rate of psychiatric disorder was found related to age at the time of the injury or to the duration of loss of consciousness.

The rate of psychiatric disorder was high in children who had an attack of epilepsy shortly after the injury, and higher still in those who developed epilepsy some time after the injury. These differences, however, were not statistically significant. Thus the presence or absence of psychiatric disorder was *not* related to the age, locus, or severity of injury.

A number of adverse family and social circumstances were found to be significantly related to the presence of psychiatric disorder. These included a broken home or unhappy marriage; contact with two or more social agencies; psychiatric disorder in the mother and high scores on her malaise inventory; psychiatric disorder in the father; and the presence of four or more siblings in the family. Not related to the presence of psychiatric disorder were such factors as social class; overcrowding in the home; one parent having had psychiatric treatment at any time in the past; and the father having psychiatric disorder. When a disadvantage scale was constructed containing five items, psychiatric disorder was strongly associated with a high score, with one point being given for each item.

Thus children who had head injuries were very likely to develop a psychiatric disorder—62 percent in this study. The presence of psychiatric disorder, however, was unrelated to either the locus of the lesion, the age at which it occurred, or its severity. The likelihood of increased psychiatric disorder in this population, however, was related to the presence of adverse environmental circumstances.

There does not appear to be evidence that one type of etiological agent causing brain damage, independent of other variables, is more likely to relate to psychiatric disorder than another agent. Studies such as Rutter's suggest that the presence of both associated intellectual retardation and abnormal physiological functioning, such as epilepsy, are likely to lead to psychiatric disorder in children with brain damage. Active brain disturbance appears to be associated more with psychiatric disorder in such children than with a loss of brain function.

What are the possible factors that interact with brain damage in children to heighten the likelihood of their developing psychiatric disorder? We will consider the following:

- Familial variables
- Academic retardation
- The social attitude of others
- Distorted social perceptions of the child

Familial Variables

The familial variables to be considered include psychiatric illness in family members and other family pathology; broken homes; social disadvantage; and family attitudes toward the handicap of the child.

In an early study, F. Grunberg and D.A. Pond showed that more epileptic children with behavior disorders came from deviant families than did those who had no psychiatric problems. They compared fifty-three epileptic children with conduct disorders to fifty-three children with none.[37] Three broad categories of possible etiological causes of the behavior disorders were considered: organic, genetic, and social. There were no significant differences between the two groups on any of the organic factors. Thirty of the fifty-three children with conduct disorder had a family history of psychiatric disorder, as opposed to sixteen in the group who did not have conduct disorder. A family history of psychopathy was the most significant finding. The greatest differences between the two groups, however, were in the social and environmental factors, particularly in those relating to "maternal attitude" and "breaks and changes" in the child's environment. Thirty-four mothers of children with conduct disorder were felt to have a disturbed attitude toward the child, as opposed to ten in the nonconduct-disorder group. A disturbed paternal attitude was found in seventeen of the fifty-three children with conduct disorder, as opposed to six with none. The conduct-disorder children also came from families in which there was greater marital discord and more breaks and changes in the environment, and from family settings in which they were more likely to be deprived of normal social opportunities. The authors compared thirty-five of the epileptic children with conduct disorder with thirty-five nonepileptic children with the same type of behavior problem. They found the same adverse social and environmental factors in both groups.

Likewise, J.A. Harrington and F.J.J. Letemendia demonstrated that children with head injuries who had a psychiatric referral had greater family pathology than those who were not referred to a psychiatrist.[38] They examined the records of children seen between 1947 and 1955 in the Children's Department of the Maudsley Hospital in London, looking for a history of head injuries in this group. Then they examined the records of children with head injury admitted to the emergency service of the University College Hospital, London, and the University Hospital in Birmingham between 1946 and 1955. Each child was then personally examined, and one parent was interviewed. There were thirty-one cases from the Maudsley psychiatric clinic population, and thirty-two from the surgical clinic population.

In looking at the psychiatric status of both groups at the time of follow up, eighteen children in the surgical clinic group were asymptomatic, as opposed to none in the psychiatric clinic group, which was to be expected. The latter group also showed more severe and varied psychiatric symptoms than did the surgical clinic group. Eighteen children in the psychiatric clinic population came from disturbed families—twelve from homes with a moderate degree of disturbance, and six from severely disturbed homes; in eight of the families there was a history of overt psychiatric disorder in one or both parents. In contrast, only ten of the surgical clinic children had disturbance in their family backgrounds—nine of a moderate degree, one of a severe degree. One or both parents were undergoing psychiatric treatment in five of the thirty-two families in the surgical group.

Finally, the investigators observed that if one used the presence and extent of a fracture, the duration of unconsciousness, and the severity of neurological sequelae as criteria of severity of head injury, the children in the surgical clinic had more severe injuries. If one assumed that the head injuries were the *major* factor in producing subsequent psychiatric problems, one would expect the surgical group to have shown an equal or greater amount of behavior disorder than the psychiatric clinic group. This was not the case, however. The authors concluded that many of the psychiatric symptoms were not *directly* attributable to the head injury alone, but were produced by other factors. As in the study by Grunberg and Pond,[39] family background seemed to be the major factor for both genetic and environmental reasons.

In Rutter's Isle of Wight study of family pathology, such as maternal depression or malaise and family quarrels, the incidence was the same in families with brain-damaged children as in those with children who had other forms of physical handicap not involving the CNS. The rate of psychiatric disorder in children with CNS damage, however, was considerably higher, so that family pathology was not solely responsible for the development of disorder in these children. Thirty-nine percent of the epileptic children with a psychiatric problem had mothers who had "nervous breakdowns," compared to only 12 percent of the children with epilepsy who had no psychiatric disorder. The incidence of maternal malaise was 67 percent in the psychiatrically disordered epileptic population, versus 26 percent in the epileptic population with no psychiatric problem; both these differences were statistically significant at the 5 percent level.

It is known that children raised in families with psychiatric disorder or with high rates of pathology and discord are at risk for the development of psychiatric problems.[40] Brain-damaged children growing up in such families are even more at risk; family pathology is one of the mechanisms by which the vulnerable brain-damaged child develops a psychiatric problem.

Broken homes were not, however, significantly more common among epileptic children with a psychiatric disorder. Psychiatric problems were significantly less common among uncomplicated epileptic children whose fathers had a nonmanual occupation. The meaning of this association with social class is not easily interpretable; no association between social class and psychiatric problems was found in the Isle of Wight study in either the general population or in children with neurological problems other than epilepsy. In fact none of the social factors investigated in that study showed any association between psychiatric disorder among brain-damaged children with conditions other than epilepsy. Father's occupation, family size, whether or not the mother worked outside the home, degree of overcrowding in the home—all were related to the development of psychiatric problems in the brain-damaged group.

Also, in contrast to the children with uncomplicated epilepsy, there was no significant increase of psychiatric disorder among the mothers of children with psychiatric disorder. But, again, in contrast to the epileptic group, broken homes were a great deal more common among brain-damaged children with psychiatric problems than among brain-damaged children with no such problems. Thus certain familial and social factors have been found to be associated with the development of psychiatric problems in children with brain damage and brain dysfunction. This area requires much further research.

One familial variable, the family's attitude toward the handicap of the brain-damaged child, is likely to play a role in the development of psychiatric problems. Little evidence is available on this point, but it seems likely that the parents' prejudice against disorders such as epilepsy may lead to the treatment of the child as "deformed" in some way. Assessing such attitudes is difficult, and research in this area is necessarily extremely complex.

Academic Retardation

The next variable to be considered is academic retardation. Many epidemiological studies have indicated that underachievement in all school subjects is associated with behavioral disturbance in children.[41]

Reading retardation is most associated with psychiatric disorder, but underachievement in other academic subjects also plays a role. The behavioral disturbance is most likely to be a "conduct" disorder rather than an "emotional" disorder, although there is a tendency toward an increased rate of all types of psychiatric disorder in children with reading retardation.

Is the presence of academic retardation one of the mechanisms of behavior disorder among brain-damaged children? In the Isle of Wight study, three times as many children with psychiatric disorders had specific reading retardation, at least two years below the expected on the basis of age and IQ, as compared with epileptic children with no psychiatric disorder. In those with brain disorder and psychiatric disorder, three times as many (64 percent) had a severe degree of specific retardation compared to the group with no psychiatric disorder. Thus it may be that, in brain-damaged children, one of the mechanisms for development of behavior disorder may be academic failure.

Social Attitudes

Some investigators such as W.M. Cruickshank believe a contributing factor to psychiatric disorder in brain-damaged children is societal attitudes toward their handicap.[42] While this seems plausible at first glance, hard evidence to support this view is lacking. While social rejection certainly may adversely affect the child's social and emotional adjustment, as a practical matter it is difficult to assess if the child is rejected *because* she/he demonstrates odd or abnormal behavior or because of some type of physical deformity. In the Isle of Wight study, for example, children were much more likely to be rejected by others because they manifested a psychiatric problem than because they were physically handicapped. Moreover, psychiatric disorder was much more common among children *with* demonstrable brain damage who were also deformed and disabled than in children *with no* CNS injury who were deformed and disabled because of orthopedic or muscular handicaps.

Distorted Social Perception

A view that has more evidence to support it is that brain injury may lead the child to have a distorted social perception. This distortion may then affect the child's pattern of social interactions, thus producing a psychiatric problem. J.J. Gallagher made a study of retarded children, comparing those who were brain injured with those who were not.[43] The brain-injured group demonstrated characteristics such as impulsive behavior and inability to defer gratification, which generated a negative attitude toward them from others in their environment; this then led to deviant behavior on their part.

Finally, U.P. Seidel and his group considered a number of these variables together. They reported a detailed psychiatric study of all crippled children between age five and fifteen who were listed on the local authority lists of handicapped children in three boroughs of London.[44] All the children had normal intelligence, defined as a tested IQ of 70 or more. Thirty-three of the children were found to have a neurological disorder above the level of the brainstem, and they were compared to forty-two who had a neurological disorder below the brainstem. There were no significant differences beween the two groups in age, sex, social class, overcrowding in the home, or background of a broken home. The diagnosis of psychiatric disorder was made from interviews with teachers, teachers' questionnaires, interviews with parents, and interviews with the children. Based on all available information, 24 percent of the group with lesions above the brainstem showed a psychiatric disorder with substantial social impairment; only 12 percent of the group with neurological disorder below the brainstem had a similar degree of psychiatric disorder. The types of disorder in the two groups were similar. Thus, among crippled children of normal intelligence, psychiatric disorder was shown to be twice as common when the neurological condition involved disease or damage to the brain.

The two groups also differed in mean IQ and in reading achievement. The mean IQ of the brain-damaged children was 90.7; that of those with a peripheral lesion was 100.8. Fifty-two percent of the brain-damaged group were found to be significantly backward in reading, compared to 15 percent of those with a peripheral lesion. This difference between the two groups with respect to reading disability held true even after the effects of IQ were parceled out. There was no association between IQ and social class in the brain-damaged group.

The investigators then looked at the following factors in relation to the presence of psychiatric disorder: degree of physical handicap; cognitive factors and schooling; and psychosocial factors. Somewhat surprisingly, psychiatric disorder was not associated with severity of physical handicap. In fact it occurred considerably less often in the children with severe physical incapacity, as judged from the parental interview. This latter finding could not be explained in terms of age, sex, type of lesion, IQ, presence of reading disability, or social class. The authors hypothesize that this finding might be due to the fact that children with a severe physical handicap adjust better to the fact that they will not be able to participate normally in society, whereas those with a mild handicap may continue to strive to do so and be continually frustrated.

There was no significant association between low IQ and the presence of psychiatric disorder, nor was it associated significantly with the presence of severe reading difficulties.

It was in the psychosocial factors that the greatest differences were found between the psychiatrically disordered group and the nondisordered group. Disorder was significantly associated with an overcrowded household; a broken home; living in a family in which there was marital discord; and psychiatric disorder in the mother.

The authors concluded that although the presence of brain damage clearly increased the risk of psychiatric disorder, the disorder was not directly caused by brain damage, but developed as a result of a combination of increased biological susceptibility and certain psychosocial factors. The psychosocial factors that were important in the genesis of the psychiatric disorder in brain-damaged children were equally important in the genesis of disorder in nonhandicapped children.[45]

SUMMARY

The data reviewed in this paper support the following conclusions. In children with definite brain damage there *is* an increased prevalence rate of psychiatric disorder. Brain damage in children does *not*, however, lead to a unique "brain-damage syndrome." In children with psychiatric disorder there is an increased prevalence rate of brain damage, but only a minority of children with psychiatric disorder have definite brain damage. In children with brain damage who do develop psychiatric disorder certain environmental factors are associated with its presence. It is difficult to tell whether or not the brain damage is *directly* responsible for the disorder, but in most cases there probably is a transactional effect between the brain damage and environmental factors to produce the disorder.

In order to advance our knowledge in this area we need the following: a reliable and valid classification system for the psychiatric disorders of childhood to help insure homogeneity of patient populations; standardized assessment procedures for the diagnosis of psychiatric disorders of childhood analogous to the SADS, DIS, PSE and others used so successfully with adults; and standardized assessment techniques for the diagnosis of brain damage and brain dysfunction in children.

NOTES

1. J. Guislain, *Abhandlung über die Phrenopathien* (Stuttgart: Rieger, 1838).
2. J.S. Werry, "Organic Factors in Childhood Psychopathological Disorders," in *Psychopathological Disorders of Childhood*, 2nd ed., ed. H. Quay and J.S. Werry (New York: John Wiley, 1979).
3. Task Force on Nomenclature and Statistics, *Diagnostic and Statistical Manual of Mental Disorders*, 3rd ed. (Washington: American Psychiatric Association, 1978).
4. *Manual of International Statistical Classification of Diseases, Injuries and Causes of Death*, 9th ed. (Geneva: World Health Organization, 1975).
5. Ibid.

6. S. Chess, A. Thomas, M. Rutter, et al., "Interaction of Temperament and Environment in the Production of Behavioral Disturbances in Children," *American Journal of Psychiatry* 120 (1963): 142; C. Wenar, "The Reliability of Developmental Histories: Summary and Evaluation of Evidence," *Psychosomatic Medicine* 25 (1963): 505.

7. D. Shaffer, "Longitudinal Research and the Minimal Brain Damage Syndrome," *Advances in Biological Psychiatry* 1 (1978): 18-34.

8. Werry, "Childhood Disorders" (See note 2).

9. Ibid.

10. Ibid.

11. Ibid.

12. D. Shaffer, " 'Soft' Neurologic Signs and Later Psychiatric Disorder—A Review," *Journal of Child Psychology and Psychiatry* 19 (January 1978): 63-66.

13. Werry, "Childhood Disorders" (See note 2).

14. Ibid.

15. J. Satterfield, D.P. Cantwell, and B. Satterfield, "Pathophysiology of the Hyperactive Child Syndrome," *Archives of General Psychiatry* 31 (1974): 839-44.

16. D. Cohen and J. Young, "Neurochemistry and Child Psychiatry," *Journal of the American Academy of Child Psychiatry* 16 (1977): 353-411.

17. R. Gittelman-Klein, "Psychological Tests and Psychiatric Diagnosis in Childhood," *Journal of the American Academy of Child Psychiatry*, in press.

18. F.K. Graham and P.W. Berman, "Current Status of Behavior Tests for Brain Damage in Infants and Preschool Children," *American Journal of Orthopsychiatry* 31 (1961): 713.

19. M. Herbert, "The Concept and Testing of Brain Damage in Children: A Review," *Journal of Child Psychology and Psychiatry* 5 (1964): 197.

20. V. Meyer, "Critique of Psychological Approaches to Brain Damage," *Journal of Mental Science* 103 (1957): 80.

21. A.J. Yates, "The Validity of Some Psychological Tests of Brain Damage," *Psychological Bulletin* 51 (1954): 359.

22. R. Reitan, "A Research Program on the Psychological Effects of Brain Lesions in Human Beings," in *International Review of Research in Mental Retardation*, ed. N. Ellis (New York: Academic Press, 1966).

23. P.E. Tanguay, "Neuropsychological Models in Child Psychiatry," in *Clinical Child Psychiatry*, ed. D.P. Cantwell and P.E. Tanguay (New York: Spectrum Medical and Scientific Publications, forthcoming).

24. M. Rutter, P. Graham, and W. Yule, *A Neuropsychiatric Study in Childhood* (Philadelphia: Lippincott, 1970).

25. Werry, "Childhood Disorders" (See note 3).

26. D.P. Cantwell, *The Hyperactive Child—Diagnosis, Management, Current Research* (New York: Spectrum Medical and Scientific Publications, 1975).

27. J.E. Hastings and R.A. Barkley, "A Review of Psychophysiological Research with Hyperkynetic Children," *Journal of Abnormal Child Psychology* 6 (1978): 413-47.

28. Cohen and Young, "Neurochemistry and Child Psychiatry" (See note 16).

29. H. Quay, "Psychopathic Behavior: Reflections on Its Nature, Origins and Treatment," in *The Structuring of Experience*, ed. I. Uzgiris and F. Weizmann (New York: Plenum Press, 1977).

30. Werry, "Childhood Disorders" (See note 2).

31. M. Rutter and E. Schopler, *Autism: A Reappraisal of Concepts and Treatment* (New York: Plenum Press, 1978).

32. Werry, "Childhood Disorders" (See note 2).

33. A. Sameroff and M. Chandler, "Reproductive Risk and the Continuum of Caretaking Casualty," in *Review of Child Development Research*, vol. 4, ed. F. Horowitz, M. Hetherington, S. Scarr-Salapatek, et al. (Chicago: University of Chicago Press, 1975).

34. M. Rutter, P. Graham, and W. Yule, "A Neuropsychiatric Study in Childhood," *Clinics in Developmental Medicine* (London) nos. 35/36 (1977).

35. Rutter, Graham, and Yule, *Study in Childhood* (See note 24).

36. Shaffer, "'Soft' Neurologic Signs" (See note 12).

37. F. Grunberg and D.A. Pond, "Conduct Disorders in Epileptic Children," *Journal of Neurology, Neurosurgery and Psychiatry* 20 (1957): 65.

38. J.A. Harrington and F.J.J. Letemendia, "Persistent Psychiatric Disorders after Head Injuries in Children," *Journal of Mental Science* 104 (1958): 205.

39. Grunberg and Pond, "Epileptic Children" (See note 37).

40. M. Rutter, *Children of Sick Parents: An Environmental Psychiatric Study*, Maudsley Monograph No. 16 (London: Oxford University Press, 1966).

41. _____, "A Child's Life," *New Scientist* 62 (1974): 763.

42. W.M. Cruickshank and H.V. Rice, *Cerebral Palsy: Its Individual and Community Problems* (Syracuse: University of Syracuse Press, 1965).

43. J.J. Gallagher, *A Comparison of Birth-Injured and Non-Birth-Injured Mentally Retarded Children on Several Psychological Variables*, Monographs of the Society for Research in Child Development, vol. 22 (Chicago: Society for Research in Child Development, 1957).

44. U.P. Seidel, O.F.D. Chadwick, and M. Rutter, "Psychological Disorders in Crippled Children. A Comparative Study of Children with and without Brain Damage," *Developmental Medicine and Child Neurology* 17 (1975): 211.

45. Ibid.

DISCUSSION

A number of French psychiatrists believe that what Cantwell describes so well as "soft neurological symptoms" may in fact not be signs of damage or lesion, but signs of slow maturation. Children's functions develop at a different rate and at a different rhythm. The most difficult cases are those who speak late, and thus speak badly, and who are therefore more vulnerable.

Attention-Deficit Disorder

If one uses the DSM-III criteria, meaning that to be diagnosed as attention-deficit disorder with hyperactivity, children have to exhibit hyperactivity, inattentiveness, and impulsive behavior as cardinal symptoms, more boys than girls have the disorder.

The phrase attention-deficit disorder (A-DD) with and without hyperactivity was chosen because of the observation that some girls, particularly the siblings of hyperactive boys, show inattentiveness and impulsive behavior. This is sometimes associated with learning disorders, but they do not exhibit the symptom of "hyperactivity." If the number of affected boys and girls in those studies are added together, it comes out about 50:50—the boys have A-DD *with* hyperactivity, and the girls have A-DD *without* hyperactivity.

Follow-Up Studies of Hyperactives

As to the future of hyperactive children, follow-up studies are relatively uniform in some respects and different in others. One of the first was that of John H. Menkes in the clinic at Johns Hopkins Hospital, where a population of eighteen children was first seen in 1941. Twenty-five years later fourteen of them were located; four of the fourteen were institutionalized with "psychosis," while the others had a variety of conduct and antisocial-type problems. That is the only long-term, follow-up study that supports to any degree the association between childhood hyperactivity and psychosis.

Most other follow-up studies indicate that there is an association between A-DD in childhood and conduct and antisocial problems in adolescence, and possibly later in life. Unfortunately these studies have not weaned out the children who have A-DD, but who also had a conduct disorder in childhood. Thus there may be an association with antisocial behavior in childhood and such behavior at a later time.

Slowness of Maturation

On the neurological question of the extent to which an examination reflects a slowness of maturation rather than a specific problem, there is no argument that indeed the functions to be measured are predominantly developmental problems appropriate at an early age that disappear with time. The logic of them is very similar to the performance of the child in cognitive skills—the levels of motor skills and cognitive skills are what one would expect.

Perinatal Risk Factors

As for measuring perinatal morbidity, there are great differences in the sophistication of fetal monitoring in many obstetrical centers, which provide relatively hard evidence of the extent to which distress of the fetus is taking place.

Paul Nichols, in a collaborative prospective American study of mothers from the beginning of pregnancy until the child was age seven, analyzed data on early prenatal and perinatal risk factors and later behavior and learning problems. As with all other associations with the hyperactive syndrome, with his large sample of 35,000 pregnancies followed prospectively, Nichols found a definitely significant but extraordinarily weak association with pre- and perinatal risk factors that were identified as they occurred—such as first trimester bleeding, the mother smoking more than three packs of cigarettes a day, and even coffee intake—as well as delivery features. The risk goes up about 3 percent for hyperactive children, as opposed to 1 percent for the controls.

One of the problems with the Nichols study is that, even with the prospective collection of data, the only behavioral measure was the one taken during a psychological test; there were *no* behavioral measures in the home or in school. The "hyperactive" children have to be hyperactive in a psychological test setting, so that diminishes the value of that study tremendously.

This still leaves a vast number of false positives and false negatives, which leads one to accept Taylor's point of view about the nonspecificity and validity of the hyperactive syndrome. As for the validity of the behavioral observations, it is true that parents' and teacher rating scales tend to correlate badly, since mothers are apt to make global judgments rather poorly. They may have one or five children and still have very little experience with observing them objectively.

Trans-Situational Groups

The most interesting group for future investigation probably consists of the trans-situational children. It is a puzzle, with the question of both soft and minor physical anomalies.

About half the published studies seem to replicate a weak association between overactives and controls, and fail to interpret this to mean there is an extraordinary low level of association, which probably accounts for the degree of diversity of findings in the literature. One is left with some weak statistical suggestion of association, but nothing that is ordinarily satisfying to general medicine.

It is rather disturbing to find that the presence or absence of soft signs in grade school children has a significant correlation with simultaneous independent ratings of psychiatric interviews for cooperation and rapport. This raises an issue worth worrying about: one does have to play the devil's advocate and suggest that a basic behavioral factor of rapport or cooperation with the examiner might conceivably account for both the early soft signs and later psychiatric disability.

As far as the low correlation of the parents' and teacher rating scales for hyperactivity, that is not surprising. In the Isle of Wight study, when the psychiatrically disordered children as a group were observed, and the parents' and teacher rating scales were examined for their relative effectiveness in picking up such children, they were equally effective. There was only a very modest correlation between the two: they tended to pick up different children. That is true not only for hyperactivity, but for psychiatric disorders in general.

There is a significant difference in the incidence of this particular problem. A small number of children are trans-situationally overactive and tend to have diminished cognitive ability, although they are not necessarily severely retarded. They do, however, have developmental delays and other kinds of problems.

We do not know whether this difference in prevalence rate is culturally determined in symptom expression, or if certain kinds of symptoms are considered "psychiatric" in one culture and not in another.

This may be true of hyperactivity. Certainly there may be a difference in the tolerance level of British teachers—considerably greater than would be the case in a typical American classroom setting. Whether that means that children are thus managed in different settings in the two countries is another matter.

There is a considerable difference in practice. The English psychiatrist does not see children referred with minor problems of inattention and hyperactivity in the classroom; the nature of the system militates against what is not usually perceived as a suitable referral problem. The kind of child who is referred is the one whom teachers perceive as being aggressive or combative.

Study of Perinatal Stress

One important American study was the work of Gerhard Werner and coworkers on the island of Kauai in Hawaii; it is one of the more impressive American epidemiological contribution of recent years. They investigated the conditions of perinatal stress over an eighteen-year period in a large cohort of children born in the same population. Perinatal stress contributes to psychiatric status if an infant begins life with an early caring environment that has deficits, primarily because of the mother's lack of caretaking ability. It is the interaction between the child's condition derived from perinatal stress and the inability of the mother to help correct that condition that sets the stage for psychiatric disorder.

What is impressive about the Kauai work is that, during the first two years of life, if there is both perinatal stress and early maternal problems the consequences for psychiatric disorder will indeed maintain themselves into adolescence.

Could this type of interaction produce the kind of findings one calls "soft neurological signs" on investigation? Could a child's incoordination or instability in neurological testing be a product of early caretaking difficulties as much as of brain damage?

The kinds of signs that discriminate are exactly those that are at quite a high level of psychological function. The implication is that this kind of process would be susceptible to impairment by factors quite other than the wiring of the brain. It might be susceptible to motivation; to the child's construct of the situation he is in; to early psychological inferences; and to early neurological inferences. That seems to be an empirical question to be investigated.

When one looks at the difficulties encountered with GSR and other autonomic measures, the extraordinary sloppiness with which most people approach such laboratory procedures is impressive. It requires an extremely meticulous laboratory environment with controlled temperature, humidity, and the like. Most people do it in a way that is likely to result in noise being recorded, not signals. For all the problems clinicians have, they often assume that highly mechanized devices are somehow free of errors. It remains to be seen whether neurometrics has any kind of external validity.

Study of "Soft Signs"

As to cooperation and soft signs, Jerome Kagan did a study in which the so-called soft signs of simultaneous perception and extinction of signs occur: the idea is to give the child double, simultaneous stimulation. That is, with the child's eyes closed the investigator touches the backs of both hands and asks the child if he has been touched in one place or two places. Up to age six or eight the children only record on stimulus.

What Kagan was looking at, in part, was the instructional setting; that in fact the children did very much better if he took them at an age at which they are not supposed to be able to respond, and said to them: "I'm going play a game with you. I'm going to touch you, sometimes on two hands and sometimes on one hand, and you let me know whether you can tell if I touched one or two.'' The report is altered by the stimulus conditions under which they are evoked. That does not mean the signs are not real, but it changes one's interpretation of them.

The differences between parents' and teachers' reports may also reflect the fact that behaviors salient for mothers and for teachers are very different. An amusing report appeared a few years ago of a comparative study of so-called hyperkinetic children in which the investigator compared an antidepressant drug, imipramine, with methylphenidate. What was astounding was that the teacher found methylphenidate calmed the child, more or less, while he was at school, but he was hell on wheels by the time he came home, which did not please the mother. The imipramine made the child semicomatose at home, which was great as far as the mother was concerned, but the teacher found it very difficult to get him to pay attention in the classroom. This was not inaccuracy in reporting, but focusing on very different behavior.

It is still true that there is a trans-situational problem with the hyperkenetic child, who is reported as such by the mother and by the teacher, but who is likely to be different in one, two, or three situations.

Early versus Late Maturation

The whole issue of early and late maturation and its impact on psychological outcomes for adolescents was looked at in a rather systematic way by Mary Kinard Jones and Paul Musin. They determined that there are highly negative outcomes as the individual becomes more discrepant; the late maturing male is the most highly discrepant individual.

When there was such confusion about the data, much of it was elucidated when the studies were analyzed by John Clausen, taking into account socioeconomic status. It turned out that the small male adolescent in a lower socioeconomic status had the most difficulty because the expectations, and in fact the demands, of that sociocultural context for largeness, high muscularity, what we lump together as "macho," were more important.

This whole arena of expectations having to do with age, rather than with biological status, has been insufficiently studied. It makes us wonder if the child in a large household has greater difficulty because the expectations are more like they are in school—there is more regimentation, for example, and the child is expected to "act his age." In that case it is chronological age, not biological age.

Research on Animals

In reading through the literature on brain damage in animals, the capacity of the mammalian nervous system to recover from damage early in life is impressive. One of the real differences between research on animals and humans is that animal work actually is exclusively on biological time, whereas some integration has to be made between biological status and expectations.

IV. PSYCHOPHARMACOLOGY

THE USE OF CHEMOTHERAPY IN CHILD PSYCHIATRY

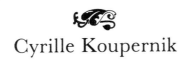

Cyrille Koupernik

The history of chemotherapy in child psychiatry is long—and full of passionate controversy. The dissension is not only over the efficacy of chemotherapy; it raises conceptual, ethical, and physiopathogenic issues. Within this wide frame, I intend to take a look at the problem that is as old as the discipline itself—psychostimulant therapy.

PSYCHOSTIMULANTS

The fist International Congress of Child Psychiatry was held in Paris in 1937, due to the efforts of the great pioneers in the field: G. Heuyer, L. Kanner, and M. Tramer. In that same year two separate papers appeared simultaneously in the *American Journal of Psychiatry*, one written by C.H. Bradley[1] and the other by M. Molitch and A.K. Eccles.[2] These two historical papers dealt with the favorable effects of a synthetic compound, Benzedrin, or dextroamphetamine.*

Beginning in 1937 research has been conducted with the objective of elucidating a not-very-well-delineated condition that afflicts children, sometimes called hyperkinesis and sometimes called minimal brain damage (MBD). Later in this paper I will discuss the very important problem of the validity of this nosological concept, which A.L. Benton defines as being a behavioral concept with neurological implications.[4] A few years later

---

* The two papers were actually inspired by one by G.A. Alles in 1933, in which he cited the stimulant effects of this substance on the central nervous system.[3]

methylphenidate, or Ritalin, was proposed as an active therapeutic agent for the same condition.

The amphetamine crusade of J.G. Millichap against restless and inattentive children[5] is still going on. It has not been proved conclusively that amphetamine is effective on a long-term basis, however, and to my knowledge no study has been made with a control group of individuals with Ph.D.'s, M.D.'s, or M.Sc.'s who, as children, had been diagnosed as hyperkinetic.

Another aspect that speaks for the therapy also has not been thoroughly investigated: not a single case of amphetamine addiction has been described among these children, although amphetamines and methylphenidate are known to provoke this condition in adolescents and adults. Finally, the appeasing action of amphetamines on excitement in children is truly paradoxical if one compares their effect on adults.

MODERN PSYCHOPHARMACOLOGY

Fifteen years after the Paris congress a new development occurred in France, which was followed by competent research in the United States, Switzerland, Belgium, and other countries. This dealt with high-class, genuine pharmacology that started with the discovery of chlorpromazine by H. Laborit, P. Huguenard, and R. Alluaume,[6] and by J. Delay, P. Deniker, and J.M. Harl.[7] This event was echoed in 1954 by the rediscovery of reserpine by N.S. Kline,[8] who four years later discovered monoamine oxidase inhibitors (MAOI).[9] In Switzerland R. Kühn reported that imipramine, although it resembled to some extent the structure of chlorpromazine, actually had a competely different effect: it was a potent tricyclic antidepressant.[10]

NEUROTRANSMITTERS

Before going on I want to stress that between the discovery of the molecule and the definition of its clinical effect one has to take into account a biochemical discovery, the first that proved to be valid in psychiatry—the reports that cerebral monoamines act as neurotransmitters.[11,12]

Three neurotransmitters are recognized as having this capacity, although there are certainly many other substances that act as neurotransmitters. Of the three, one is an indolamine-serotonin, or 5HT, and two are catecholamines, dopamine (DA) and norepinephrine (NE). Although these facts are very well known they are still disputed in an emotional and irrational manner by those who are unwilling to admit there is a biochemical basis for psychic phenomena.

What can we learn from these data? They remind us of other discoveries in neurology, namely, the depletion in dopamine of central grey nucleii, which is the basis of Parkinson's disease; the fact that the blood-brain barrier cannot be crossed by neurotransmitters, but is permeable by their precursors; and that the precursor of the catecholamines is L-dopa, while that of seratonin is 5-hydroxy tryptophane or 5HTP.

At this point we might stop and take into account the fact that Parkinson's disease is an illness of senescence—a degenerative process. Should we not therefore be cautious about applying to child psychiatry concepts that may not be akin to its biological equipment?

Be that as it may, the discovery of these drugs had led to a very fruitful hypothesis in terms of schizophrenia and mania, that is, the major tranquilizers, which we in France call neuroleptics, are active against these two conditions. In spite of the fact that their chemical structures are radically different, they produce side effects similar to extrapyramidal Parkinsonism. This would seem to favor the dopaminergic theory of these two psychoses, and it is to some extent probable that the difference between them lies in the different neuronal sets that are the site of the disorder of dopamine metabolism.

TOWARD A NEW NOSOLOGY

First, one may believe there is a true dichotomy between manic-depressive psychosis, on the one hand, and schizophrenia, on the other. But in the light of modern chemotherapy such an approach is not feasible: schizophrenia and mania are obviously both improved by neuroleptics—phenothiazines, butyrophenones, and sulpiride, to name the most widely used drugs— and aggravated by antidepressants, be they tricyclic or MAOI. Nevertheless, as mentioned earlier, from a clinical standpoint schizophrenia and mania are obviously not the same disease. The difference in underlying mechanisms may be topographical, involving a different dopaminergic neuronal set, for example, mesolimbic on the one side and mesocortical on the other,[13] or biochemical: according to R. Tissot the levels of 5HT and NE are low, while that of DA is high; in mania all three neurotransmitters have a high level.[14]

Second, one might expect to find a catecholaminergic (DA or NE) pathology, on the one hand, and a serotoninergic (5HT) on the other.

Where this is not the case it seems that the same drug may act on both NE and 5HT. This may be an intraneuronal inhibition of MAOI produced or secreted by mitochondria, for MAOI destroy all the cerebral monoamines (5HT, NE, and DA) that circulate in a free form toward the synapse.

The so-called recapture of the neurotransmitters at their synaptic levels by the secreting neuron is characteristic of tricyclic antidepressants. One way or the other the same biological end result is obtained, that is, a rise in the level of NE and/or 5HT at the synaptic level. It may be that the same effect exists for DA, due to the action of the new dopaminergic compounds claimed to have antidepressant potentialities.

I now wish to mention three other aspects of the antidepressants. One is physiological: 5HT is probably the main agent of the so-called "slow-pattern sleep," while NE controls the paradoxical sleep, which explains why tricyclic antidepressants interface with sleep. The second aspect has to do with difficulties in micturition; we will deal with this in the section on treatment of enuresis. The third aspect concerns cardiotoxicity, which has to be placed in the general framework of the potential danger involved in giving potent drugs to children.

LITHIUM

Lithium is the third great type of therapeutic agent of psychiatric chemotherapy, with only one indisputable therapeutic indication—a state of manic excitement. This is so, even though its effect is not as potent as that of neuroleptics, and its main activity is prevention of periodic episodes of manic depressive psychosis, and, to a lesser degree, of unipolar depression and the schizoaffective* variety of schizophrenia.

Those are the weapons of modern chemotherapy.

THE INDICATIONS

We must now ask ourselves the following questions:
- Is MBD susceptible to the benefits of well-codified treatment?
- Is it feasible to consider that the psychoses experienced by the adolescent and adult also affect the child?
- Can the uncontrolled agitation of low-grade, mentally deficient children benefit from chemical sedation?

---

* Schizoaffective is the term used for recurrent or cyclic varieties of schizophrenia.

- Can enuresis be treated by tricyclics?
- Are there unjustified indications?
- What are the risks of iatrogenesis?

I. CONSISTENCY OF THE CONCEPT OF MBD

I have written on the subject of MBD and I confess I consider it to be a dubious entity.[15] In fact no two investigators can agree on symptomatology: some even describe the syndrome as hyperactivity *sine* hyperactivity.[16] Nor is there agreement on the reliability of the so-called "soft" neurological symptoms, such as hyperactivity of deep reflexes, clumsiness, hypotonia, or the characteristics of EEG, namely, very intense reactions to hyperventilation.

Moreover, opinions vary widely as to incidence: while some American epidemiological data provide the mean figure as between 5 and 10 percent, the study by M. Rutter, P.H. Graham, and W. Yule concluded that only two children in 2,189 could be considered hyperkinetic;[17] and M. Bax in his study of 1,200 children on the Isle of Wight found not a single one.[18]

There is an equal discrepancy concerning pathogenesis. P.H. Wender claims there is a well-established correlation between MBD and cerebral damage and/or genetic factors—this way of presenting concepts is very eloquent—but at the same time he admits that the majority of children at risk do not have the MBD syndrome.[19]

The relative weakness of the arguments in favor of the existence of brain damage has led to the adoption of the less compromising label of dysfunction, as indicated in the report of the Oxford Seminar on Minimal Brain Dysfunction in 1962.[20] After that report was published, supporters of the syndrome, especially Wender, tried to formulate it in modern physiological terms, referring to the phenomenon of arousal of the reticular substance. In his 1972 paper, however, Wender stated on one page that these children are in a state of hyperarousal, and on the next page that they are in a state of hypoarousal.[21]

Attempts to explain MBD in terms of the biochemistry of neurotransmitters are to my mind just as unsatisfactory; they refer to the chemical similarity of amphetamines and catecholamines, which in itself is not sufficient.

What is left, then, of the new formulation of MBD (the D now meaning dysfunction) and of the syndrome of the hyperkinetic child? The answers will probably vary according to what one believes to be the goals of psychiatry. I have always had the impression that the MBD syndrome and the energy invested in its correction were mainly due to irritation on the part of people in the child's milieu, be they parents or teachers, and that the objective of therapy was to some extent to make these children conform more to the wishes and expectations of the adults who share their lives. I do not support such an orientation.

At the same time there is no reason to charge our American colleagues with a lack of intellectual rigor; after all, they have been our masters and our models in many fields. I would therefore suggest a parallel study be made to try to explain the reason (probably a physiological one) dextroamphetamine and methylphenidate have a paradoxically sedative action on the child—contrary to what happens in the adult; a study should also be made of why no case of addiction has been observed in children, even though prepubertal children may become alcoholics and heroin addicts.

II. ADULT-TYPE PSYCHOSES IN CHILDREN

I will now take up the second question, namely, can adult-type psychoses be exhibited by children?

In regard to manic-depressive psychosis, opinions differ. Some investigators claim they have never seen a manic episode before puberty, and I share this view. I even wonder whether such episodes in very young adolescents are not an atypical variety of onset schizophrenia. This brings us back to the problem of dopaminergic resemblance between mania and schizophrenia. S.C. Feinstein has described three very precocious cases: one, a girl, experienced the first episode at age three and a half; during the second episode she was treated successfully with 900 mg. lithium carbonate.[22] M. Dugas and colleagues have also observed cases of mania in children.[23] O.S. Jorgensen limits himself to citing a historical case of mania in a prepubertal boy,[24] originally described in 1960 by J. Anthony and P. Scott.[25]

B. Lena believes lithium may be usefully prescribed for impulsive and aggressive children or adolescents even when they have no mood disorders, which is the main indication in the adult. On the contrary, a periodic or recurrent rhythm reinforces indications for use of the drug. At the same time, however, Lena maintains one should not try to superimpose an adult nosological concept on the prepubertal or recently pubertal individual; because of possible metabolic complications, she favors short-term treatment, the average duration being six months.[26]

I have never seen a case of endogenous melancholia in children, and I have never prescribed tricyclic antidepressants for children, with the exception of those with enuresis. I am also cautious about prescribing these two groups of antidepressants for adolescents for the following reasons:

• Suicide among young children is rare, and there is therefore less need for chemotherapeutic intervention.

• A young child is capable of swallowing large doses of tricyclics, mistaking them for candy. K.M. Goel and R.A. Shanks saw sixty such cases over a seven-year period; forty-two of the children were between age two and four, and one died.[27]

• Adolescents are usually strongly opposed to chemotherapy. They label all psychotropic drugs as a chemical straitjacket, whereas psychedelic drugs are considered to be the pathway to freedom.

• Adolescents are, however, prone to take large amounts of psychotropic drugs in attempts to commit suicide* and thus draw attention to their distress during this difficult period of their lives.

Schizophrenia presents a somewhat different situation. We in Europe used to refer to the few cases of dementia praecocissima described by Sancta de Sanctis,[28] which was a truly exceptional diagnosis. In the United States, on the other hand, the very frequent diagnosis of childhood schizophrenia due to the use of psychodynamic criteria has led to the rather frequent formulation of this diagnosis; that is probably less true today. Other authors tend to equate the terms schizoid and schizophrenia.

Of the three nosological entities—infantile psychosis, infantile schizophrenia, and infantile Kanner's syndrome (autism)—only the last is valid, in my opinion. But apparently there is no pathogenic similarity between Kanner's syndrome and juvenile and/or adult schizophrenia. The condition never develops into paranoid schizophrenia, which is the main indication for neuroleptics in adolescents and adults. In the experience of B. Fish the use of trifluoperazine in autism has been far from successful.[29]

Nevertheless, I. Kolvin describes varieties of infantile schizophrenia as late onset psychosis.[30] Dugas and coworkers observed 111 psychotic children, fifty-six of whom were between age fourteen and eighteen; thirty-two of these were treated successfully. The action was less obvious in twelve of the children who were in a latency state; it was even less so in those with infantile psychosis. In eighteen of forty-three cases only those with hyperkinesis showed improvement.[31]

III. CONTROL OF STATES OF AGITATION

Therapeutic treatment with neuroleptics seems justified to me in children who are very restless, and at the same time severely retarded from the intellectual standpoint. Some of these children may have low-grade mental

---

* So-called "parasuicide."

deficiency or extensive brain lesions, and thus exhibit very disturbed behavior; others may be autistic.

Neuroleptic therapy may allow some of these children to remain with their families; others may have to be placed in institutions that can provide various kinds of therapies. In prescribing, one should determine the minimal dosage that will provide sedation while allowing the child to remain alert. The most frequently used neuroleptic drugs are the phenothiazines (propericiazine and trifluoperazine) or butyrophenones (haloperidol). The parenteral method of administration should seldom be used, however, because of our lack of knowledge of future effects of the drugs; this is true also of the depot phenothiazines. The effect of an injection lasts from fifteen to thirty days. Benzodiazepines (diazepam, dipotassium, chlorazepate) have less serious side effects, but are probably less effective.

IV. TREATMENT OF ENURESIS

Tricyclics are being tried in the treatment of childhood enuresis because micturitional difficulties have been observed in adults. On the whole, the results are satisfactory. Dugas and his colleagues instituted a posology of 0.5 to 1.0 mg./kg. body weight for a period of two to three months and observed no side effects; in their opinion tolerance to tricyclics is fairly good.[32]

If we compare these results with that of coercion, which was used before World War II, the failure of various medications, including amphetamines, and the systematic use of psychoanalytical therapy, we may conclude that treatment of enuresis with tricyclics is worthwhile. They probably act through the smooth muscles of the bladder, but also, because of their central action, on sleep patterns.

V. DEBATABLE INDICATIONS

With few exceptions benzodiazepines should not be prescribed as tranquilizers for children, as they are for adults; and one should never prescribe hypnotics for regular use in a child who has problems sleeping. Nor should one use neuroleptics, especially butyrophenones, for tics, despite the fact that they are effective in the treatment of Gilles de la Tourette's *maladie des tics*.

I find it difficult to understand why MAOI have been prescribed for mentally deficient children, as reported by M. Beaujard and E. Revol[33] and by F. Licenziati and V. Rossolini;[34] or tricyclics, as reported by M. Linnoila and colleagues;[35] or lithium for hyperkinetic or psychopathic children. Such treatments are not only unsuccessful, they may be dangerous.

VI. SIDE EFFECTS AND TOXICITY

Some side effects are so well known I will not attempt to describe them here, but merely say that, in treating children, if the chances of success are not certain one is not empowered to take risks.

Cases of tardive, permanent dyskinesia have been mentioned recently as being caused by the use of neuroleptics, especially after the drug has been withdrawn. To my knowledge, however, no report has described this disorder in a child.* Dugas and his group have cited a case of a child with photosensitivity, which may leave a lasting pigmentation;[37] this has also been observed in adults, as has gynecomastia with hypertrophy of the clitoris. The first symptom, at least, is explainable by the well-known action of neuroleptics on prolactin.

D.J. Safer and coworkers have reported that dextramphetamine and methylphenidate inhibit growth hormone: the weight and height of children who have undergone such therapy are below normal.[38] B.G. Winsberg has described a case, first cited by J.S. Werry and R.L. Sprague,[39] that was characterized by a delusional state, ataxia, and dyskinesia due to methylphenidate;[40] three others have been mentioned by A.R. Lucas and M. Weiss in which psychosis was also induced by methylphenidate.[41] Winsberg himself has observed a psychotic child in the course of treatment with methylphenidate, and another with orofacial and branchial dyskinesia.[42] It is of some interest to note that A.B. Bremness and J. Sverd also recently described a methlyphenidate-induced Gilles de la Tourette syndrome in a child age nine and a half. The child had no tic before treatment; the syndrome showed a 90 percent improvement when the medication was stopped; but five weeks after discontinuation of the drug the tic reappeared.[43]

It is well known that methylphenidate and amphetamines act on the postsynaptic dopaminergic receptor in a way antagonistic to that of neuroleptics. It should be noted that from time to time one sees amphetamine addicts with schizophrenic-like psychosis indistinguishable from genuine schizophrenia. Amphetamines will also produce abnormal compulsive movements in animals.

---

* Editor's note: Since submitting this chapter for publication Dr. Koupernik has read a report that describes such a case[36] and refers to four prior publications on the same subject.

In conclusion, it is far from obvious that chemotherapy has the same wide field of indications in the child as it has in the adolescent or the adult. This may be additional proof that one does not actually observe the serious psychotic processes until a child reaches puberty, which may mean that the metabolism of the three well-known neurotransmitters is different in the child. From a practical standpoint, chemotherapy in the child should remain purely symptomatic.

NOTES

1. C.H. Bradley, "The Behavior of Children Receiving Benzedrine," *American Journal of Psychiatry* 94 (1937): 577-85.
2. M. Molitch and A.K. Eccles, "Effect of Benzedrine Sulfate on Intelligence Scores of Children," *American Journal of Psychology* 94 (1937): 587-90.
3. G.A. Alles, "The Comparative Physiological Actions of d,l-Beta-Phenyl-Isopropyl-amines," *Journal of Pharmacology and Experimental Therapeutics* 47 (1933): 339-54.
4. A.L. Benton, "Minimal Brain Dysfunction from a Neuropsychological Point of View," in *Minimal Brain Dysfunction*, ed. F.F. de la Cruz, B.H. Fox, and R.H. Roberts (New York: New York Academy of Sciences, 1973): 23-97.
5. J.G. Millichap, "Drugs in the Management of Hyperkinetic and Perceptually Handicapped Children," *Journal of the American Medical Association* 206 (1968): 1527-30.
6. H. Laborit, P. Huguenard, and R. Alluaume, "Un Nouveau Stabilisateur Neurovég-étatif, le 4,560 R.P.," *Presse Médicale* 60, no. 10 (13 February 1952): 206-08.
7. J. Delay, P. Deniker, and J.M. Harl, "Utilisation en Thérapeutique Psychiatrique d'une Phénothíazine d'Action Élective Centrale (4,560 R.P.)," *Annales Médico-Psychologiques* 110, no. 2 (June 1952): 112-17.
8. N.S. Kline, "Use of Rauwolfia Serpentina Benth in Neuropsychiatric Conditions," *Annals of the New York Academy of Sciences* 59 (1954):107-32.
9. _____, "Clinical Experience with Iproniazid (Marsilid)," *Journal of Clinical Experimental Psychopathology* 10, no. 2 (1958): 72-78.
10. R. Kühn, "Du Traitement des États Dépressifs par un Dérivé de l'Imidobenzyle (G 22355)," *Journal Suisse de Médecine* 89 no. 35-36 (1957): 1135-40.
11. B.B. Brodie and E. Costa, "Some Current Views on Brain Monoamines," in *Monoamines et Système Nerveux Central*, ed. J. de Ajuriaguerra (Paris: Masson & Cie, 1962).
12. J. Glowinski and R.J. Baldessarini, "Metabolism of Norepinephrine in the Central Nervous System," *Pharmacological Review* 18 (1966): 1201-38.
13. J.P. Tassin, L. Stinus, H. Simon, et al., "Quantitative Distribution of Dopaminergic Terminals in Various Areas of Rat Cerebral Cortex. Implications of the Dopaminergic Mesocortical System with the So-Called 'Ventral Tegmental Area Syndrome'," in *Advances in Biochemical Pharmacology*, ed. G. Gessa and E. Costal (New York: Raven Press, 1977): 21-28.
14. R. Tissot, "Le Concept Hypothétique: l'Unité Physiopathologique des Psychoses Monoaminergiques," *Encéphale* I, no. 4 (1975): 289-339.
15. C. Koupernik, R. MacKeith, and J. Francis-Williams, "Neurological Correlates of Motor and Perceptual Development," in *Perceptual and Learning Disabilities in Children*, vol. 2, *Research and Theory*, ed. W.M. Cruickshank and D.P. Hallahan (Syracuse: University of Syracuse Press, 1975): 103-35.
16. G. Weiss, K. Minde, J.S. Werry, et al., "Studies on the Hyperactive Child: Five-Year Follow Up," *Archives of General Psychiatry* 24 (1971): 409-14.
17. M. Rutter, P.H. Graham, and W. Yule, *A Neuropsychiatric Study in Childhood* (London: Heinemann, 1970).

18. M. Bax and R. MacKeith, eds., *Minimal Cerebral Dysfunction* (London: Heinemann, 1963).

19. P.H. Wender, *Minimal Brain Dysfunction in Children* (New York: John Wiley, 1971).

20. Bax and MacKeith, *Minimal Dysfunction* (See note 18).

21. P.H. Wender, "The Minimal Brain Dysfunction Syndrome in Children," *Journal of Nervous and Mental Diseases* 155 (1972): 55-71.

22. S.C. Feinstein, "Diagnostic and Therapeutic Aspects of Manic-Depressive Illness in Early Childhood," *Early Child Developmental Care* 3, no. 1 (1973): 1-12.

23. M. Dugas, J. Velin, C. Guériot, et al., "L'Utilisation de Nouvelles Chimiotherapies en Psychiatrie Chez l'Enfant (Neuroleptiques d'Action Prolongée, Anti-Dépresseurs et Lithium)," *Cahiers de Médecine* 14, no. 9 (1973): 711-16.

24. O.S. Jørgensen, "Pharmacological Treatment for Psychotic Children. A Survey," *Acta Psychiatrica Scandinavica* 59 (1979): 229-38.

25. J. Anthony and P. Scott, "Manic Depressive Psychosis in Childhood," *Child Psychology and Psychiatry* I (1960): 53-72.

26. B. Lena, "Lithium in Child and Adolescent Psychiatry," *Archives of General Psychiatry* 36 (1979): 854-55.

27. K.M. Goel and R.A. Shanks, "Amitriptyline Poisoning in Children," *British Medical Journal* 1, no. 5902 (1974): 261-63.

28. S. de Sanctis, cited in J. de Ajuriaguerra, *Manuel de Psychiatrie de l'Enfant* (Paris: Masson & Cie, 1970).

29. B. Fish, "Longitudinal Observations of Biological Deviations in a Schizophrenic Infant," *American Journal of Psychiatry* 116 (1959): 25.

30. I. Kolvin, "Psychoses in Childhood: A Comparative Study," in *Infantile Autism, Concepts, Characteristics and Treatment*, ed. M. Rutter (Edinburgh and London: Churchill, Livingstone, 1971): 7-26.

31. Dugas, Velin, and Guériot, "Nouvelles Chimiotherapies" (See note 23).

32. Ibid.

33. M. Beaujard and E. Revol, "Medicaments Psycho-Analeptiques et Arriération Mental," *Journal de Médecine de Lyon* 44 (1963): 1313-18.

34. F. Licenziati and V. Rossolini, "L'Azione della Nialamide sui Ritardi Mentali nella Scuola, "*Gazzetta Internazionale di Medizina e Chirurgia* 70, no. 1 (1965): 75-79.

35. M. Linnoila, "Characteristics of Therapeutic Response to Imipramine in Hyperactive Children," *American Journal of Psychiatry* 136, no. 9 (1979): 1201-03.

36. L.K. Petty and C.J. Spar, "Haloperidol-Induced Tardive Dyskinesia in a 10-Year-Old Girl," *American Journal of Psychiatry* 137, no. 6 (1980): 745-46.

37. Dugas, Velin, and Guériot, "Nouvelles Chimiotherapies" (See note 23).

38. D.J. Safer, R.P. Allen, and E. Barr, "Growth Rebound after Termination of Stimulant Drugs," *Journal of Pediatrics* 86, no. 1 (1975): 113-16.

39. J.S. Werry and R.L. Sprague, cited in B.G. Winsberg, M. Press, I. Bialer, et al., "Dextro-Amphetamine and Methylphenidate in the Treatment of Hyperactive/Aggressive Children," *Pediatrics* 53, no. 2 (1974): 236-41.

40. Winsberg, Press, Bialer, et al., "Dextro-Amphetamine" (See note 39).

41. A.R. Lucas and M. Weiss, "Methylphenidate Hallucinosis," *Journal of the American Medical Association* 217 (1971): 1079.

42. Winsberg, Press, Bialer, et al., "Dextro-Amphetamine" (See note 39).

43. A.B. Bremness and J. Sverd, "Methylphenidate-Induced Tourette Syndrome," *American Journal of Psychiatry* 136, no. 10 (1979): 1334-35.

DIAGNOSTIC SIGNIFICANCE OF DRUG RESPONSE IN CHILD PSYCHIATRY

Judith L. Rapoport

INTRODUCTION

One of the most interesting concepts in the field of psychopharmacology is that of "pharmacological dissection" of behavioral syndromes. In child psychiatry, where diagnosis has been muddled in conception and for the most part poorly validated, the notion that drug response might confirm clinical syndromes has been particularly attractive. Such an idea is prominent in the concept of a "paradoxical" response to a stimulant drug; is present in some theorizing about the antieneuretic effect of antidepressants; and has been invoked concerning the partial response of autistic children to antipsychotic medication.

With some minor qualifications, however, the pharmacological approach to syndromal identification has not held in child psychiatry. On the other hand, "dissection of drug response" may in itself be of considerable interest, albeit at a locus closer to the site of drug action and relatively removed from the original clinical concept of specific clinical response.

This paper will discuss the nonspecificity of drug response on clinical grounds, and then review other aspects of drug response as exemplified by the differing affective responses to stimulants among children and adults, or the tolerance to tricyclics, which may provide the basis for "dissection" of syndromes through an understanding of the mechanism of drug action.

CLINICAL SPECIFICITY OF STIMULANT DRUG RESPONSE

The human behavioral response to stimulants holds considerable interest for general psychiatry. In depressed patients mood improvement with stimulants has been found to predict clinical response to tricyclics;[1-3] in acute schizophrenic patients stimulants have been reported to worsen psychosis.[4] In child psychiatry the useful effects of stimulants on hyperactive/conduct-disordered children[5,6] have been used to support other evidence that these children are hypoaroused.[7,8] Similarly, beneficial drug effects have been hypothesized to occur through reversal of attention deficit,[9,10] presuming that vigilance effects occur chiefly via reversal of a deficit state.[11]

There has been extensive speculation that age and diagnostic differences in stimulant drug response provide clues to understanding the pathophysiology of the hyperactive child syndrome. No comparison has been made, however, of stimulant drug effects in normal children, hyperactive children, and normal adults under the same experimental conditions. Questions of the specificity of the hyperactive child's response to stimulants, and of the qualitative or quantitative differences in amphetamine response between children and adults cannot be answered until such a comparison is made.

A recently completed study at the National Institute of Mental Health (NIMH) investigated the cognitive, electrophysiological, and behavioral responses to d-amphetamine of normal and hyperactive boys and of normal adult males—the latter given either the same *per weight* dose (0.5 mg./kg.) of amphetamine as the children, or a lower dose (0.25 mg./kg.), which more closely approximates that used in other studies with adults and is close to the *absolute total* dose commonly given to children. This study was a unique attempt to test the direction and amplitude of drug effects on children and adults under identical circumstances, using a variety of behavioral, cognitive, and physiological measures.[12,13]

Specific questions addressed were: Is the amphetamine response different in normal and hyperactive children? Is the decreased motor activity in hyperactive children a "paradoxical effect" with respect to either pathological state or age?

The group of fourteen normal boys was selected from professional families living in the area; all were considered free of learning and behavior problems: none had previously been exposed to amphetamines. The fifteen hyperactive boys were referred by local practitioners and clinics; all had long-standing behavior and learning problems and were considered restless and inattentive both at home and at school.

Area universities and colleges were contacted to obtain a total sample of thiry-one males between age eighteen and thirty who had no history of childhood learning or behavior problems, current psychiatric illness, or regular drug use; they were divided into two groups on the basis of dosage. The first group (N = 15) received the same per weight, single dose of amphetamine elixir as the children (0.5 mg./kg.), with a maximum of 35 mg. ("high dose" group); the second group (N = 16) received half the children's dose, namely, 0.25 mg./kg. of amphetamine elixir ("low dose" group), with a maximal dose of 17.5 mg./kg.

The study took place over three mornings—Monday, Wednesday, and Friday—of a given week between 8:30 A.M. and 12:00 noon. One subject was tested each week, and all were asked to get their usual amount of sleep the night before each test session. Procedures were identical for children and adults.

Measures included:

• Motor activity was measured for a two-hour period, commencing one-half hour after drug administration, by an acceleration-sensitive device with a solid-state memory that can store data on number of movements per unit time over a forty-eight-hour period.[14]

• Skin conductance was monitored continuously during a session consisting of a three-minute rest period; eight 75 decibel (db) tones to which no response was required; and a reaction-time task, which consisted of twenty trials—ten with a fixed four-second preparatory interval, followed by ten with a ten-second interval.

• The Rosvold Continuous Performance Test[15] was modified to allow a greater performance range in normal subjects. A sequence of single numerals was presented to the subject on a light-emitting diode (LED) display with a stimulus duration of 100 msec. The subject was requested to push a button if a 4 appeared, if, and only if, the button for a number outside the critical sequence was a commission error.

• Children were read aloud a modification of the Van Kammen-Murphy Mood Scale,[16] which has been shown to be sensitive to single-dose amphetamine effects. Adults completed both the original adult mood scale and the child's version of the scale. The scales, which were completed for baseline, drug, and placebo sessions by all subjects, consisted of items to which a subject had to check, or answer, "not at all," "a little," "some," or "a lot." The items were discussed with the children during the practice session and they were asked to give examples of situations in which they might respond "feel sad," "feel like crying," "feel happy," and so on; all gave appropriate responses, which suggested a good grasp of these concepts.

In addition, learning task and speech and language measures were obtained, and behavioral ratings were made of affect and motor activity. The results were interesting, both for the similarities and for the differences between the groups. The similarities were most striking with respect to activity.

Figures 1, 2, and 3 show total trunkal motor activity during the two hours of testing—placebo and drug conditions—of children and adults. Both normal and hyperactive boys showed a significant decrease in activity after administration of amphetamine.

In the adults the 0.5 mg./kg. dose produced a nonsignificant decrease in mean activity, while the lower dose of 0.25 mg./kg. produced a *significant decrease* in motor activity (p <.03). Reaction time decreased in both groups of children on the drug, and in one of the adult groups.

On the placebo, hyperactive children had significantly longer reaction time than the other three groups; normal children differed from the high-dose adult group only for the long preparatory interval (PI). No group differed significantly from any other with respect to conductance. Following amphetamine, reaction time for the short PI decreased significantly for normal and hyperactive boys; reaction time for the long PI decreased only for hyperactives. Skin conductance to reaction-time stimuli decreased for the normal children only.

The low-dose adult group had a significant decrease in reaction time for the long PI, and a trend toward a decrease in skin conductance amplitude.

The continuous performance test (CPT) showed significant improvement on one or more vigilance measures—either errors of commission or omission, or in decrease in interstimulus interval—for both groups of children and the high-dose adult group.

Normal children had significantly decreased omission errors on amphetamine; hyperactive children showed a trend toward a decrease in omission errors.

Affective response, on the other hand, was strikingly different. Both groups of children reported no "euphoric" responses on amphetamine. The only significant drug effect on the self-report scale for the normal group was for the item "feel funny"; the hyperactive children were more likely to report "feel funny," and to rate themselves as "more tired or cranky." In contrast, both adult groups showed significant euphoria with both doses, and reported feeling *less* tired on the drug, although this effect was more marked in the high-dose group.

The difference in the effect of stimulants on the self-report scale among children and adult groups is of considerable interest. Hyperactive children do not exhibit euphoria on stimulants, and a persistent dysphoria is

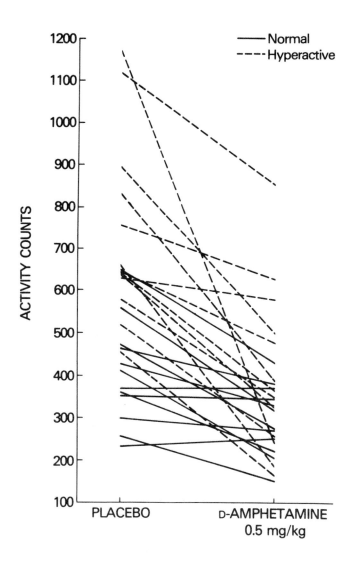

Figure 1. Motor activity during two-hour test sessions following placebo or amphet-amine.

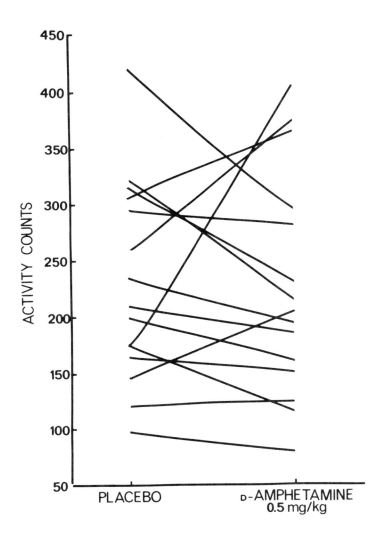

Figure 2. Motor activity during two-hour test sessions of normal adults. High dose
N = 15.

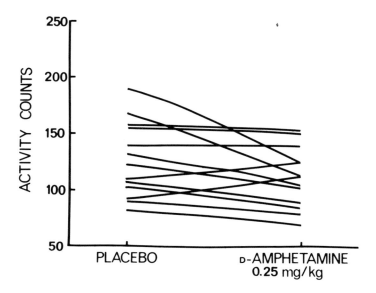

Figure 3. Motor activity during two-hour test sessions of normal adults. Low dose N = 13.

common among chronically treated hyperactive children—a side effect of the medication that often troubles the child's family.[17,18] In contrast, with both doses of stimulants, both experienced and drug-naive adults found amphetamine to be mood elevating. One possibility that must be considered, however, is that these results could have been due to the decreased reporting of subjective effects by children.

We speculate that this difference in mood-altering effect may be of fundamental importance, and that the differential response to the drug may imply a differing underlying chemical mediation of mood between prepubertal children and adults.

Normal and hyperactive children and normal adults exhibited many similar responses to stimulants, including vigilance; improved cognitive performance; and, for all but the high-dose adults, decreased motor activity during cognitive testing.

In both hyperactive and normal children the vigilance, CPT, and reaction-time tasks showed significant improvement due to amphetamine;

the data for the adults are less consistent, but where significant or borderline differences were found, they were also in the direction of improvements. Quantitatively, on both tasks the greatest improvement was shown by the hyperactive group, which can most conservatively be explained by their more impaired placebo values. The generally greater effects of the drug on the children compared to the adults admits of a similar explanation. Studies using psychomotor and attentional tasks in adults have been hard pressed to demonstrate improvement due to stimulant drugs in the absence of some impairing factor such as sleep deprivation, fatigue, or boredom.[19,20] The present data suggest that childhood and hyperactivity have stimulant-reversible attention impairments, and that these effects are additive.

In summary, ignoring the issue of statistical significance or magnitude of drug effect after amphetamine, all four groups showed decreased motor activity, faster reaction time, and enhanced memory. Normal and hyperactive children, and at least one adult group, showed improved vigilance and reaction time. Since these behaviors are all target symptoms in hyperactive children, our data does not strongly support the concept of a unique stimulant drug response in that clinical group.

Moreover, differences in stimulant drug effects between normal and hyperactive children are much less striking than they are between hyperactive boys and adults. Speculations about the pathophysiology of the hyperactive syndrome based on drug response have suffered from the lack of such a control group. The data are more consistent with a model of a relative deficiency ameliorated by amphetamine, or a nonspecific symptomatic relief by amphetamine.

The generally similar response to amphetamine of the normal and hyperactive children may explain the lack of consistent prediction of stimulant drug response among different studies and the variety of children who "respond," as outlined in recent reviews.[21,22]

CLINICAL RESPONSE TO TRICYCLIC ANTIDEPRESSANTS IN CHILD PSYCHIATRY

The pediatric age group offers a rich and varied clinical population in which to study the psychopharmacology of tricyclic antidepressants. A brief overview will summarize the four clinical conditions of childhood and adolescence in which tricyclics have been studied systematically: hyperkinesis, enuresis, school phobia, and, most recently, depression. What little is known about the unique aspects of the pharmacology of these drugs in childhood, such as tolerance to drug effect and the time course of clinical response, will be discussed.

Two pediatric conditions have been shown to respond to tricyclic treatment, at least on a short-term basis: enuresis and hyperkinesis. Reports on the treatment of these disorders—which represent all but two of the controlled studies with tricyclics in children—share in common an established, immediate clinical effect often seen following the first dose; and a wearing-off of efficacy for many patients with chronic (two to five weeks) drug administration.

In contrast, few studies suggest a probable *delayed* effect of tricyclics in school-phobic and clinically depressed children.

Enuresis

Following the initial brief report of R. McLean,[23] and a controlled clinical trial by A. Poussaint and D. Ditman,[24] more than thirty double-blind studies demonstrated the symptomatic efficacy of tricyclic medication in enuresis, with a bedtime dosage of from 25 to 125 mg. While improvement was noted in 60 to 80 percent of most samples, total remissions were reported in only 10 to 50 percent during drug treatment for this condition, which has a significant placebo remission rate. The literature has been reviewed extensively by B. Blackwell and J. Currah, who concluded that the case for the cure of enuresis by tricyclics is not proven, and that most children resume wetting when medication is stopped.[25]

Most drug studies of enuretic children have not used the same dose of tricyclics, similar populations, or similar diagnostic criteria. For that reason it has been difficult to make a statement about the comparative effectiveness of various tricyclics, or to define "good responders." In general, institutionalized, retarded, older enuretics, and those who are daytime wetters, seem to show a less favorable response.

In a recent study twenty disturbed and twenty nondisturbed severely enuretic boys were shown to respond equally well to both imipramine (IMI) and desmethylimipramine (DMI).[26] The only partial predictor of clinical response was the plasma concentration of tricyclics, *not* behavioral disturbance in the child. The antienuretic response was not simply related to plasma level, however, as decreased effectiveness occurred in some children in spite of the adequate plasma concentration of the drug. In the same study the lack of effectiveness of methscopolamine indicates that peripheral anticholinergic mechanisms of action are not basic to antienuretic effect. Nonetheless a central anticholinergic mechanism could still be operative.

Alternatively, the equivalence of DMI and IMI in the study might indicate a noradrenergic antienuretic mechanism. Moreover ephedrine, a sympathomimetic amine that activates α and β receptors, significantly reduced the number of wet nights in a population of enuretics, although it was less effective than IMI.[27] The inefficacy of both methylphenidate and amphetamine,[28,29] however, might be used to argue against an adrenergic mode of action. It would be of great interest to compare the antienuretic effect of IMI with that of the presumed new antidepressants such as Iprindol, Mianserin, or Zimelidine, as an as yet unknown mechanism of tricyclics may be important in the treatment of enuresis. A recent comprehensive review of the physiology of micturition stresses the uncertain role of the sympathetic nervous system and the problems in interpreting pharmacological results.[30]

Hyperkinetic Behavior Disorders

Shortly after tricyclics began to be used for enuresis, reports on the use of drugs in hyperactive/aggressive children claimed therapeutic effects similar to those obtained with stimulants.[31,32] More recently, controlled trials have generally confirmed these initial open studies and have shown the beneficial effect of tricyclics in doses of from 2 to 5 mg./kg. for children exhibiting restless, antisocial behavior.[33–38] The response is immediate and in some cases dramatic; most of the studies, however, have shown methylphenidate or amphetamine to be superior to tricyclics.

All these controlled studies are short term—of durations of four weeks or less; the long-term usefulness of tricyclics for these disorders remains controversial. In an open study, R. Gittelman-Klein indicated that an initial response to a daily dose of 150-300 mg. of IMI seen at two weeks was not maintained at twelve weeks.[39] Similarly, in a one-year follow up, significantly more hyperactive children had discontinued tricyclic medication than had discontinued methylphenidate, even when both groups had shown an initial response after six weeks.[40] The author's experience is that long-term treatment of conduct-disordered or hyperactive children with tricyclics is unsatisfactory; this point deserves further study. Attempts to predict IMI response in hyperactive children on the basis of clinical examination or history have been unsuccessful.* For example, while about

* P. Quinn and J. Rapoport: unpublished observations.

25 percent of a sample of hyperactive boys showed some depressive symptomatology, this subgroup was not differentially responsive to tricyclic medication; neither was a positive family history of depressive disorder predictive of response.

Separation Anxiety

A single double-blind study has shown that IMI benefits the separation anxiety associated with school phobia.[41] The effect was seen six weeks after an average daily dose of 152 mg., but the authors stress that the anticipatory anxiety associated with school return did not seem altered. More studies are needed to confirm the usefulness of tricyclics in school phobics. There are questions as to the safety of the drugs, since the doses said to be required are high and have been associated with one fatality. This study is of great interest, however, as it probably indicates a delayed effect—not seen at three weeks—in contrast to that seen with enuresis or hyperkinesis. This latter point is not completely certain, as the dose was increased over the six-week period; thus dose-effect may be confounded with treatment duration.

Depressive Disorder

The difficulty of defining depressive disorder in childhood has been reviewed elsewhere;[42-44] it will not be discussed here except to note the apparent rarity of true adult-type depression in childhood, and to state that the overuse of vague diagnostic labels such as "masked depression" or "depressive equivalent" has been detrimental to research in this area.

In uncontrolled studies IMI has been described as useful for a variety of possible depressive symptoms such as learning disabilities, irritability, dysphoria, insomnia, nightmares, and somatic manifestations, for example, headaches and stomach aches. Some of these studies are particularly suggestive of true antidepressant action.[45-47] The children observed, described as having social withdrawal, deteriorating school performance, and self-destruction of recent onset, seem to benefit from tricyclic medication. Most of these studies, however, lack clear clinical description; objective behavior ratings; independent diagnostic ratings; or proper controls for time and placebo effects.

J. Puig-Antich and coworkers have completed an open trial of IMI with eight children who met the adult Research Diagnostic Criteria for depressive disorder;[48] behavior rating and clinical evaluation, using standardized scales, indicated that six of the eight improved on the drug. This is the first methodologically adequate study of the antidepressant efficacy of a tricyclic in prepubertal children. Too few children have completed the double-blind protocol to form any conclusions; clinical response appears to be delayed, however, occurring after only two weeks or so of treatment.

The interesting point here is that immediate clinical effects of tricyclics seen in children with hyperactivity or enuresis, conditions often regarded as "developmental delays," are probably mediated by a different mechanism than the delayed clinical effect seen after two to four weeks in depressed or school-phobic children, that is, those with "neurotic" disorders. The latter conditions are *not* associated with hyperactivity and enuresis, and in fact occur more usually in children with no signs of neurological immaturity. The differing time course of the drug effect may help validate these broad nosological categories. It may be that the immediate effects of the drug, such as reuptake blockade of norepinephrine, are crucial for enuresis and hyperactivity, while alteration in receptor sensitivity is necessary for efficacy in school phobia or depression.

While the specificity of drug response has not yielded any simple answers, two new and intriguing areas of pharmacological "dissection" should be covered as they represent new areas of investigation that may be promising: the lithium response of offspring of lithium-responding parents; and the treatment of obsessive-compulsive disorders with chlorimipramine (Anafranil, Ciba-Geigy). The former suggests a new means of grouping patients by family history of drug response, possibly independent of syndromal identification; the latter represents a last bastion of "specificity of drug response" of a well-known but poorly understood symptom pattern.

Childhood Obsessive-Compulsive Disorders

Childhood obsessive-compulsive disorders are found in only 1 to 2 percent of the childhood psychiatric population. The chronicity and "purity" of the disorder, however, and its relative resistance to treatment make it an important diagnostic entity for child psychiatrists to understand.[49]

Childhood obsessive-compulsive disease has held an analogous position to that of Gilles de la Tourette's syndrome. Although the onset of symptoms of at least half the patients with Tourette's syndrome occurs during childhood, diagnosis is typically not made until age eighteen.[50] Investigators describing the clinical picture of obsessive-compulsive disease in adolescence acknowledge that their patients frequently give retrospective histories of identical symptoms beginning as early as age three or four. A cumulative review suggests that one-third of 357 cases were ill before age fifteen.[51] Others have cited the onset of obsessive disorder in childhood: P. Janet, for example, reported a case of obsessional neurosis in a five-year-old;[52] the "rat man's" symptoms appeared at age six or seven.[53] Some of Janet's cases were probably the Tourette syndrome, however, since tics are one of the earliest signs of obsessive disorder. S. Freud cited age six to eight as the usual age at which obsessive predisposition occurs,[54] and E. Kringlen noted that about half his ninety-one adult patients had become ill before age twenty, and one-fifth of them before puberty.[55]

The recent upsurge of interest in obsessive disorders has been due in part to the claims that chlorimipramine, a tricyclic antidepressant with relative specific potency for blocking the reuptake of serotonin, is specifically useful for this disorder.[56]

In contrast to sporadic trials of other agents, there have now been many reports of the usefulness of chlorimipramine for compulsive disorder in adults.[57-60] Can one say that the serotonin system is involved in obsessive-compulsive disease?

Of more than fifty citations in the literature, only two were controlled, double-blind studies; several controlled studies are currently in progress in Europe and the United States. In an ongoing study at the NIMH of chlorimipramine treatment of obsessive-compulsive children and adolescents, preliminary data suggest there may be a differential benefit from that drug compared with DMI or a placebo in a double-blind comparative study.

Many questions of course remain, such as the relationship of clinical change to the antidepressant activity of the drug. These findings need to be extended and replicated. Nevertheless these observations may provide a rare example of specific drug treatment response of a particular behavioral syndrome that has great interest for child psychiatry.

Lithium-Response Syndrome

A.L. Annell has reported extensive use of lithium in children and adolescents who manifested a variety of symptoms, including flagrant psychosis, but who had in common a periodic course: in one series, eleven of twelve children responded with marked clinical change.[61,62] L.F. Gram and O.J. Rafaelsen, in a double-blind, controlled study of eighteen inpatients with the diagnosis of psychosis since at least age five, found that many symptoms responded to lithium compared to a placebo, but the results were by no means dramatic.[63]

Two controlled studies did not find lithium useful for hyperactive children, although possible responses for individual cases were suggested.[64,65] In a search for a lithium-responsive subgroup, W.L. Dyson and A. Barcai reported two cases of hyperactive children who had a lithium-responding parent.[66] Their clinical data are not convincing: one child required concomitant continued use of stimulants, and no control periods were observed.

The idea of a drug-responsive subgroup selected on the basis of positive parental treatment response may, however, be a useful model for future studies, and may prove more rewarding than subgrouping by symptoms. But it must be stressed that although lithium may be effective in a variety of disorders, positive response should not be equated with a diagnosis of manic-depressive disease in childhood.[67]

Leon Cytryn and Donald McKnew of the NIMH are conducting a sixteen-week, double-blind study of the lithium response of prepubertal offspring of lithium-responding, bipolar, affectively ill parents. This is a unique attempt to study alternate, four-week placebo and drug periods in a group of children with mixed symptomatology—some are hyperactive/behavior disordered, while others appear depressed or highly anxious. Preliminary data from the seven children who have completed the study indicate that some of them are clearly lithium responders; it is too early to see whether or not there is any particular behavioral pattern in this sample associated with positive response. This study may represent one important approach to pediatric psychopharmacological research and to validation of diagnosis in childhood.

In summary, major diagnostic categories of "depression" or "hyperactivity" are not validated in any simple fashion by clinical drug response to a particular class of agents. Careful study of drug response, however, particularly *pattern* of response, may still provide answers to the underlying pathophysiology of some childhood psychiatric disorders.

NOTES

1. J. Fawcett and V. Siomopolous, "Dextroamphetamine Response as a Possible Predictor of Improvement with Tricyclic Therapy in Depression," *Archives of General Psychiatry* 25 (1971): 247-55.

2. J. Fawcett, J. Mass, and H. Dekirmenjian, "Depression and MHPG Excretion: Response to Dextroamphetamine and Tricyclic Antidepressants," *Archives of General Psychiatry* 26 (1973): 246-51.

3. D.P. Van Kammen and D.L. Murphy, "Prediction of Imipramine Antidepressant Response by One-Day D-amphetamine Trial," *American Journal of Psychiatry* 138 (1978): 1179-84.

4. D. Segal and J. Janowsky, "Psychostimulant-Induced Behavioral Effects; Possible Models of Schizophrenia," in *Psychopharmacology, A Generation of Progress*, ed. M. Lipton, A. Dimascio, and K. Killam (New York: Raven Press, 1977): 1113-23.

5. C. Bradley, "The Behavior of Children Receiving Benzedrine," *American Journal of Orthopsychiatry* 94 (1937): 577-85.

6. C. Bradley and M. Bowen, "Amphetamine (Benzedrine) Therapy of Children's Behavior Disorders," *American Journal of Orthopsychiatry* 11 (1941): 92-103.

7. J. Satterfield, D. Cantwell, and B. Satterfield, "Pathophysiology of the Hyperactive Children Syndrome," *Archives of General Psychiatry* 31 (1974): 839-43.

8. C. Kornetsky, "Psychoactive Drugs in the Immature Organism," *Psychopharmacologia* 17 (1970): 105-36.

9. V. Douglas, "Stop, Look and Listen: The Problem of Sustained Attention and Impulse Control in Hyperactive and Normal Children," *Canadian Journal of Behavioural Science* 41 (1972): 259-83.

10. V. Douglas, D. Sykes, and G. Morgenstern "Sustained Attention in Hyperactive Children," *Journal of Child Psychology and Psychiatry* 14 (1973): 213-20.

11. D. Sykes, V. Douglas, and G. Morgenstern, "The Effect of Methylphenidate on Sustained Attention in Hyperactive Children," *Psychopharmacologia* 25 (1972): 263-74.

12. J. Rapoport, M.S. Buchsbaum, T.P. Zahn, et al., "Dextroamphetamine: Cognitive and Behavioral Effects in Normal Prepubertal Boys," *Science* 199 (1978): 560-63.

13. _____, "Dextroamphetamine: Cognitive and Behavioral Effects in Normal and Hyperactive Boys and Normal Adult Males," *Archives of General Psychiatry*, in press.

14. T.M. Colburn, B.M. Smith, T. Guarini, et al., "An Ambulatory Activity Monitor with Solid State Memory," *ISA Transactions* 15 (1976): 149-54.

15. H. Rosvold, A. Mirsky, I. Sarason, et al., "A Continuous Performance Test of Brain Damage," *Journal of Consulting Psychology* 20 (1956): 343-50.

16. D.P. Van Kammen and D.L. Murphy, "Attentuation of the Euphoriant and Activating Effects of D- and L-Amphetamine by Lithium Carbonate Treatment," *Psychopharmacologia* 44 (1975): 215-24.

17. C. Whalen, B. Hentker, B. Collins, et al., "Peer Interaction in a Structured Communication Task: Comparison of Normal and Hyperactive Boys and of Methylphenidate (Ritalin) and Placebo Effects," *Child Development* 50 (1979): 388-401.

18. C.K. Conners, "Discussion," in *Depression in Childhood: Diagnosis, Treatment, and Conceptual Models*, ed. J. Schulterbrandt and A. Raskin (New York: Raven Press, 1977): 101-06.

19. B. Weiss and V.G. Laties, "Enhancement of Human Performance by Caffeine and the Amphetamines," *Pharmacology Review* 14 (1962): 1-36.

20. V.G. Laties and B. Weiss, "Performance Enhancement by the Amphetamines: A New Appraisal," in *Proceedings of the 5th International Congress of Collegium Internationale Neuropsychopharmacologicum* (Amsterdam: Excerpta Medica, 1967): 800-08.

21. B. Fish, "The 'One Child-One Drug' Myth of Stimulants in Hyperkinesis," *Archives of General Psychiatry* 25 (1971): 193-203.

22. R. Barkley, "Predicting the Response of Hyperkinetic Children to Stimulant Drugs: A Review," *Journal of Abnormal Child Psychology* 4 (1976): 327-48.

23. R. McLean, "Imipramine Hydroxychloride (Tofranil) and Enuresis," *American Journal of Psychiatry* 117 (1960): 551.

24. A. Poussaint and D. Ditman, "A Controlled Study of Imipramine (Tofranil) in the Treatment of Childhood Enuresis," *Journal of Pediatrics* 67 (1965): 285-90.

25. B. Blackwell and J. Currah, "The Psychopharmacology of Nocturnal Enuresis," in *Bladder Control and Enuresis* (Clinics in Developmental Medicine #48/49), ed. I. Kolvin, R. MacKeith, and S. Meadow (London: Heinemann, 1973).

26. J. Rapoport, E. Mikkelsen, A. Zavadil, et al., "Enuresis. II: Psychopathology, Plasma Tricyclic Concentration and Antienuretic Responses," *Archives of General Psychiatry*, in press.

27. General Practitioner Research Group, "Sedatives and Stimulants Compound in Enuresis," *Practitioner* 204 (1970): 584-90.

28. E. Breger, "Hydroxyzine Hydrochloride and Methylphenidate Hydroxychloride in the Management of Enuresis," *Journal of Pediatrics* 61 (1962): 443-47.

29. W. McConaghy, "A Controlled Trial of Imipramine, Amphetamine, Pad and Bell Conditioning and Random Awakening in the Treatment of Nocturnal Enuresis," *Medical Journal of Australia* 2 (1969): 237-39.

30. J. Stephenson, "Physiological and Pharmacological Basis for the Chemotherapy of Enuresis," *Psychological Medicine* 9 (1979): 1-15.

31. J. Rapoport, "Childhood Behavior and Learning Problems Treated with Imipramine," *International Journal of Neuropsychiatry* 1 (1965): 635-42.

32. A. Krakowski, "Amitryptyline in Treatment of Hyperkinetic Children: A Double Blind Study," *Psychosomatics* 6 (1965): 355-60.

33. J. Waizer, S. Hoffman, P. Polizos, et al., "Outpatient Treatment of Hyperactive School Children with Imipramine," *American Journal of Psychiatry* 131 (1974): 587-91.

34. B. Winsberg, I. Bialer, S. Kupietz, et al., "Effects of Imipramine and Dextroamphetamine on Behavior of Neuropsychiatrically Impaired Children," *American Journal of Psychiatry* 128 (1972): 1425-32.

35. J. Rapoport, P. Quinn, G. Bradbard, et al., "Imipramine and Methylphenidate Treatment of Hyperactive Boys," *Archives of General Psychiatry* 30 (1975): 789-94.

36. L. Greenberg, A. Yellin, C. Spring, et al., "Clinical Effects of Imipramine and Methylphenidate in Hyperactive Children," *International Journal of Mental Health* 4 (1975): 144-56.

37. L. Yepes, E. Balka, B. Winsberg, et al., "Amitryptyline and Methylphenidate Treatment of Behaviorally Disordered Children," *Journal of Child Psychology and Psychiatry* 18 (1977): 39-52.

38. S. Kupietz and E. Balka, "Alterations in Vigilance Performance of Children Receiving Amitryptyline and Methylphenidate Pharmacotherapy," *Psychopharmacology* 50 (1976): 24-33.

39. R. Gittelman-Klein, "Pilot Clinical Trial of Imipramine in Hyperkinetic Children," in *Clinical Use of Stimulant Drugs in Children,* ed. C. Conners (The Hague: Excerpta Medica, 1974): 199-201.

40. P. O. Quinn and J. Rapoport, "A One-Year Follow-Up of Hyperactive Boys Treated with Imipramine or Methylphenidate," *American Journal of Psychiatry* 132 (1975): 241-45.

41. R. Gittelman-Klein and D. Klein, "Controlled Imipramine Management of School Phobia," *Archives of General Psychiatry* 25 (1971): 204-07.

42. C. Conners, "Classification and Treatment of Childhood Depressive Equivalents," in *Depression: Behavioral, Biochemical, Diagnostic and Treatment Concepts,* ed. D. Gallant and G. Simpson (New York: Spectrum, 1976): 181-96.

43. P. Graham, "Depression in Pre-Pubertal Children," *Developmental Medicine and Child Neurology* 16 (1974): 340-49.

44. J. Rapoport, "Pediatric Psychopharmacology and Childhood Depression," in *Progress in Psychiatric Drug Treatment,* ed. D. Klein and R. Gittelman-Klein (New York: Brunner Mazel, 1976).

45. W. Ling, G. Oftedal, and W. Weinberg, "Depressive Illness in Childhood Presenting as Severe Headache," *American Journal of Diseases of Children* 120 (1970): 122-24.

46. W. Weinberg, J. Rutman, L. Sullivan, et al., "Depression in Children Referred to an Education Diagnostic Center: Diagnosis and Treatment," *Journal of Pediatrics* 83 (1973): 1065-72.

47. E. Frommer, "Treatment of Childhood Depression with Antidepressant Drugs," *British Medical Journal* 1 (1967): 729-32.

48. J. Puig-Antich, S. Balu, N. Marx, et al., "Prepubertal Major Depressive Disorder: A Pilot Study," *Journal of the American Academy of Child Psychiatry* 17 (1979): 695-97.

49. R. Elkins, J. Rapoport, and A. Lipsky, "Childhood Obsessive-Compulsive Disorder: A Biological Viewpoint, *Journal of the American Academy of Child Psychiatry*, submitted.

50. A. Shapiro, E. Shapiro, R. Bruun, et al., *Gilles de la Tourette Syndrome* (New York: Raven Press, 1978).

51. H. R. Beech, *Obsessive States* (London: Methuen, 1974).

52. P. Janet, *Les Obsessions et la Psychiasthenia*, 2 vols., 2nd ed. (Paris: Bailliére, 1903).

53. S. Freud, *Notes on a Case of Obsessional Neurosis*, stand. ed. 10 (London: Hogarth Press, 1903): 153-318.

54. _____, *The Disposition to Obsessional Neurosis* (London: Hogarth Press, 1913): 311-26.

55. E. Kringlen, "Obsessional Neurotics," *British Journal of Psychiatry* 111 (1965): 709-22.

56. A. Todrick and A. Tait, "The Inhibition of Human Platelet 5-Hydroxytryptamine Update by Tricyclic Antidepressant Drugs," *Journal of Pharmacy and Pharmacology* 21 (1969): 751-60.

57. F.E. Cordoba and J.J. Lopez Ibor Alino, "Monochlorimipramine in Psychiatric Patients Resistant to Other Forms of Treatment," *Acta Luso-Españalas Neurologica y Psyquiatrica* (Madrid) 26 (1967): 119-47.

58. N. Capstick, "Chlorimipramine in Obsessional States," *Psychosomatics* 12 (1971): 335.

59. J. Wyndowe, L. Salyom, and J. Anarth, "Anafranil in Obsessive-Compulsive Neurosis," *Current Therapeutic Research* 18 (1975): 611-17.

60. J.A. Yarura-Tobias, F. Neziroglu, and L. Berman, "Chlorimipramine for Obsessive-Compulsive Neurosis: An Organic Approach," *Current Therapeutic Research* 20 (1976): 541-48.

61. A.L. Annell, "Lithium in the Treatment of Children and Adolescents," *Acta Psychiatrica Scandinavica* 207, suppl. (1969): 19-30.

62. _____, "Manic-Depressive Illness in Children and Effect of Treatment with Lithium Carbonate," *Acta Paedopsychiatrica* (Basel) 36 (1969): 292-301.

63. L.F. Gram and O.J. Rafaelsen, "Lithium Treatment of Psychotic Children and Adolescents," *Acta Psychiatrica Scandinavica* 48 (1972): 253-60.

64. P.L. Whitehead and L.D. Clark, "Effect of Lithium Carbonate, Placebo and Thioridazine on Hyperactive Children," *American Journal of Psychiatry* 127 (1970): 824-25.

65. L.L. Greenhill, R.O. Rieder, P.H. Wender, et al., "Lithium Carbonate in the Treatment of Hyperactive Children," *Archives of General Psychiatry* 28 (1973): 636-40.

66. W.L. Dyson and A. Barcai, "Treatment of Children of Lithium-Responding Parents," *Current Therapeutic Research* 12 (1970): 286-90.

67. M. Schou, "Lithium in Psychiatric Therapy and Prophylaxis: A Review with Special Regard to Its Use in Children," in *Depressive States in Childhood and Adolescence*, ed. A.L. Annell (New York: John Wiley & Sons, 1972): 479-87.

DISCUSSION

Children and Drugs

How can we explain the difference in effect between addictive drugs taken in childhood, which do not lead to drug addiction in postadolescence or adulthood, and sedatives taken in early infancy, which expose the child to a higher risk of drug addiction later on?

Many factors must come into play. One could wonder, for example, whether parents who systematically give sedatives to their children are not themselves very disturbed. People who take amphetamines are looking for a harmless treatment of a given symptom. Psychostimulant drugs act as a kind of vaccination. That of course is rather a strange philosophy for medicine, but it is interesting. It is advisable to do longitudinal studies of children who take drugs at different ages to see how they evolve.

Campaigns in France

Systematic campaigns against drug use in France are overdone because they prevent people from treating basic dysfunctions. But, at the same time, a philosophy that implies that children should not have access to drugs and medicines is a good one; the fewer drugs or medicines children take the better off they are.

Experimental Drugs

With regard to work with experimental drugs, it would appear that their effect on hyperactivity in children mobilizes the noradrenalin sources.

Clonidine is a very interesting drug because of its direct agonist properties. One problem is that it seems as if very low doses may have a precipitant effect and higher doses a postsynaptic effect. It is a very difficult drug to interpret or to work with.

The person in America who has used clonidine the most is giving it to children with Giles de la Tourette syndrome, most of whom have behavioral disturbances. Judging from reports there is no immediate action, but there is some improvement over a period of weeks or months. The doses range considerably, so it is not clear whether one is predicting an increase or a decrease in augmenting effects.

Use of Amphetamines

It is difficult to convey the ray of light that was felt when Rapoport published some studies on drug use in normal children and had the courage to go ahead. Many people had thought of it, but for some reason or another had had reservations about using children. The data show the apparent difference in mental response, that is, the lack of euphoria. The reason preadolescents do not go on to become amphetamine addicts when given this drug for the treatment of hyperkenesis is this lack of a euphoric response.

Children on amphetamines may look depressed. One child had unexplained spells of crying. When the psychiatrist discussed with him the desirability of stopping the drug because it made him cry, he said: "Please don't. I'm doing so much better in school. I don't mind crying." The crying episode stopped after a fairly short period of time; it was a symptomatic response.

Pre- and Postadolescent Use

How does one account for the difference reported by Rapoport in postadolescent and preadolescent use. Something is different—"I feel funny"— but it is not interpreted as feeling good. One could argue that most of the time children feel so much better than adults that there is a different threshold to begin with. Perhaps children are already so euphoric there is no place to go. The most obvious difference has to do with some hormonal mediation.

A number of quite normal and well-functioning people admit they have been using absolutely minute amounts of amphetamines or Ritalin for a number of years without any sign of addiction or abuse in the usual sense—and 5 mg. a day over twenty years cannot be considered abuse. So there is a whole world of subtle use that never comes to clinical attention: it is only as a researcher in this area that one becomes the recipient of these bits of information; the situation is very poorly understood.

Reactions to Drugs

One of the questions we have to ask is what adults know about experimentation. Many people think that reactions to drugs are learned, that you have to know what an amphetamine is going to do before you respond to it properly. That is an important methodological point.

In Rapoport's study it might have been more of a pressing issue some time ago if experiments were being done on very smart, upper-middle-class youngsters who knew they were going to get speed or a placebo; many were well aware of the reactions their older brothers and sisters had had from speed.

Ten years ago one could not have said the groups were in any way comparable. They are still not really comparable, but they were enough so that there was no obvious difference. In fact many of the youngsters said it was very interesting to have been in the study, but they were extremely disappointed because they did not like the drug much. They said they wanted to be in another study, but they did not want to get the same substance.

About the lack of a euphoric response, in Rapoport's study, it is interesting that both groups of children, hyperactives and normals, did not have any, whereas the adults, who apparently were normal, did.

Different Responses of Adults and Children

Paul Wender is doing a series of studies in Utah with adults who are psychiatrically disturbed, but who do not meet any criterion for schizophrenic, manic-depressive, or any other major disorder. They tend to be a hodge-podge of patients who were hyperactive as children. These people, in their thirties, live in an area near Salt Lake City that nobody moves to or leaves, so there are three generations of families, and the parents are still around to report on what the adults were like as children.

In a series of double-blind studies with methylphenidate, Tofranil, and Dexedrine, Wender finds they do not get a euphoric response and do not become tolerant over time, but do exhibit a marked improvement in their various types of psychiatric statuses.

On the same kind of issue, that is, determinant of the difference in activity responses in children and adults, there should be a differential appreciation of the context of the two groups. Perhaps the situation in which you are in can determine the intensity of the emotion partly produced by the arousal capacity of the drug. One wonders whether it is that kind of presence that might differentiate the children and the adults.

Some peer group interactional studies that Barbara Henker and colleagues are doing at the University of California, Los Angeles, indicate that children who are stimulated by methylphenidate, compared with a placebo, make more negative statements about themselves in doing play tasks with peers. They in fact look more dysphoric on the drug.

Rate Dependency

What is closer to the naturalistic setting? The question of rate dependency is intriguing. Of course if one looks at the data in the animal literature on different strains of guinea pigs and rats, it in fact does seem that the base rate can even predict the direction of effect.

Taking a very simple-minded approach, there is a rather powerful case against rate dependency, in that extremely sedentary adults in the Rapoport study who received the low dose of the stimulant looked for all the world like the group in this auditorium—just adults sitting quietly with little or no motion observable. It was quite astonishing to find there was a .03-P value for decrease in activity, and, similarly, that the normal children who were usually well-behaved and quiet were performing way beyond their years. In the vigilance test these groups became less active.

In other words, rate dependency seems an attractive notion. Robins, a psychologist in California, has done a good deal of work on rate-dependency stimulant effects, and has now reanalyzed them in a normal child group, a hyperactive child group, and an adult group. He has been able to establish some relationship between base rate and drug effect, and to salvage something that was very meaningful. As an outsider it seems to be a totally antirate-dependency effect, in the sense that the subjects were quieter, more attentive folk, but Robins does not see it that way.

Response to Lithium

Rapoport was asked whether, in three of the eight children who were lithium-responders, there are any biological markers in the families that suggest a subgroup might be responding. There has been a report recently on red blood cell permeability to lithium.

One cannot stress the psychosocial attributes too much. Researchers should be warned about dealing with manic-depressive, lithium-responding parents and their children. The parents tend to see their children as extensions of themselves, and are absolutely intent on having the children respond to lithium. It is only by the most elaborate ruse—by keeping the blind absolutely blind, by not telling them it is a four-week period, and by changing the number every single week—that one can gain any idea of whether or not the drug is useful. No markers were used, in part because Elliot Gershon, who has been studying adults, was very skeptical about those differences being specific and suggested they not be used.

Previous Experience with Drugs

The question was raised as to whether there was any evidence in Rapoport's work of previous experience on the part of adults who displayed euphoria. In a sense adults are accustomed to taking things to make them feel good, so they may take pills with a certain expectation—one does not usually take them to feel bad.

Also, was there a previous history of drug ingestion, perhaps in terms of acquired enzymes that may cross over? If the subjects had been taking barbiturates or other drugs that might have an effect, that would eliminate certain depressive aspects or produce other pathways that would give a euphoric effect.

The adults were asked that question and the investigators were relieved to find that approximately half of the thirty adults said they had never used stimulants or other drugs before. The reason for this astonishingly high rate of 50 percent of college students who were drug naive is that normal volunteer students are sent to the NIH by rather fundamentalist religious groups whose college-age children do this as part of a religious contribution or to earn money. The data for drug-wise and drug-naive subjects were analyzed separately, and there were no differences between the groups in that respect.

There are several studies showing a fairly good prediction from a single dose in response to a several-week response with hyperactive children, but this was a single-dose study. The experiment was not repeated because permission could not have been obtained from the Human Subject Commission.

Responses of Males and Females

It took Rapoport two years to do the study, which was very difficult in terms of recruiting purposes—getting the right comparable sample. As a result an effort was made to get subjects of the greatest interest. There is controversy about the use of stimulants in hyperactive adolescents, although they probably are useful. The investigators wanted to pick the closest contrast groups. Therefore, because these were grade school boys with a mean age of ten, for whom the effects of stimulants in hyperactivity had been demonstrated, they were the most convincing group of normals.

There is no evidence that drug responsiveness is different in girls, or that hyperactive girls are very different. But this was a difficult enough study to do, and the purpose was to simplify things, so only boys were used.

Propriety of Experimentation with Lithium

The question was raised as to the propriety of using a drug in children with as vague a justification as lithium in view of the very disturbing reports from the Scandinavian countries, still to be verified elsewhere, on the high rate of induction of adrenal pathology visible on biopsy. American nephrologists do not quite know what to make of the findings, but they are disturbing. Given this fact, one questions the use of lithium in children, even for relatively short periods of time. One assumes that developing organs may be more vulnerable. There is no evidence as far as the kidney and lithium is concerned, but Scandinavian reports in *The Lancet* and elsewhere concerning renal pathology secondary to lithium are distressing.

Clinical Practice

Rapoport's research is not intended to generalize to general practice. In view of the reports of poisoning with tricyclics, although her group was extremely interested, theoretically, in the tricyclic treatment of enuresis, that was not considered the treatment of choice; the data suggest that if the families are supportive, the bell and pad is the treatment of first choice.

Her study of the effect of amphetamines in normal children is edifying from the viewpoint of understanding mechanisms, but it is confusing from the viewpoint of clinical practice. Do Rapoport's findings in abnormal children have any implications or indications for the use of amphetamines in clinical practice? And what is her current advice as far as the indications for the use in overactive children, in terms of which symptoms, what types of disability, and so on, she would regard as being most crucial in coming to a decision about whether or not to prescribe these drugs?

Responsiveness to a pharmacological agent is highly respectable in clinical medicine. Insulin would lower the blood sugar of anybody in this room, and yet it is of course a crucial treatment in diabetes. Digitalis has a similar effects on normal and abnormal heart muscles. Perhaps more to the point, diuretics, which may be lifesaving in congestive heart failure, are operating on normal kidneys. Fluid retention occurs at a different point in the pathophysiology of the disorder, and yet diuretics are an important and extremely respectable part of the armamentarium. The nonspecificity suggests that the drug actions are perhaps further down a common causal chain, possibly in terms of biogenic amines.

There are, of course, examples of specific action of drugs. Tricyclics have relatively little mood effect on nondepressed people, and the phenothiazines do not improve the thinking of nonpsychotic individuals.

So there are both kinds of drugs—drugs that have, as Don Klein says, a thermostat-regulating effect, and those that are entirely nonspecific. The latter are among some of the most respectable drugs clinical pharmacology has to offer medicine.

Rapoport's study was in no way an antidrug study. The use of stimulants in hyperactivity remains a very difficult puzzle. It is hard to believe that a drug with such dramatic short-term effects has no long-term benefit, but the few studies that have addressed the long-term benefit do not seem to show it yet; the right study could not of course be done for legal, political, and strategic reasons.

Did Rapoport observe inattention or distractability, and what are the implications for the use of the drugs? Should one largely be guided by the level of complaint of the social agencies concerned about these types of behavior?

It is not fair, from the viewpoint of a researcher, to compare that situation with the life of a practitioner. Perhaps more to the point, the practitioner always has to weigh the benefits and risks in an individual case when giving any sort of treatment. The practitioner faces the situation where a child is out of control, where the trial of behavioral treatment has not worked. The better the comparative studies are done on stimulants and behavior modification, the more disappointing, unfortunately, behavioral approaches seem to be.

In those situations stimulants still seem to be clinically sensible and useful. It is a complicated issue, the question of what is referred to in America as pharmacological hedonism. Following the normal trial of drug studies, Rapoport was unnerved when one of the professional parents said of his son, "He really did better on Dilatine." She wondered what they had in mind, because their sons were already paragons; thus there were all sorts of public health aspects involved.

Tests with Caffeine

Of course there was no question of giving stimulants to normal children, but tests have been made with caffeine in normal children, because that is a dietary substance of wide interest—about 10 percent of an American middle-class, white suburban sample reported the daily use of a great deal of iced tea and cola beverages. Increased vigilance is being observed, at least in that area, and increased restlessness with the intake of caffeine. It may well be that the question is more applicable in a broad public health sense than was intended.

V. INTERGROUP TENSIONS
AND CHILD DEVELOPMENT

THE FUNCTION OF PLAYGROUPS IN NORTHERN IRELAND

Margaret E.R. Morrow

The birthright of every child is to be loved and to be happy. According to a well-known psychiatrist in Belfast *all* children in Northern Ireland are *at risk* because they are members of a divided community.

Morris Fraser in *Children in Conflict* tells of a Belfast headmaster who decided to prohibit from his school all references to the disturbances and to ban all riot games and toy guns. The effect was remarkable: attendance at that school remained at 90 percent. Local vandalism fell dramatically. Two other schools adopted the same course with similar results.[1] This was one way of protecting children from the effects of violence on the streets.

There is also something to be said for removing children from troubled areas for short periods, but this should be done at a time of quiet; to send them away when riots are taking place only gives rise to anxiety. Short-term integration projects such as camps, outings, or the twinning of schools are thought to be of doubtful value. Children may learn tolerance and unlearn myths from encounters with children of the "other side," but their new tolerance is little appreciated when they return home to communities where myths are gospel and sectarian hatred is the first of the commandments.

It is very sad to see three-year-olds, at an age when they should be singing nursery rhymes, show their hatred of the "other side" by spitting, shouting abuse, using four-letter words, or singing party songs with great gusto, but with no understanding of whom they hate or whose side they are on. Their play consists of throwing, hitting, and kicking, on the one hand, and, on the other, a withdrawn, apathetic lack of interest in play. These are indeed "children at risk."

Tense situations create tense people; there is nothing more inhibiting to sound, wholesome growth than tension—which must be relieved. Given playgroup activities, a tense child may become more relaxed and easier to live with and thus may make the parent-child relationship more satisfying. Alternatively, the parent who is relieved for a time each week of the constant pressure created by a particular child may become less tense, and so open the way for a more harmonious relationship with that child.

We believe playgroups play a vital part in the prevention of the "emotionally battered child." Parents and children in Northern Ireland have special problems that place on them a greater strain than they can normally be expected to bear without help, and our playgroups play a significant role in this area, also.

CHILDREN IN A PLAYGROUP

The following are but a few examples that illustrate what living in a troubled area means for both children and parents.

• Little Deirdre is completely withdrawn and her mother is distressed. Due to explosions, nearly all the windows in Deirdre's home have been blown out on six different occasions, mainly at night. With a patient, caring, one-to-one relationship in a playgroup Deirdre has learned how to cope with her fears and anxieties, and her mother has become more relaxed, so a happier relationship exists.

• On the ninth floor of a block of flats is a young mother with three young children; her husband is interned. Each time there is a knock on the door, they ask themselves: Who is it? It could be the army on a "search raid." The only safe place the mother and children know of is the playgroup.

• A father newly released from jail answers the door with a newborn baby in his arms and a three-year-old behind him. A man shoots the father in the knees because he decided not to become involved in the movement again. Hysterics are all around—nightmares galore for the three-year-old—apprehension and anxiety for parents. Next morning the whole story, with floods of tears, is told to the playgroup leader, who gives comfort and support.

• Because of the general anti-army feeling in the area a bonny three-year-old girl stamps her foot and spits at the soldiers standing on guard at the barrier near the playgroup. The same little girl, a few weeks later, when the anti-army feeling has subsided somewhat in the area, shares her sweets with the soldiers on duty. How can parents cope when they live in such communities? They need a lot of support in providing consistency and stability within the family.

- A child arrives at playgroup with deep bite marks on her legs and arms. The mother says "a big boy in the street did it." Later in the morning, while having a cup of tea with the playgroup leader, the mother confesses it was she who made the marks on the child: "You ring me each time you feel like that and I will help you," replies the leader. This arrangement, along with help from a social worker, helps that mother to control her feelings, and child battering is thus prevented.

- About nine months ago a three-year-old who had recently been diagnosed as a hemophiliac, was admitted to one of our Belfast playgroups. Because of his condition, both parents were afraid to let the child out of their sight, and he was not allowed outdoors except under supervision. The mother was very possessive, and also extremely indulgent with the child, who was never chastised in any way because of his condition.

The mother had a history of nervous depression, and she was expecting a second child in about eight months. She was very worried that the second child might also be a hemophiliac, and this made her even more apprehensive.

She and the boy came to playgroup in a taxi, and she stayed until the end. When she could not come she sent the father, who was a shift worker. The playgroup staff found the child was not able to share or to play in a group. He smacked staff members and kicked when asked to do something he did not want to do. His mother gave the staff no backup in disciplining the child.

As her pregnancy advanced to the seventh and eighth months the playgroup leader was worried that the child would be taken from the playgroup when his mother found herself no longer able to accompany him. The leader spoke to the father, who agreed that this could happen. The outcome was that the next time the mother attended the antenatal clinic the father sent the boy to the playgroup, unaccompanied, in a playgroup taxi. When his mother arrived home she became hysterical and phoned the playgroup about four times that day seeking reassurance that the child was safe.

Since that day the boy has come to the group alone, not because his mother was convinced, but because the father insisted. She very gradually stopped rushing out to the taxi, and stopped standing watch at the window waiting for the taxi to arrive home. The child is now beginning to play with other children and to accept rules of behavior without a tantrum each time.

The new baby, a little girl, arrived six weeks ago. The mother is now much less tense and accepts the fact that the first child must be allowed to live a full life and to learn to live with his illness.

• Michael arrived at playgroup when he was age two, but he looked like a ten-month-old. He did not walk or talk, he was pale and thin, and had a "little-old-man" face.

His mother was wounded in cross-fire shooting between a soldier and a sniper when Michael was age four months. There were ten children in the family, and the oldest girl age eighteen took on the role of mother, but Michael failed to thrive. The health visitor, who was concerned about Michael's failure to meet the normal milestones, felt that the stimulation of the playgroup might help him.

One day while changing Michael's socks the playgroup leader noticed that his feet were "gathered up," and on closer examination found his toenails had grown into the underflesh of his toes. The health visitor was alerted and the matter was dealt with.

Michael began to walk and talk, and he was toilet trained in the playgroup. He is now five and a place has been reserved for him in a special care school. Michael will cope much better for having had the playgroup experience. His eighteen-year-old sister did her best, but she needed help and support.

ROLE OF PLAYGROUPS

Playgroups are for preschoolchildren under age five, and, besides providing appropriate opportunities for the children to play, they may be providing them with their first experience of the larger society outside the home. It may also be the first "help" experienced by the mother in rearing her child.

People who have worked with difficult or disturbed children realize that play allows for the expression of many difficult and painful feelings, and that through such expression their damaging or restricting effects can be lessened. If observed by an adult with therapeutic skills and knowledge, the children may be helped to express their feelings more fully. Eventually their attitudes towards important people in their environment, such as their parents, may undergo change because they have been helped through play to express their anxieties, fears, and tensions and to gain a measure of control over them. Playgroups are all about attitudes and relationships, experiences and learning, caring and supporting the child and family. They are nonpolitical and nonsectarian. Integration is often experienced and enjoyed, but, sadly, short-lived, due to the pattern of sectarian schooling that exists in Northern Ireland.

We know that children are the sum of their experiences, and it is therefore hoped that the enriching environment presented to both parents and children will spinoff into the family and eventually into the community.

A playgroup leader gave me the following information regarding the children attending her group at that time:

Karen: Being observed at present by National Society for the Prevention of Cruelty to Children (NSPCC) social workers; child always hungry.

Kelly: Social problems; mother recently lost baby boy.

Lisa: Caring family background.

Tommy: Caring family background.

Lydia: Mother works as assistant in the playgroup; good caring family background.

Lisa and Jim: Both children seek constant attention; father in jail.

Thomas: Very upsetting family background; mother leaves home regularly and leaves children with father, who is very unsuitable.

Jackson: Family connected with NSPCC since 1970; mother inflicts cruelty.

Trevor: Mother attending psychiatrist; is expecting baby soon.

Norman: Good stable relationship in family.

Gordon: Mother has split personality; father suffered slight brain damage in accident and has brain storms.

Marilyn: Good relationship with parents.

One might ask who needs the most support in this group: the children? the parents? the playgroup staff?

A playgroup is an environment so structured as to promote the full growth of the young child—physically, socially, intellectually, and emotionally. Because the wholesome growth of the young child depends in large measure upon the understanding and growth of the parents, playgroups are for both child and mother—and father, too, when this is possible.

• A child age three and a half, in conversation with another child in the playgroup: "My mummy sleeps with a hatchet under her pillow and she will kill anybody who tries to get her." The father is in jail and the mother lives in fear of the paramilitary group that wants her to cooperate with them—she has refused financial assistance from them.

• One child to another: "If a policeman came through that door I'd shoot him."

• Four little boys pushing another boy age three on a trolley; when asked what was happening: "He's been shot and we're taking him to the morgue."

• A child painting nothing but crosses: "They are all dead people; they have been shot."

Children with problems can become problem children unless the adults recognize the distress signals and do something about it. This is where the playgroups can offer help to both parents and children. They are a preventive and supportive factor in a situation where violence is experienced daily.

To quote Morris Fraser again: "A great deal was once made of setting a child 'an example.' Now we talk about 'providing behavioral cues,' but the principle is exactly the same. What is more, it has turned out to be just as valid and as important as the Victorians said it was."[2]

Playgroups in Northern Ireland are playing a definite part in the social strategy that affects children.

- "I've learned to enjoy my children in playgroup," say many mothers.
- "My wife is a different person since going to playgroup," say many fathers.
- "Life is better for me since I started playgroup," I am sure would be the comment from many children if they could put their feelings into words.

William Van Der Eyken in *The Pre-School Years* states that playgroups, which began as a minor movement, are now a major social influence.[3] Parents help playgroups; playgroups help parents. This exchange is a great new contribution the playgroup movement makes to the community. Young children have a right to grow up in an environment that favors their development. They have a right to grow up in a social climate in which they can play freely with others. They have a right to live free from violence, from the imposition of the adult world on their own, and they have a right to be respected for what they are—people who happen to be very young.

NOTES

1. Morris Fraser, *Children in Conflict* (New York: Basic Books, 1977).
2. Ibid.
3. William Van Der Eyken, *The Pre-School Years*, 4th ed. (Harmondsworth, England: Penguin, 1977).

CHILDREN UNDER FIRE: ISRAEL

❦

Alfred M. Freedman

For the past six years I have been involved in several projects in the Middle East, including a study of psychological aspects of Arab-Israeli tension, and, more recently, efforts to build bridges by bringing together Egyptian and Israeli psychiatrists. As time has passed I have grown more and more concerned about the psychological consequences of the decades of tension, interrupted by open warfare, on children who are born and raised—and who die—in this ambience. Other questions that come to mind include the possible transmission of hostility from generation to generation, and how these children, upon achieving adulthood, will shape society. Such experiences and resulting issues are, of course, not unique to the Middle East.

Recently I had a visit from a young man who two years ago completed his residency in general psychiatry and child psychiatry at the New York Medical College. His country of origin was Nicaragua, and he was one of the best residents we have had in the past several years. He told me that during the uprising against General Anastasio Somoza-Debayle he had served as general medical officer in a hospital on the Costa Rican border. After the conflict subsided he was sent to the United States to get medical aid, as well as advice on how to deal with the anticipated mental health problems.

With reference to the latter mission he turned to me first. When he asked where I thought the very limited resources of Nicaragua could be directed to alleviate mental health problems, I immediately responded that my first priority would be the plight of the children, particularly those who had been orphaned or whose family lives had been severely disrupted. He received my suggestion warmly and described the great many children who had been orphaned or who were completely out of touch with their families in the midst of the chaos that still prevailed. Even more shocking was the fact that possibly as many as half the Sandinist guerillas were between the ages of eleven and fifteen. He described how jolting it was when one first saw a child on patrol who has killed people with a machine gun. We wondered together what the possible consequences of such early experiences with violence could mean in later years.

The experiences of the children of Nicaragua and of the Middle East could be multiplied by those of many other children in other places and at different times; they are by no means unique in this century.

PAUCITY OF RESEARCH

Since 1914 we have lived through almost continuous tension, cold war, armed conflict, genocide, concentration camps, death camps, terrorism, guerrilla warfare—an endless succession of disasters. Children have been exposed to these catastrophic events directly, as well as indirectly through the tensions and anxieties of the adults around them. Surprisingly enough, however, there is a paucity of well-designed research on children who have been exposed to these horrors.

Apparently, because of the overriding concern about winning wars, no time could be spent in worrying about their effects on children. It was not until World War II, when technological advances made bombing almost a daily occurrence in cities such as London, that any serious studies were undertaken. These included investigations of the behavior of children under the stress of wartime bombing, as well as the effects of evacuation, which often meant separation from parents.[1-5]

Reports of these studies indicated that during shelling or bombing there was little evidence of increased anxiety or panic in children. When anxiety did appear, investigators explained it as being related to anxiety in the adults around the children. Thus D. Burlingham and A. Freud wrote: "Cases in which nervousness, bedwetting and other symptoms . . . persisted after air raids were attributable to the over-anxious reactions of parents."[6] It was therefore concluded that small children can experience physical danger without serious traumatic effects; what does traumatize them is separation from their parents or reactions of fear in their mothers or other adults.

Some reports indicated the negative influences of shelling. For example, M.I. Dunsdon, in a World War II study of 8,000 children in Bristol, observed that those who remained in the city and came under fire showed an eightfold greater incidence of psychological disturbances than children who were evacuated from the city. He also found that, in the first stage of the shelling, symptoms of apathy appeared in the children, and subsequently there were further indications of reactive depression.[7] In Finland, T. Brander reported that children under fire showed signs of activity inhibition, marked startle reactions, and severe terror states at night.[8]

It must be emphasized that all these studies were essentially observational. There were rarely any comparison groups, and little use was made of psychological instruments to examine the influence of wartime stress conditions on children. The bulk of the investigations appear to indicate that, apart from separation from the mother, and panic or anxiety in parents or other close adults, children cope with wartime conditions without too much difficulty. Possibly the changes are more subtle and of a more general behavioral type. The investigators were mainly looking for the resulting manifestions of major psychiatric syndromes.

I am reminded of the remarks of a European colleague who was in secondary school during the time his country was occupied by the Nazis. In the long period I had known him he had rarely spoken of those years, but the last time I saw him—in anticipation of this conference—I asked him more directly and persistently about his wartime experiences. "Oh yes," he said, "it was my first experience with death all around me. When I'd go to school in the morning I got used to seeing a man lying in the gutter who had just been shot, or someone hanging on a busy corner. I got used to it, you know. After that I never felt anything until my first child was born." This statement would not emerge as the result of testing on an anxiety scale.

STUDIES IN ISRAEL

The opportunity to deal scientifically and professionally with the effects on children of war-related stress and tension emerged as a result of the thirty-one years of war or uneasy truce in the Middle East since the founding of the State of Israel in 1948. Virtually all the studies in existence have been done in Israel, possibly because of its abundance of professional workers and research scientists in the behavioral and social sciences and in education. In spite of these resources, however, there was until 1974 a paucity of such research. According to N.A. Milgram, this was a result of the enormous preoccupation with overwhelming day-to-day problems, such as coping with hundreds of thousands of European refugees prior to the war and survivors of the holocaust after the war.[9]

Over 300,000 immigrants arrived in Israel from Europe during the 1930s; after the opening of immigration in 1948 several hundred thousand more European refugees and migrants arrived, many of them survivors of concentration camps. Since the early 1950s over half a million new migrants have poured in from the Arab countries.

The 1957 Sinai campaign and the Six-Day War in 1967 produced very few casualties, and the latter conflict in particular produced a state of euphoria and prosperity. Professionals were so preoccupied with medical problems and rehabilitation, however, they largely ignored psychological issues.

The 1973 Yom Kippur War stimulated great interest in the effects and consequences of war tensions. The initial success of the Egyptian and Syrian armies, the successful surprise attack, and the ambiguous conclusion of the war, as well as the revolution in thinking on the part of the Israelis regarding the realities of life in the Middle East, resulted in a new social awareness of war-related psychological stress and the importance of coping with it effectively. The war also generated concern over how stress was affecting children. The relatively large number of casualties for a small country—2,500 dead and over 10,000 injured—had its impact on children, many of whom lost fathers or siblings. Depression and anxiety—on a personal level, as well as over the survival of their nation—became evident. Illustrative of this state of mind was a decision taken in December 1973, one month after the end of the war, to hold an international conference on psychological stress and adjustment in times of war and peace. This conference, held in 1974, was reconvened three and a half years later.

In 1969–70, during the War of Attrition, and since the conclusion of the 1973 war there have been constant raids and shellings, particularly along the Lebanese border, and these episodes caused concern in regard to their effects on children.

EFFECTS OF BOMBARDMENT

Abner Z. Ziv and his colleagues have carried out several studies on the effects of bombardment on children in Israel. In one study Ziv and R. Israeli compared 103 children from seven kibbutzim subject to frequent shelling with ninety children from seven kibbutzim that never came under fire. The groups were similar in terms of age and sex distribution, and the investigators hypothesized that the manifest anxiety scores of children in shelled kibbutzim would be higher than those of the other children. Anxiety levels were measured by a Hebrew version of the Child's Manifest Anxiety

Scale, and administered at a time when all the border kibbutzim were under almost constant fire. It is of interest that the hypothesis that children in shelled kibbutzim would have higher levels of anxiety was not supported. It was also hypothesized that, as this and other tests indicated that girls usually have higher anxiety levels than boys, the gap between these levels in boys and girls in shelled kibbutzim would be greater than in kibbutzim not subject to shelling. This hypothesis was also not supported by the study.[10] The authors offer as a possible explanation an adaptation level theory that maintains that adapation level is represented by the stimulus to which the individual either does not respond or responds in an indifferent or neutral manner.[11] In the words of D. Mechanic:

> To the extent that an individual acquires the tools capable of dealing with difficult life situations, that which in some circumstances might be a threatening situation can become routine and ordinary.[12]

When shelling first began the children were awakened during the night and had to run to shelters. According to observers this caused confusion and anxiety. Subsequently, when permanent shelters were built with special places to sleep, the situation became more acceptable and less frightening. The shelter became a regular, safe, and familiar place in which to live, and as a consequence it is believed the children's adaptation level to shelling increased. Further, when they remained with a group during this fear-producing situation, anxiety decreased.[13] This fits with S. Schachter's theory of affiliation, since the kibbutzim represent an ideal social framework for constant reinforcement of a need affiliation.[14].

In addition to the mutual support they received in the shelled kibbutzim, the children were given great encouragement and attention, not only from the adults in their immediate environment, but from the general population. Their courage was publicized widely in the mass media, and this became a source of pride to the children, who often announced proudly: "Again they talked about us on the radio."[15] As in all such studies, of course, it might well be that the measuring instruments did not detect the higher anxiety levels of the children who were shelled. It has been suggested that the potentiality for anxiety symptoms may persist for a long time, and only manifest itself when subsequent stress is encountered.

EFFECTS OF STRESS

Observing the apparent resilience of children under conditions that would appear stressful, Ziv, W.W. Kruglanski, and S. Shulman undertook an investigation of the processes mediating the reactions of the children to these circumstances.[16] Some have argued that wartime shelling, as such, is not perceived as stressful by children, possibly because they cannot comprehend the negative consequences. This might be true of young children, but the authors felt it would be less plausible for older children, that is, from grade school on, and set up a study to examine such a group. It is important to note that their study did not address itself to pathological symptoms or to immediate reactions to air raids or other stress.

The research involved 818 children in grades IV through VIII. The stress group, consisting of 521 children, were from two Israeli settlements that had been exposed to frequent shellings from across the border. At the time the study was carried out the settlements in the stress group had had a year and a half of relative calm, but there was no assurance that shelling might not be resumed at any moment. The nonstress group, consisting of 297 children, came from two comparable Israeli settlements that had never been shelled. Otherwise the children had similar socioeconomic and cultural backgrounds, and the length of their parents' residence in the respective settlements was about the same. The test battery for all the children consisted of:

• A general questionnaire inquiring into the children's attitudes toward their locale of residence, their preferred dreams, aggressiveness toward the enemy, and their sociometric choices as to the reasons for these feelings.

• A questionnaire about attitudes toward the war.

• Rosenzweig's Picture-Frustration Test.

In summary, it was found that the shelled children exhibited a greater degree of local patriotism, a greater degree of covert aggression, and a greater appreciation of the personality trait of courage than did the nonshelled controls. There were no differences, however, between the shelled and nonshelled groups with respect to attitudes toward the war, desire for peace, and overt aggression toward the enemy.

The children in the stress group tended to prefer aggressive dreams, and, in particular, dreams involving defeat of the enemy. The authors interpreted these findings in terms of an active process of coping with stress. For example, stress could produce increased group cohesiveness, resulting in their placing a higher value on the locale of residence. In the stress group there were no escape dreams about abandoning the place of residence. The covert aggressiveness evident in the Rosenzweig Test and in the dreams could be interpreted as an endeavor to combat actively the felt threat. The greater desirability of courage as a personal trait might be seen as a successful mastery of the child's fears, and is considered a highly desirable accomplishment under stress.[17]

It is noteworthy that in both groups there was an equal desire for peace and resistance to overt expressions of hostility toward the Arabs, including terrorists. The authors' preferred interpretation was in terms of a coping process activated by the children's exposure to prolonged shelling and affected in its expression by prevailing social norms.[18] An alternative interpretation might be that these results could be a consequence of the mediating influence of parental behavior rather than stress per se. Further, this study did not distinguish between transient situation-bound behavior and more profound effects on the children's personalities.

Another recent study on the effects of war stress on children was made by L. Baider and E. Rosenfeld, stimulated by the pioneering studies of Freud and Burlingham on the behavior of children during the blitz in London and after they were evacuated from the city and separated from their mothers. Their research indicated that the critical issue was separation from parents or reactions of fear on the part of their mothers and other adults around them.[19]

EFFECTS OF PARENTAL FEARS

Baider and Rosenfeld undertook to study the effects of parental fears on children in wartime Israel.[20] They observed that parental fear reactions were especially traumatic for a small child when parents deny the facts of war in order to protect the youngster. In addition, parents often attempted to mask their own unhappiness and anxiety by pretending everything was normal. It was then necessary for the child to find out what was really going on, utilizing her/his own resources, and to determine what her/his own role and place in the traumatic events might be. This study took place in an urban center during the Yom Kippur War in 1973. The situation differed from the study of Ziv, Kruglanski and Shulman, in which there was constant shelling and the sound of war was quite evident.

In the 1973 war fathers left suddenly without any warning; there were two brief air raid alarms; and for the first three weeks there were blackouts at night. Only on television was the civilian population exposed to the sounds and sights of war. But there was another kind of strain—an almost complete absence of news from the two fighting fronts, accompanied by a wave of notifications to families of those who had been killed, wounded, or missing. There was a constant scrutiny of Egyptian and Syrian newspapers in a painful search for photographs of prisoners of war.

Otherwise life went on essentially unchanged—children attended school, mothers worked, if they were working mothers, shops were open, and the crowds in the street were as before. The opportunity for mothers and other adults to shield the children from the reality of war was inviting and seemed effortless. A child's questions were either ignored or diverted. On the other hand, the child sensed the mother's extraordinary tension, preoccupation, inattentiveness, or overindulgence.[21]

The authors illustrated their points with some case histories. One describes a two-and-a-half-year-old boy whose father suddenly put on his uniform and left the house on the afternoon of Yom Kippur. Although he was stationed in a relatively safe area and telephoned home every few days, the child cried constantly, clung to his mother, and wanted to eat incessantly. He slept poorly, cried at night, rejected his toys, and tried to drag his mother to his father's car; his mother responded by pulling him away. When she sought help, the mother said to the therapist: "How can I explain? He doesn't understand."

The therapist, however, told the child directly what his father was doing, where he was, and why he was there. He instructed the mother not only to explain, but, when soldiers were encountered, to point out that the child's father was doing similar work, and, in addition, to arrange for the child to speak to his father on the phone. The child's behavior improved, and some days later when the father came home on leave for a few hours and took the child out for a ride he appeared quite happy and did not cry when the father left. In another instance, while visiting a department store the child noticed a toy gun, pointed to it, and said, "Daddy, daddy," identifying his father through the gun.

Another case describes a four-and-a-half-year-old girl whose father did not go to war. Although her parents watched television news and heeded blackout precautions, they tried to maintain an atmosphere of "everything as usual" and made no mention of the war. The child began to exhibit signs of regression, particularly bedwetting, and showed concern because her father was not in the army. After consultation, the mother was advised to be frank with the child and have the father explain that he worked in an industry essential to the war. The girl's tension and anxiety, as well as the bedwetting ended, but it is noteworthy that she never seemed to recover trust in her mother, and always put questions to her father.[22]

The authors speculate that one reason so many parents were afraid to be frank with their children was their awareness that Israel had been in a state of war for some twenty-five years and that there had been deaths in many of the families. There were feelings of despair and guilt among parents of small children, not only for having allowed the state of war to continue, but for bringing up generation after generation to face war after war. They quoted a popular song that emerged from the Yom Kippur War, which has the following refrain:

> I promise you
> My little daughter
> That this will be
> The last war.

The person who wrote that song, and those who sang it or listened to it, were fully aware that fighting might break out again at any moment. As a result of the guilt the parents felt, they might have been closing off the one avenue that could give them and their children the strength to face reality together.[23]

RISE IN ANXIETY LEVELS

The foregoing studies appear to demonstrate that if social supports are sufficiently strong, and if children are not separated from their parents, there is little increase in anxiety among children subject to war stress. In contrast, other studies offer somewhat different data. R.M. Milgram and N.A. Milgram, for example, also investigated the effects of the Yom Kippur War on anxiety among Israeli children and found that the postwar level was almost double that measured before the war.[24]

In May 1973, some five months before the October war broke out, they administered the Sarason General Anxiety Scale and the Tennessee Self-Concept Scale to a group of eighty-five children—42 boys and 43 girls—in the fifth and sixth grades of two Tel Aviv schools, one upper-middle class and the other lower-middle class. The tests were readministered, along with the war stress questionnaire, in December 1973, two months after the war. At that time, however, the Israeli army was still completely mobilized and a wartime atmosphere prevailed.

The investigators not only found a notable increase in the levels of anxiety, but those children who had the lowest peacetime levels were found to have the highest postwar levels. Thus boys who scored lower in anxiety than girls in peacetime reversed positions and were higher in anxiety in the December testing. Similarly, upper-middle-class children who showed less anxiety than lower-middle-class children in the May testing reported more in December. The investigators concluded that neither the amount of personal involvement in the war nor self-concepts were associated with the rise in anxiety. Although these were urban children, not involved in or subject to the direct effects of war, they were not insulated from its realities. They were aware, for example, that 2,500 men had been killed, and shared the community's general apprehensions.

A possible explanation offered by the investigators was that the children initially highest in trait anxiety, that is, anxiety characterized over time, or how the child usually feels, were certain lower-middle class girls. It is speculated that they found in the objective stress of war a reality focus for disturbed feelings, thereby reducing anxiety in much the same way the development of phobias may relieve intense feelings of previously free-floating anxiety.[25]

The authors also speculated that children who viewed the world as relatively anxiety-provoking, and who were thereby accustomed to high levels of anxieties even in peacetime, reacted with less additional anxiety to war than did children who did not view the world as threatening and who were relatively unaccustomed to feelings of apprehension. This is offered as an explanation of the reversibility of anxiety levels.

On the average, at least one family member of each child was mobilized, but no deaths were reported in this population, although there were a number of injuries. It appeared that the actual impact of the war on a given child was not measured simply by summing up the objective facts of the family's military involvement.[26]

In another investigation Akiba Cohen and Hanna Adone studied children's fear responses to television clips from the Yom Kippur War. They reported greater fear among girls than boys, and greater fear to a clip with authentic background sounds than to the identical clip with an announcer's voice-over.[27]

Yacov Rofe and Isaac Lewn studied youths in a northern development town exposed to shelling and attack with youths in a comparable town in central Israel as controls. Differences were reported on such variables as personality structure, political attitudes, dreaming, and daydreaming.[28]

Of interest in regard to later developments in children is the report of a team of psychologists and obstetricians that the tension of war and physical proximity to possible attack were associated with such physiological changes in pregnant women as increased blood pressure, and disturbances such as premature births, low birth weight, or death of the baby at birth.[29]

I have not been able to find any published material on the responses of children to war tensions in Egypt. In conversations with Egyptian colleagues, however, I was able to gather some anecdotal material. Mohammed Shaalan is collecting tapes of conversations with village children about their attitudes toward war, peace, Israelis, and Jews.* In essence, their experiences are similar to those of children in Israel, and for that matter to experiences reported during World War II. No distinct pathology can be ascribed to the tensions of the war and, since at no time was there

---

* Professor Mohammed Shaalan: personal communication.

any necessity to evacuate Egyptian children and separate them from their parents, no resulting anxiety from this cause was observed. Further, no areas were subjected to constant shelling or bombardment. Yet feelings of great dependence on parental attitudes, as well as on the social norms of the community, were clearly evident. Concern was also expressed about the transmission of hostility. Feelings of having been humiliated and the need for vengeance were also described.

Surveying the literature on children under fire I have the uneasy feeling that one might draw the conclusion that as far as they are concerned war is acceptable, particularly if they can remain with their mothers and if both parents are urged to be open and honest with their children. The literature describes the remarkable resilience of children and their ability to cope, particularly in situations in which the social norms are those of courage, stoicism, and group allegiance. This would indicate that, at best, exposure to bombardment and constant shelling does not produce distinct psychopathology, and, at worst, it contributes toward an increase in anxiety in most children.

My uneasiness stems from two considerations:

SUBTLE EFFECTS OF WAR

First, the effects of war and tension on children may be very subtle, and discernible in social behavior only in later years. Throughout the world we are concerned about the alienation of our youth, and the widespread feelings of hopelessness and powerlessness that may contribute largely to the development of the drug culture and the culture of narcissism—the so-called "me" generation. The future is viewed with despair, which results in the pursuit of immediate gratification.

To what extent are these attitudes the consequence of conditions of tension and anxiety in the environment of these young people? To what extent are hostility, resentment, vengeance, and fear of destruction inculcated in children whose parents have undergone similar experiences, or who were raised in a climate of expectation of disaster?

Second, children should enjoy life while they are growing up. Whatever their ultimate psychological states when they reach adulthood it is outrageous that children should have to live in constant terror of bombardment; sleep in bomb shelters for months at a time; be raised with insufficient food; and be orphaned—that they should be living joyless lives. "A familiar and safe bunker" is still a bunker. Seeing people shattered, hung, or starving may become "routine and ordinary," but can we countenance a civilization in which such cruelty is viewed as "routine and ordinary"?

In the early 1960s, during the period when there was heightened concern about educating the culturally deprived, attempts were made to justify this because such children would get better jobs, contribute more taxes to the national coffers, and be deterred from delinquency. Children should be educated because it is their right, and it is our duty to assure them an education. The goal should be to find the best way to do this and not wait for a study proving that education necessarily results in a better job. With the high rate of unemployment among young minority members in the United States one might conclude that education is not worthwhile. Obviously an absurd idea!

The tension and anxiety generated by wartime stresses in children are incompatible with a decent upbringing. I most strongly urge research on the immediate and long-range effects of chronic tension and war stress on children. Such research should be of two kinds: in-depth, longitudinal studies of individual children or cohorts of children until they reach adulthood; and studies of how children raised in an ambience of stress, tension, and death will, as they grow older, influence our major social institutions, mores, beliefs, and interpersonal practices.

This is not to minimize the necessity for research on the consequences of various other forms of stress and deprivation on children. One should not, however, wait for proof that the later effects are detrimental before resolving in this International Year of the Child to take action to prevent the stresses of cold war and armed conflict. We must contribute to creating a world where all children, not just a few, live in peace and harmony. Can one remain complacent when children in one part of the world can play and frolic in the sun, while others starve; live in bomb shelters; flee, with or without their parents, from the ravages of war only to be turned back at the nation's borders to face death; or are born and live in concentration camps?

In the words of Elizabeth Barrett Browning:

> Do you hear the children weeping,
> Oh my brothers . . . the young children
> Oh my brothers, they are weeping bitterly,
> They are weeping in the playtime of the others.

NOTES

1. A. Freud and D. Burlingham, *Young Children in Wartime* (London: George Allen and Unwin, 1942).

2. R. Solomon, "Emotional Stress under Air Raids," *American Journal of Psychiatry* 7 (1942): 142-49.

3. J.L. Despert, "Preliminary Report on Children's Reactions to the War, Including a Critical Survey of the Literature," (New York: Cornell University Medical College, 1942).

4. T. Brander, "Psychiatric Observations among Finnish Children during the Russo-Finnish War of 1939—40," *Nervous Child* 2 (1943): 313-19.

5. F. Bordman, "Child Psychiatry in Wartime," *British Journal of Educational Psychiatry* 35 (1944): 293-301.

6. Freud and Burlingham, *Children in Wartime* (See note 1).

7. M.I. Dunsdon, "A Psychologist's Contribution to Air Raid Problems," *Mental Health* 2 (1941): 37-41.

8. Brander, "Finnish Children" (See note 4).

9. N.A. Milgram, "Psychological Stress and Adjustment in Times of War and Peace: The Israeli Experience as Presented in Two Conferences," *Israel Journal of Psychiatry* (1979): 327-38.

10. A. Ziv and R. Israeli, "Effects of Bombardment on the Manifest Anxiety Level of Children Living in Kibbutzim," *Journal of Consulting and Clinical Psychology* 40 (1973): 287-91.

11. Ibid.

12. D. Mechanic, *Students and Stress* (Glencoe, Illinois: Free Press of Glencoe, 1962).

13. Ibid.

14. S. Schachter, *The Psychology of Affiliation* (Palo Alto, California: Stanford University Press, 1959).

15. Ziv and Israeli, "Children in Kibbutzim" (See note 10).

16. A. Ziv, W.W. Kruglanski, and S. Shulman, "Children's Psychological Reaction to Wartime Stress," *Journal of Personality and Social Psychology* 30 (1974): 24-30.

17. Ibid.

18. Ibid.

19. Freud and Burlingham, *Children in Wartime* (See note 1).

20. L. Baider and E. Rosenfeld, "Effects of Parental Fears on Children in Wartime," *Social Casework* 55, no. 8 (October 1974): 497-503.

21. Ibid.

22. Ibid.

23. Ibid.

24. R.M. Milgram and N.A. Milgram, "The Effect of the Yom Kippur War on Anxiety Level in Israeli Children," *Journal of Psychology* 94 (1976): 107-13.

25. Ibid.

26. Ibid.

27. A. Cohen and H. Adone, quoted in Milgram, "Israeli Experience" (See note 9).

28. Y. Rofe and I. Lewn, quoted in Milgram, "Israeli Experience" (See note 9).

29. Milgram, "Israeli Experience" (See note 9).

IMMIGRANT CHILDREN: A MINORITY AT RISK

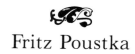

Fritz Poustka

My remarks are intended to draw attention to some issues arising from the migratory movement within Europe—especially to the Federal Republic of Germany.

In spite of many statements of good will and the creation of model programs—such as one to ensure better integration of children into the school system—they are often planned and implemented haphazardly. In addition, the lack of research in this field and the dearth of precise demographic data mean that there are few indices to demonstrate the severity of the problem at the present time, not to speak of the future.

Children of migrant workers, whether they are born in the host country or brought there at an early age, have to cope with a variety of problems in adapting to a new social environment, and this is compounded by linguistic difficulties in the process of acquiring an education. The physical and psychic health of these children is sometimes described as unsatisfactory, and they do not always have easy access to agencies, social or medical, that could help them.

It is estimated that some 10 million foreigners, adults and children, are now working and living in Western European countries. Who are these people, and from which countries do they come? As far as is known, most come from distant regions where the sociocultural milieu is very different from that of the host countries; some, however, find the new conditions familiar.

It is this heterogeneity that makes it so difficult to define the issues. For example, West Indians and Asians move to the United Kingdom; Africans from the Mahgreb and other regions to France; Turks to

Germany; Yugoslavians to Austria; Irish to England; Finns to Sweden; and southern Italians to the north of Italy.

Even within one country, the problems immigrant families face depend on a variety of conditions related to the fact that they usually belong to so-called minority groups; have different social and legal statuses in terms of their cultural backgrounds; find it hard to gain access to schools and to the labor market; and have difficulty with the process of assimilation or acculturation. The amount of time they are permitted to stay is very much influenced by these factors, and often depends on the predominating political tendencies of the host country.

The variety of patterns that exist within one country has been described for the Netherlands by A.L. Th. Verdonck. That country has been the recipient of 300,000 people repatriated from former colonies in the East Indies such as Surinam and the Antilles; 32,000 Moluccans; 115,000 from other countries in the European Economic Community (EEC); and 180,000 from Mediterranean countries. When Indonesian children were excluded, in 1976 there were some 100,000 children age zero to fourteen who were not Dutch nationals; 25 percent of these children lived in Amsterdam, the Hague, and Rotterdam. Fifty percent of all foreign children in the Netherlands come from Mediterranean countries.[1]

One of the important aspects of the modern migratory movement is that at first the migrants came to the host country to work for a specific length of time, not to become assimilated into its social structure. The exceptions were entire families who came, for example, from Surinam to the Netherlands before official policy changed or those countries attained independent status. In a better legal position, also, are Italians who go to other EEC countries (Table 1).

The overwhelming proportion of foreign workers who moved during the 1960s and early 1970s were supposed to return home under the rotating principles then in effect. They were employed in industrial plants in the developed regions of Europe where they received training qualifications that enabled them to increase their incomes and send remittances to their families at home. They also of course made up for the shortage of manpower in the countries to which they moved.

According to the *Continuous Reporting System on Migration* of the Office of Economic and Cultural Development (OECD), in 1978 foreigners constituted the following percentages of the populations of the following countries: Germany, 6.3; France, 6.1; Switzerland, 15.2; Sweden, 4.3; Belgium, 7.1, and the Netherlands, 2.1.[2]

For a number of reasons it is now clear that the rotation process has not and will never work. Since 1973, after the recruiting of foreign workers

TABLE 1. ESTIMATED NUMBER OF FOREIGN WORKERS IN WESTERN EUROPEAN COUNTRIES, 1977

From	Migrated To							
	Austria	Belgium	France	Germany	Luxemburg	Netherlands	Sweden	Switzerland
Algeria	—	2,400	331,100	—	—	—	200	—
Austria	—	3,700	—	75,000	—	—	2,400	24,100
Finland	—	—	—	2,900	—	—	103,000	—
Greece	—	9,600	—	162,500	—	1,900	9,200	4,800
Italy	2,100	106,400	199,200	281,200	10,800	10,000	2,800	253,100
Morocco	—	22,200	152,300	15,200	—	29,200	600	—
Portugal	—	3,000	360,700	60,200	12,900	5,200	1,000	4,800
Spain	—	27,300	204,000	100,300	2,200	17,500	1,900	62,700
Tunisia	—	1,900	73,000	—	—	1,100	400	—
Turkey	27,000	17,000	31,200	517,500	—	42,400	4,200	14,900
Yugoslavia	131,000	—	42,400	377,200	600	8,000	25,800	25,400
Other	28,800	111,900	190,600	296,600	22,600	21,000	73,800	103,000
Total	188,900	305,400	1,584,500	1,888,600	49,100	136,300	225,300	492,800

SOURCE: *Continuing Reporting System on Migration (SOPEMI), 1978 Report* (Paris: Office of Economic and Cultural Development, 1979).

to the north of Germany was halted, the families of workers in that region began to arrive in large numbers. It is now estimated that most of these families will not return home. They will stay in Germany and other host countries, which will have to change their policies toward integration and even assimilation, especially for the second generation.

So, since almost none of the developed European countries have yet officially changed their policies, the present time could be called a period of transition, especially for the children of the migrants.

Again according to the OECD, the numbers of foreign children age zero to fourteen were estimated at 8.3 percent in Germany in 1978—of the 11.6 million German children in that age group, almost 1 million were foreign born; 7.7 percent in France; and 19.8 in Switzerland.[3] It has to be kept in mind, however, that these figures represent great heterogeneity. Some of these children came to be reunited with their families; were the products of different kinds of educational systems; and most speak only their native language. Others began school in the host country, and some were born there. These children are influenced by their present sociocultural backgrounds and by their parents' position in the host country.

To demonstrate this more clearly, I shall concentrate mainly on the situation of foreign children in West Germany at the present time. To better understand the problems I shall first describe the backgrounds of these children.

THE BORDERLINE LIFE OF MIGRANT PARENTS

Of the 4 million foreigners now in West Germany, about 2.85 million were brought from such so-called typical recruitment countries as Turkey, 1.12 million; Yugoslavia, 630,000; Italy, 570,000; Greece, 328,000; and Spain, 201,000. These guest workers live in industrial regions, primarily in urban districts. The state (*land*) of Baden-Württemberg has 827,000 foreigners, about 9 percent of its population. The state with the highest proportion of foreigners is North-Rhine-Westphalia, with 1.228 million, or 7.2 percent of its population. Foreigners constitute 9.5 percent of the population of Berlin—some 182,000.[4]

According to the *Ausländer-zentralregister* in Baden-Württemberg, despite the halt in the recruitment of new workers in 1973 the number of foreigners in that state has not decreased because the families of the workers still come to join them. In Baden-Württemberg 24.1 percent of the foreigners are Turkish; 22.7 percent, Yugoslavian; and 21.9 percent, Italians. Two-hundred and fifty-two thousand of these are children, which means that one-quarter of all foreign children in the Federal Republic of Germany live in Baden-Württemberg.

What are their parents' qualifications? What future hopes do they have? Under what conditions do they live? How long are they willing to stay? These are questions that are receiving serious attention at the present time, but not much research has been undertaken except for that carried out by M. Borris in 1973,[5] and A. Kudat and colleagues in 1974.[6] Extensive investigations by E. Gaugler and coworkers were conducted in Baden-Württemberg in 1979.[7] Studies made in the mid-1970s were summarized in 1978 by R.C. Rist, who described the political policies of Germany as preventing foreign employees and their families from opportunities to advance their situation.[8]

In describing the condition of foreign workers I shall rely mainly on the findings of Gaugler and coworkers in Baden-Württemberg, for their research is the most comprehensive and current.[9]

WHERE DO THE FOREIGN WORKERS COME FROM?

Most of the foreigners do not come from underdeveloped regions of their home countries. While 86 percent of Italians in Baden-Württemberg come from rural southern Italy, about 66 percent of the Spanish, 75 percent of the Yugoslavians, and 96 percent of the Turks come from the most developed regions of their respective countries and did not move from one part to another before going abroad.

This means that despite their low levels of education and vocational qualifications, in comparison with German workers, they represent skilled and well-trained workers in their countries of origin. In Baden-Württemberg, however, 16 percent of the Turks, 14 percent of the Spanish, 11 percent of the Yugoslavians, and 6 percent of the Greeks and Italians have had no schooling. Compulsory education in their respective countries had, however, benefited 79 percent of the Greeks and Yugoslavians; 71 percent of the Turks; 54 percent of the Italians; and 46 percent of the Spanish. Compared to German standards of vocational training, the Yugoslavians have the highest level, 40 percent, followed by 21 percent of Italians, 20 percent of Greeks and Turks, and 18 percent of the Spanish.

The selection procedures of the former recruitment offices run by the German Federal Employment Service (*Bundesanstalt für Arbeit*) until 1973 were responsible for these relatively high qualifications. Selection was not made by local officials.

According to a 1975 OECD report cited by Rist,[10] 55 percent of all skilled Yugoslavian workers, for example, were employed in other countries during that year. This has had a serious effect on the economic development of their homelands, and has been harmful in terms of the investment made to train the workers who subsequently left for employment elsewhere.

H.-J. Hoffman-Nowotny has coined the term *Unterschichtung*, which means that, despite their superior qualifications, foreign workers create a social stratum at the lowest level of society, thus causing new problems by not participating in the general development of the host country.[11]

About 49 percent of foreign workers and their families typically live in inferior city housing, compared to 5 percent of Germans, and they usually have to pay higher rents; this is also true when they are not concentrated in urban areas. Some 30 percent of the Turks and between 15 and 17 percent of other foreigners live in what might be called ghettoes.[12]

This means the beginning of the well-known invasion-succession cycle, as only a small number of economically deprived Germans live in such circumstances. Housing conditions are deteriorating; foreign stores and agencies, travel agencies, for example, are being opened; and kindergartens and schools are under pressure to cope with the high concentration of foreign children. So the segregation of foreigners in ghettoes may be anticipated in many German towns and cities.

Furthermore the foreigners are inhibited in their contacts with Germans. They lack fluency in the language, and they do not have the opportunity to obtain additional vocational training that would make vertical mobility possible. Lack of knowledge of the language also causes a lack of communication with Germans in the industrial plants, and this condition is not improving as the foreign workers extend their stay: a great many plan to remain fifteen years or more, and 54 percent have their families with them.

The situation of these parents has a great deal of influence on the minds and aspirations of their children. C. Wilpert's investigation of children in grades V to VIII in West Berlin schools indicated that the offspring of foreign parents had a higher level of aspiration in terms of schoolwork and vocational training than a group of German controls. Although Turkish girls, for example, did not have as high a level of aspiration as Turkish boys, their level was still higher than those in the German female control group. This seems to be a particularly unrealistic attitude because they will not be given the same opportunities as their German peers. In Wilpert's interviews, the second generation of children of foreign guest workers did not believe they had the same opportunities as German children; the most doubtful were the Turkish children, especially those who had lived more than five years in Germany and who had been educated in segregated classrooms.[13]

GUEST WORKERS' CHILDREN IN SCHOOL

In a study conducted in 1975 by V. Boos-Nünning and M. Hohmann of German teachers of the children of guest workers, they pointed out three factors:

• The uneven level of education of foreign children, which causes a great many to fail.

• Behavioral problems caused because the children do not understand the content of what they are being taught, and thus lose interest.

• The marginal social position of the children in school and in society.

The most serious problem was that even in higher grades the children had difficulties with the German language. Boos-Nünning and Hohmann concluded that there is a special methodological challenge in reaching these children, but that the teachers were not prepared to accept it. Even though the teachers revealed no racist feelings or prejudices, they felt uncertain because they had difficulty in understanding the children based on cultural and linguistic factors. The children's socioeconomic backgrounds, which might also have had a strong influence, was not considered by the teachers. As a consequence they did not feel the necessity to take postgraduate training in order to be in a better position to solve the problems of the students.[14]

Research was not initiated in this field until H.R. Koch began his work in 1970,[15] and there are still no data available to indicate the level of knowledge of the German language of foreign children entering German schools, even though this is described as one of the most serious obstacles to learning.

The number of foreign students in German schools is increasing, however. In the 1978−79 school year, excluding vocational schools, 486,300 foreign children were enrolled, 51,800 more than the previous year, and a fourteen-fold increase over the 1965−66 school year. Over 80 percent of these children are from countries in southern Europe (Table 2).[16]

The proportion of foreigners in relation to the total enrollment of students in elementary, special, and high schools is shown in Table 3. In Baden-Württemberg, for example, in 1978−79 the proportion in schools for subnormal children was 12.3 percent. According to demographic data on the child population of Germany, foreigners are overrepresented by approximately 50 percent in such special schools.[17]

TABLE 2. FOREIGN STUDENTS IN SCHOOLS IN THE
FEDERAL REPUBLIC OF GERMANY
(PERCENTAGES)

From	1974−75	1975−76	School Year 1976−77	1977−78	1978−79
Greece	14.2	13.1	12.2	11.1	10.3
Italy	18.2	17.0	16.3	15.6	14.5
Portugal	2.7	3.1	3.4	3.5	3.4
Spain	8.0	7.4	6.7	6.0	5.3
Turkey	29.2	32.4	34.4	37.3	41.3
Yugoslavia	9.2	9.2	9.5	10.0	10.2
Total	81.5	82.2	82.5	83.5	85.0

SOURCE: Secretariat of the Standing Conference of the Ministry of Public Worship
and Education of the States of the Federal Republic of Germany, 1979.

TABLE 3. FOREIGN STUDENTS IN VARIOUS TYPES OF SCHOOLS
IN THE FEDERAL REPUBLIC OF GERMANY
(PERCENTAGES)

Type of School	1970−71	1976−77	1977−78	1978−79
Elementary (Grund- und Hauptschulen)	2.2	5.6	6.2	7.4
For subnormals (Sonderschulen)	1.2	3.7	4.5	5.4
Advanced training (Gymnasien)	0.9	1.5	1.5	1.6
Advanced training (Realschulen)	0.6	1.3	1.3	1.5

SOURCE: Secretariat of the Standing Conference of the Ministry of Public Worship
and Education of the States of the Federal Republic of Germany, 1979.

The high rate of underachievers among foreign students has led to controversial discussions about sociocultural influences, the impact of lack of fluency in the German language, and testing procedures for selecting pupils for special schools.[18,19] But, again, few reliable statistics are available and theoretical estimates cannot substitute for lack of empirical data.

Given the statistical data available, however, one has to be skeptical about, for example, the number of foreign students who complete their studies, even at the lowest level of secondary school (*Hauptschulen*). In the school year 1975—76 only 25.7 percent of foreign students completed secondary school. School in Germany is compulsory until age eighteen, and adolescents then go on at least to a vocational school. Here the situation is even worse: one out of two foreign students between age fifteen and eighteen cannot find employment as apprentices.

One in five foreign students attends classes in which 20 percent of the students are foreigners. Repeated grades are associated strongly with nationality, so that, for example, there is a strong negative correlation for Yugoslavians and a strong positive one for Turkish children. But if all these data are compared with those for Germans of low socioeconomic status, many more similarities can be shown. So the social distance they experience at school cannot be discussed in terms of language alone.

These statistics, provided by R. Burkard for schools in Baden-Württemberg in 1977,[20] led to discussions in the Parliament of that state. In response, the Ministry of Education stated that it no longer keeps a record of foreign children in grades V through X; 40 percent of foreign students are classified as "other livings," however, and it is assumed that they have returned to their countries of origin. Given the fact that these children are not counted, 80.6 percent of foreign students completed elementary secondary school in 1979.[21]

Several types of schooling have been proposed as best suited to introduce foreign children to the German school system. First, there are the so-called national preparatory classes of one or two years' duration for those who have to learn German; they participate with German students in areas such as music and sports, where language is assumed to be of little importance. Other foreign children attend classes where varying amounts of time are devoted to teaching in German and in the students' mother tongues. There are such schools in Hamburg with a four-year course; in North-Rhine-Westphalia with a six-year course; and in Bavaria, where classes are taught in the children's native language for nine years.[22] The curriculum includes an introduction to the host country's history and geography; sometimes instruction in the religion of the country of origin is provided by foreign teachers who may be employed by the German government or by the consular authorities of their respective countries.

As Rist has pointed out, two extreme models of education may be observed: one based on the rotation principle, which prepares foreign children to return to their countries of origin; the other, "the Berlin approach," is based on the theory of full integration of the children into the German school system.[23] Because of the high percentage of foreign pupils in many schools—in some, there is even a majority—both models lead to further segregation of the children. Finally, because neither busing nor shifting school boundaries provides a solution, the school system at the present time cannot cope with the dimensions of the issue.

The extent of the problem in the German schools cannot be realized unless one looks at it from the point of view of the various foreign school systems. Compulsory schooling in countries of southern Europe vary from five years in Turkey, to six in Greece and in Italy, to eight in Yugoslavia and in Spain. But there are many other differences.[24] Analogies may be seen in the research in the United Kingdom by P. Barnes[25] and by J.S. Dosanjh[26] on child rearing practices and patterns of discipline among immigrant families from the Punjab and the West Indies. They are so different from the practices of English families that they lead to an aversion to current primary school ethos on the part of the migrants and to a tendency to teach children at home. A similar pattern was found among foreign parents in an industrial town in Baden-Württemberg who were asked why their children did not attend kindergarten: less than 50 percent of Italians and Yugoslavians did so, and only 10 percent of Turks, compared to approximately 90 percent of Germans.[27]

Ghetto-like living conditions; a high percentage of foreign students being taught in their mother language part of their day or in segregated classes during normal school hours; foreign teachers out of contact with their German counterparts and partly under the control of their consular officials; high levels of aspiration on the part of both parents and children, thwarted by the great social distance experienced in the school system; no source to help them take advantage of opportunities offered by school authorities to do schoolwork at home; limited interaction with German families; a sometimes very restrictive education, especially for Turkish girls, which inhibits contacts with peer groups and opportunities to learn German—these are only some of the links in the chain of problems that cannot be resolved in the near future. These are the reasons the term "social bomb" was coined. Rist argues that neither "Germanization" nor the principle of rotation, which educates foreign children to return to their own countries—even when they are born in Germany!—can solve the dilemma.[28] It is a plea for the creation of a pluralistic society. This would be quite a new situation in Germany.

It should be kept in mind that in 1966 the *land* of North-Rhine-Westphalia was the first to require compulsory education for foreign children. Official changes to open up access to educational facilities, not guided by the principle of rotation, became the chief concern when new worker recruitment was stopped; but families continued to arrive in Germany to be reunited. Germany has not, however, changed its legal position toward defining itself as an immigrant country.

One has to keep in mind, also, certain features of the historical background of rotation: there has been a migratory movement to Germany since the 1860s and 1880s. German workers from eastern Prussia, together with Polish and Italian workers, came mainly to the industrial regions of the Ruhr. Of the 800,000 foreign workers who arrived before World War I, some 70 percent were from eastern Europe and 16 percent from Italy. By 1910 foreigners constituted about 25 percent of the workers in the industrial areas.

At that time Max Weber, among others, expressed anxiety about the possible dangerous influence Polish workers might have on the German way of life, especially through the school system.[29] Between 1890 and 1900 it was forbidden to teach Polish or to establish Polish private schools. According to M. Heinemann special classes were established for Polish children to teach them German and to imbue them with a spirit of German nationalism.[30] Laws enacted in 1901 excluded foreign children from compulsory education. This was also the case during the period between the two world wars. Education in their own language was available only for a minority of foreign students who attended private schools.

At the end of World War II, 18 million Germans from the eastern part of the former German Reich had to be integrated with the population of the Federal Republic. Since 1961 between 200,000 and 300,000 people have migrated each year from the Democratic Republic.

According to H.D. Walz there were some 72,000 foreign workers in Germany in 1954; after the Berlin Wall was constructed in 1961 the number of foreign workers increased suddenly and explosively.[31]

Some local authorities had taken the first step toward the creation of a pluralistic society and the integration of cultural aspects of Turkish, Greek, Yugoslavian, and Italian societies with those of Germany. Attempts are being made to experiment with making the mother tongues of foreign pupils a second language, but only in certain selected schools. To diminish the social distance between foreign parents and the German school system, this should begin in kindergarten.

FOREIGN CHILDREN AND BILINGUALISM

A. Verdoot has drawn attention to the distinction between

> bilingualism, which is essentially a characterisation of individual linguistic behaviour, and diglossia, which is a characterisation of linguistic organisation at the social-cultural level. Diglossia is, indeed, a widely accepted social consensus as to which language is to be used between which interlocutors when given topics are discussed under given conditions. Diglossia and bilingualism need not necessarily co-vary, as there may be monolingual individuals in a society which is essentially diglossic (ex. Luxemburg), and, vice versa, bilingual individuals in an essentially monoglossaic society (ex. France).[32]

Some distinctions can be made concerning migrant workers and their children. Diglossia without bilingualism occurs, for example, when the migrants lack opportunities to acquire the language of the host country because they cluster in homogeneous districts inhabited only by other migrants. When no progress is made in learning the new language, and when the mother tongue is not used constantly, they may become functionally illiterate in both languages. It may be argued that the parents are unable to communicate with their children in either German or their mother tongue because they are so divorced from the customs of daily living; furthermore they are unable to deal with school authorities and other educational establishments that provide postgraduate qualifications for the workers in the plants.

In a recently completed, but not fully analyzed, study by the author and his colleagues in Mannheim, virtually all Turkish and Italian adolescents, age thirteen and fourteen, and their parents reported that their native tongues were used in family conversations, but that the children themselves communicated mainly in German. In another systematic examination of the children's knowledge of German, school reports seem to depend on a more sophisticated and abstract level in every-day conversation.

R.E. van Dervoort's studies of the reading performance of bilingual English-German first-graders support the view that intensive remedial language instruction for balanced bilinguals is counterindicated; the best method of teaching a second language to children age five and six is for them to have intensive contact with their peers, from whom they learn colloquial German, including the identical grammatical mistakes that teachers have to deal with when the youngsters begin to go to school.[33]

THE HEALTH OF GUEST WORKERS' CHILDREN

Some data are now available on the incidence rates of mortality and morbidity among the children of guest workers in a few German cities. According to E. Schmidt, the mortality rate of infants born to foreign mothers under age twenty is lower than the rate of those born to German mothers of the same age.[34] The reason perhaps concerns the problem of unmarried mothers: 35 percent of German mothers age fifteen to nineteen are not married, compared to 11 percent of foreign mothers in that age group. The mortality rate for infants born to unmarried mothers is 17 percent higher than for those born to married mothers. The perinatal mortality rate of babies born to foreign mothers is slightly higher than that of German babies. Casualties, skull fractures, bronchitis, influenza, and diarrhea occur at a significantly higher rate among foreign children.

In an investigation of a representative group of children in Düsseldorf, J. Collatz and coworkers found that 70.9 percent of Germans attend preventive medical centers for children; the rate for Turks is 52.2 percent and that for people from Mediterranean countries 46.9 percent. Among the Turkish population, 31 percent do not bring their infants to the center for check-ups after their birth in a hospital. This does not mean that these children are healthier than German children, but that, again, the barrier of communication intervenes.[35] Arrangements should be made for medical or social workers to visit the homes of these families.

In terms of the socioeconomic status of foreign workers and German workers, Collatz and colleagues have shown that the children of foreigners are taken to preventive medical centers significantly less frequently than the matched German population.[36] So socioeconomic status alone is not responsible. Factors that do have a strong influence are: living conditions, for example, a high density of people per dwelling; high rate of working mothers among foreigners: full-time jobs are held by 35 percent of Mediterranean mothers and 18 percent of Turkish mothers, compared to 9 percent of German mothers; lack of neighborhood services; lack of education; a higher proportion of households with more than three children; a widespread aversion to visiting doctors under any condition; and a lack of information, or misinformation, about how to apply for insurance benefits. Moreover, E. Majewski and coworkers contend that diagnostic and therapeutic rehabilitation procedures do not reach foreign children to the same extent that they do German children.[37] Some of these factors are equally applicable to other European countries such as Denmark.[38]

Psychiatric Problems

Although psychiatric problems associated with the migration of families is of great concern in many countries, little is known about the mental health problems of children of guest workers in developed European countries. In his review of the literature in 1975, W. Böker came to a similar conclusion about psychiatric disorders among adult guest workers.[39] H.B.M. Murphy contended in 1974 that the mental health of immigrants is usually poorer than that of nonimmigrants, even allowing for such factors as age and level of education; he draws attention, particularly, to the much more frequent and important minor mental disorders.[40] In 1977, however, Murphy stated that this is not always true, and that hypotheses about social selection and social causation have lost much of their significance.[41]

R. Cochrane in 1979 presented data on Asian and West Indian children, and came to the conclusion that Asian children show lower rates of behavioral deviance and have lower rates of admission to mental institutions than do British children; the children of West Indian immigrants exhibit no differences, but do have higher rates of mental hospital admissions. The pattern for adults, incidentally, is similar to that of children.[42]

A.M. Kallarackal and M. Herbert describe the well-being of Indian immigrant children in a study made in Leicester. Compared to a control group of English youngsters they showed a five-fold rate of maladjustment on parents' questionnaires compared to a two-and-one-half-fold higher score on teacher rating scales.[43]

A representative patient population was analyzed recently by H. Häfner, who could find no indication of a higher frequency of psychiatric disorders among immigrant workers age fourteen and over when the unusual age and sex composition of this group was controlled. He concludes there is a lack of evidence to suggest that migrant workers display an above-average susceptibility to emotional crises.[44] Other investigations carried out in Germany express doubt as to whether behavioral deviance or psychiatric disorder among younger children of foreign workers really show similar patterns.

In 1975, in a study of admissions to child psychiatric hospitals in the previous thirteen years, K.J. Ehrhardt and M.M. Schmidt also found a low incidence rate: foreign children were underrepresented twenty- to fortyfold.[45] A field survey based on questionnaires carried out by A. Röhrig and colleagues in Mannheim indicated that emotional disorder, but not antisocial behavior, was significantly higher than in the German control group.[46]

Other investigations, such as those of A. Izquierdo[47] and H.-P. Schmidtke,[48] are of questionable value because of methodological limitations. No estimation of the prevalence of psychiatric disorder in Germany has been obtained from epidemiological studies of a general population using interview methods—nothing comparable to the studies of M. Rutter and colleagues in London in 1974.[49] In interviews with parents they found no difference in the rate of psychiatric disorder among West Indian and nonimmigrant children, nor did the immigrant children display different behavior at school than nonimmigrants.

CONCLUSIONS

It seems clear that comparisons of various countries are of limited value because of the heterogeneity of the respective social, legal, and political conditions of the host countries and the immigrant populations.

It has been clearly demonstrated that immigrant children will continue to be at risk in terms of education, health care, and such societal aspects as acculturation and assimilation. There is no evidence at the present time that mental health or antisocial behavior are more evident among immigrant children than among the indigenous population, although very little research has been done in this area to date. But many potential threats can be foreseen, such as high unemployment rates among foreign youth.

The second generation of immigrants also is at risk in the future— their number is increasing: some industrial towns such as Mannheim have a 12 percent population of immigrants, but the annual birth rate of immigrant children is about 35 percent; one in three children under age six is a "foreigner." The economic future of worker-immigrants tends to be negative because of the great numbers of children born to the soon-to-be-retired workers. E. Gehmacher has analyzed costs and profits of guest workers in Vienna, taking into account integration versus the principle of rotation.[50] But this kind of analysis should not predominate at the present time or in the future.

Y. Charliet has reviewed the problems of children who did not migrate with their families, as well as those of children who went back to their home countries.[51]

To conclude with a quotation from Max Frisch:
"We called for manpower and human beings arrived."

NOTES

1. A.L. Th. Verdonck, "Children of Immigrants: Social Position and Implied Risks for Mental Health" (Paper presented at the World Congress on Mental Health, Salzburg, 8-13 July 1979).

2. *Continuous Reporting System on Migration, 1978 Report* (SOPEMI) (Paris: Office of Economic and Cultural Development, 1979).

3. Ibid.

4. *Statistisches Jahrbuch für die Bundesrepublik Deutschland* (Wiesbaden: Statistische Bundesamt, 1978 and 1979).

5. M. Borris, *Ausländische Arbeiter in Einer Großstadt* (Frankfurt am Main: Europäische Verlagsanstalt, 1973).

6. A. Kudat and C. Wilpert, *International Labor Migration: A Description of Preliminary Findings* (Berlin: Wissenschaftszentrum, 1974).

7. E. Gaugler, W. Weber, et al., "Forschungsverbund: Probleme der Ausländerbeschäftigung," Mimeographed (Bonn: Integrierter Endbericht, Bundesministerium für Forschung und Technologie, July 1979).

8. R.C. Rist, *Guest Workers in Germany* (New York: Praeger, 1978).

9. Gaugler, Weber, et al. "Forschungsverbund" (See note 7).

10. Rist, *Guest Workers* (See note 8).

11. H.-J. Hoffmann-Nowotny, *Soziologie des Fremdarbeiterprobleme* (Stuttgart: np, 1973).

12. Gaugler, Weber, et al. "Forschungsverbund" (See note 7).

13. C. Wilpert, *Zukunftsaspirationen und das Adaptive Verhalten der Zweiten Generation Ausländischer Arbeitsmigranten* (Königstein: Athäneum, forthcoming).

14. V. Boos-Nünning and M. Hohmann, "Zur Situation Deutscher Lehrer von Kindern Ausländischer Arbeitnehmer. Ergebnisse einer Qualitätiven Untersuchung," *Bildung und Erziehung* 28, no. 1 (1975): 43-52.

15. H.R. Koch, *Gastarbeiterkinder in Deutschen Schulen* (np: Königswinter, 1970).

16. Der Schulbesuch Ausländischer Schüler in der Bundesrepublik Deutschland, 1965–66–1978–79," Mimeographed (Bonn: Sekretariat der Ständigen Konferenz der Kultusminister der Länder in der Bundesrepublik Deutschland, 10 August 1979).

17. *Lehrerzeitung Baden-Württemberg*, no. 22 (1977): 604.

18. H.-P. Schmidtke, "Ausländerkinder und Sonderschule," *Zeitschrift für Heilpädagogik* 28, no. 3 (1977): 170-75.

19. A. Sander, "Entgegnung zu Schmidtke: Ausländerkinder und Sonderschule," *Zeitschrift für Heilpädagogik* 28, no. 3 (1977): 176-80.

20. R. Burkard, "Mehr Chancen für die Zweite Generation?" *Baden-Württemberg in Wort und Zahl* 25, no. 8 (August 1977): 218-23.

21. "Hauptschulabschluß Ausländischer Schüler" *Landtag von Baden-Württemberg* 7/6681 (12 May 1979).

22. H. Reich, "Education of the Children of Migrant Workers in the Federal Republic of Germany: Cooperation between Foreign and German Teachers," in *Educational Culture*, Second Seminar of the Council of European Teachers (np: Council of Europe, 4 November 1979): 12-16.

23. Rist, *Guest Workers* (See note 8).

24. V. Boos-Nünning and M. Hohmann, eds., *Ausländische Kinder, Schule und Gesellschaft im Herkunftsland* (Düsseldorf: Schwann, 1977).

25. P. Barnes, "A Comparative Study of Punjabi and English Child Rearing Practices in the English East Midlands" (Paper presented at the Ninth International Congress of the International Association for Child Psychiatry and Allied Disciplines, Melbourne, Australia, 23 August 1978).

26. J.S. Dosanjh, "Comparative Styles of Child Rearing and Patterns of Discipline in English and Immigrant Families" (Unpublished manuscript, 1979).

27. W. Liprecht. "Ausländer zum Kindergartenbesuch ihrer Kinder" (Stadt Mannheim, Büro für Städtentwicklung, unpublished manuscript, 1979).

28. Rist, *Guest Workers* (See note 8).

29. M. Weber (1895), cited in H.D. Walz, "Jugendliche Gastarbeiter" (Mimeographed thesis, 1978).

30. M. Heinemann, "Die Assimilation Fremdsprachiger Schulkinder durch die Volksschule in Preußen seit 1880," *Bildung und Erziehung* 28 (1975): 53-61.

31. H.D. Walz, "Jugendliche Gastarbeiter" (Mimeographed thesis, 1978).

32. A. Verdoot, "Educational Policies on Languages: The Case of the Children of Migrant Workers, in *Language, Ethnicity and Intergroup Relations*, ed. M. Giles (London: Academic Press, 1977).

33. R.E. van Dervoort, "Bilingualismus und Lesen Lernen: Untersuchungen an Deutsch-Amerikanischen Schülern," *Psychologie, Erzeihen, Unterricht* 27 (1980): 73-80.

34. E. Schmidt, "Morbidität und Mortalität der Kinder Ausländischer Arbeitnehmer in der Bundesrepublik Deutschland," in *Die Kinder Ausländischer Arbeitnehmer,* ed. Th. Hellbrügge (München: Urban und Schwarzenberg, 1980).

35. J. Collatz, M. Hecker, P. Malzahn, et al., "Psychosoziale Momente der Nutzung der Gesetzlichen Früherkennungsuntersuchungen für Säuglinge und Kleinkinder durch Ausländische Eltern," in ibid: 225-47.

36. J. Collatz, J. Natzschka, and D. Schwoon, "Krankheiten, Einweisungshäufigkeit und Krankheitsverläufe bei Ausländischen Kindern im Krankenhaus," *Öffentlich Gesundtheitlich-Wesen* 39 (1977): 746-58.

37. E. Majewski, J. Collatz, and M. Maneke, "Probleme der Versorgung Behinderter und von Behinderung Bedrohter Kinder Ausländischer Arbeitnehmer," in Th. Helbrügge, ed., *Die Kinder Ausländischer Arbeitnehmer* (München: Urban und Schwarzenberg, 1980).

38. S. Kleback, *Immigrant Children—Danish Children: Equal Living Conditions?* (Copenhagen: University of Copenhagen, Institute for Social Medicine, Publication no. 8, 1978).

39. W. Böker, "Psychiatrie der Gastarbeiter," in *Psychiatrie der Gegenwart*, ed. K.P. Kisker, I.-E. Meyer, C. Müller, et al. (Berlin, Heidelberg, New York: Springer-Verlag, 1975).

40. H.B.M. Murphy, "Mental Health: Guidelines for Immigration Policy," *International Migration*, XII, no. 4 (1974): 333-50.

41. ———, "Migration, Culture and Mental Health," *Psychological Medicine* 7 (1977): 677-84.

42. R. Cochrane, "Psychological and Behavioral Disturbance in West Indians, Indians and Pakistanis in Britain: A Comparison of Rates among Children and Adults," *British Journal of Psychiatry* 134 (1979): 201-10.

43. A.M. Kallarackal and M. Herbert, "The Well-Being of Indian Immigrant Children," *New Society* (26 February 1976): 322-24.

44. H. Häfner, *Psychiatrische Morbidität von Gastarbeitern in Mannheim—Epidemiologische Analyse einer Inanspruchnahmepopulation* (np: *Nervenarzt,* forthcoming).

45. K.J. Ehrhardt and M.M. Schmidt, "Psychiatrische Erkrankungen bei 'Gastarbeiter-Kindern.' I. Zur Häufigkeit und Verteilung," in *Therapien in der Kinder und Jugendpsychiatrie, Kongressbericht*, Vol. 2, ed. F. Poustka, W. Spiel, et al. (1975): S. 1251-55.

46. A. Röhrig, W.G. Bayer, V. Gärtner-Harnach, et al., "Psychische Störungen bei Ausländischen Arbeitnehmern in der Bundesrepublik Deutschland," in ibid: S. 1247-50.

47. A. Izquierdo, "Anpassungs-, Persönlichkeits-, und Schulproblematik von Spanischen Arbeitnehmerkindern in der BRD. Eine Vergleichsuntersuchung, Diplomarbeit," Mimeographed (Heidelberg: 1975).

48. H.-P. Schmidtke, *Förderung Verhaltensauffälliger Ausländerkinder* (Düsseldorf: Schwann, 1978).

49. M. Rutter, W. Yule, M. Berger, et al., "Children of West Indian Immigrants. Rates of Behavioural Deviance and Psychiatric Disorder," *Journal of Child Psychology and Psychiatry* 15 (1974): 241-62.

50. E. Gehmacher, "Probleme einer Kosten-Nutzen-Analyse der Gastarbeiterbeschäftigung," *Europäische Rundschau* 3, no. 4 (1975): 91-105.

51. Y. Charliet, ed., *Children of Migrant Workers and Their Home Countries* (Paris: International Children's Centre, 1979).

DISCUSSION

Need for Research

Is there a role for research in the climate that prevails in Belfast and other major cities in Northern Ireland? There is a wealth of material for investigators in Belfast, but Morris Fraser's book, *Children in Conflict*, is the only study that attempts to portray what is happening to the children.[1] Perhaps investigators are afraid to go there; something is keeping them away.

There is a great need for research, but it must be of a special kind; it has to be in much greater depth and much more subtle than it has been up to now—not merely studies of the increase in the levels of anxiety or the presence of psychopathology, but of people's attitudes toward themselves and toward others around them.

Long-Range Effects of Tension

We seem to be returning to a rather Hobbesian view of society: man against man. To what extent has this been produced by generations raised in a state of tension? Very soon all the leaders of social institutions in the United States will be individuals who were children or adolescents during World War II. In what way will the continuing state of tension since then influence the nature of American society?

There have to be studies of another order—studies of the structure of society and how this determines attitudes of groups of individuals; and, beyond that, how people who were children during World War II reacted to the tension, the helplessness, and the fear of nuclear bombardment that threatened to destroy the world. In what way are our global problems at the present time related to that?

What is the legitimate interest of research? Protestants are hating Catholics; Jews and Arabs are violating precepts that almost every religious group would agree a priori are those on which life is based.

Is it necessary to demonstrate that hatred leads to psychopathology, to nervousness, or bed-wetting, in order to say that people should not hate? Do we have to demonstrate that air raid drills make children nervous in order to try to find ways of obliterating war?

Is it necessary to demonstrate that children bloated by starvation will suffer from subsequent brain damage in order to mobilize resources to feed them? These are really issues that mental health professionals and physicians in general have to address.

Pseudospeciation

Erik Eriksen has made the point that one of the greatest ills of mankind is what he calls pseudospeciation, that is, the insistence that some races are less than fully human members of our single species of homo sapiens.

Perhaps what we are dealing with are moral issues, where research is to some extent irrelevant. The essential issue in Northern Ireland or in Israel is to bring about a political solution, so that all people will have to worry about is the same poverty they had before, without, for example, the added Catholic-Protestant hatred and killings.

There is a need for research on adaptive mechanisms people undergo during times of stress. A greater understanding of these mechanisms is of considerable importance.

We live in a world that ascribes tremendous importance and status to scientific activity. In Britain the attention of the public has been drawn to mental handicap, for example, because scientists have been taking a serious interest in this disorder. The work done in showing that community methods of dealing with the handicapped are superior to hospital care, in terms of language development and other factors, is not very convincing, but the publicity the mentally handicapped has received is different from that given by the mass media; it has been a very important factor in convincing the government to act on this issue.

Moral Development of Children

The notion that moral development is of no concern to scientists is questionable. The field of moral development in children is one to which psychiatrists and others have given too little attention.

One of the areas very pertinent to the point about living in regions where human life is regarded as unimportant is that of the effect of such a vicious and cruel ambience on the moral development of children. If a twelve-year-old is an active guerilla, is killing a disturbing or a banal act to that child? This is another important area for research.

VI. ADOLESCENT DEVELOPMENT: EPIDEMIOLOGY OF DRUG USE AND ABUSE

EPIDEMIOLOGY OF ADOLESCENT DRUG USE AND ABUSE*

Lee N. Robins

The epidemiology of adolescent drug use and abuse can tell us how prevalent drug use is at a particular time in a particular place, and how that prevalence changes over time. It can provide information about the distribution of drug use in the population, which may give us clues as to etiology. It can also tell us what the natural history of drug abuse is, including at what age it usually begins; how long it typically lasts; what the most common symptoms are; and how many abusers come for treatment. The natural history one obtains in surveys presents a very different picture from that obtained from treated cases. Users in the general population tend to be younger and the disorder tends to be milder.

In the last few years a vast amount of work has been done in surveying the use of illicit drugs among American children. Most of this work has been funded by the National Institute on Drug Abuse. Although we now probably know more about children's drug use than we do about any other type of adolescent psychopathology, it is still not clear to what extent illicit drug use *is* psychopathology. This paper will review what we now know about the frequency with which various types of drugs are used by young people, and then raise the question of the extent to which drug use appears to be pathological, either in terms of its predictors or its consequences.

In describing the distribution of drug abuse, I will rely particularly on the recently published data obtained in 1978 by Lloyd Johnston and colleagues from a nationwide cohort of high school seniors,[1] the fourth such cohort they have studied. This study not only gives the overall prevalence

* Supported in part by USPHS Grants DA 00013, DA 00259, MH 31302, MH 18864, and DA 4RG008.

rate of drug use, but its distribution by geographic region, city size, and sex of the user. It also provides information about the natural history of drug use, including the typical age of first use, and how many of those who have ever used drugs continue that use to the present time. Because the study has covered four cohorts, we can learn from it how drug use by young people has changed over time.

While the study is unique in having data for four years for a large national sample, its drawback is that it covers only that portion of young people in school through grade XII. The degree to which omitting high school dropouts affects the results can be estimated by comparing Johnston's data with those obtained by John A. O'Donnell and coworkers from a national sample of young men,[2] as well as results of our own studies of adolescent drug use among young blacks[3] and Vietnam veterans.[4] In addition to our work, follow-up studies done by Denise Kandel in a sample of New York State high schools,[5] by Richard and Shirley L. Jessor of Colorado high school and college students,[6] and by Gene M. Smith of Boston elementary and high school students[7] provide information about users prior to their taking drugs, and thus may give us clues as to the causes of drug abuse.

Studies of high school and college students tell us more about the use of drugs than about their abuse; the number of abusers found in samples of young people is usually too small to allow statistical analysis. Further, the development of the problems usually requires time. Since the onset of illicit drug use usually occurs toward the end of adolescence, drug use problems are more common among young adults than among adolescents. If we stretch our definition of adolescence to age nineteen to twenty, we can take advantage of our study of veterans—who had extraordinary exposure to marijuana, opium, and heroin while in Vietnam—to learn something about predictors of addiction in a high-risk setting.

AGE AT FIRST USE

The purchase of even legal drugs by children is generally forbidden in the United States. While the age of legal purchase is determined at the local level, and therefore differs from one region to another, the purchase of cigarettes is usually not legal before age sixteen, and that of alcohol not before eighteen or twenty-one. The first *use* of legal drugs, however, almost always occurs before the age at which they can be purchased; and the use of illicit drugs is almost always preceded by the use of legal drugs. It is also true that although the public is much more concerned about the use of illicit than legal drugs, alcohol, a legal drug, causes adolescents greater difficulty. (Of course the same is true of adults.)

Table 1 shows the growing proportion of students who have ever used licit or illicit drugs as they progress through school. The cumulative percentages underlined indicate the median age of first use by students who will ever use drugs before completing high school. Half of those who will use alcohol or cigarettes will have done so before finishing grade IX, that is, before age fifteen. Only one category of illicit drugs is used as early as the legal drugs—the inhalants (glue and gasoline); on the average, others are first used a year later, at about age fifteen. The only drug typically first used later than fifteen is cocaine, probably because it is expensive and therefore may not be affordable by younger children, and because its popularity is recent. New drugs are usually tried first by more experienced users who are familiar with most previously available drugs and who have experimented widely.

POPULARITY OF DIFFERENT DRUGS

The bottom line of Table 1 indicates the drugs most popular among adolescents, regardless of when they were first used. Alcohol is by far the most common, having been used by 93 percent of adolescents before they finish high school. Marijuana is the most frequently used of the illicit drugs; it is now being used by 59 percent of high school seniors. Next is the other legal drug, cigarettes, used daily by almost one-third of students before graduation.

This pattern of popularity of various drugs is not unique to high school seniors. Table 2 compares Johnston's figures for male high school seniors[8] with O'Donnell's results from a national survey of men age twenty to thirty selected from draft registration records regardless of level of education.[9] The first year of Johnston's study, 1975, is cited in the comparison because that was the year O'Donnell's data were collected. The rank order of drugs by popularity of use is remarkably similar in the two samples, although rates of *illicit* drug use are somewhat lower in the O'Donnell study, probably because the older men in the latter sample were less exposed to the drug epidemic that began in the late 1960s. O'Donnell's study—as does our survey of Vietnam veterans and nonveteran controls[10]—finds that the age of risk of using drugs for the first time usually ends at about twenty-five.

In Kandel's survey of high school students she found that the popularity of drugs reflected the order in which they were taken, with the more frequently used being adopted before the less frequently used; thus drug

TABLE 1. 1978 HIGH SCHOOL SENIORS: CUMULATIVE EXPERIENCE WITH DRUGS BY AGE AND GRADE

Grade	Age	Alcohol	Cigarettes (Daily)	Inhalants	Marijuana	Stimulants	Sedatives	Opiates
				Cumulative Percentages of Ever Used				
By Grade VI	11	9	4	2	2	<.5	<.5	<.5
By Grade VIII	13	32	13	5	14	2	2	1
By Grade IX	14	56	20	8	28	7	6	3
By Grade X	15	74	26	9	43	13	10	6
By Grade XI	16	87	30	11	54	19	14	8
By Grade XII	17	93	32	12	59	23	16	10

NOTE: The cumulative percentages *underlined* indicate the median age of first use by students who will ever use drugs before completing high school. Half of those who will use alcohol or cigarettes will have done so before finishing grade IX, that is, before age fifteen.

SOURCE: L. Johnston, J.G. Bachman, and P.M. O'Malley, *Drugs and the Class of '78: Behaviors, Attitudes and Recent National Trends* (Rockville, Maryland: National Institute on Drug Abuse, 1979).

TABLE 2. ANNUAL PREVALENCE OF DRUG USE AMONG MALES

	Johnston's Male High School Seniors[1] 1975 (N = 9,400) (Percent)	O'Donnell's National Sample of Men Age 20–30[2] 1974–75 (N = 2,510) (Percent)
Alcohol	87	92
Marijuana	45	38
Hallucinogens	14	7
Stimulants	16	12
Sedatives	13	9
Cocaine	7	7
Heroin	1	2
Opiates other than heroin	6	10

SOURCES: 1) L. Johnston, J.G. Bachman, and P.M. O'Malley, *Drugs and the Class of '78: Behaviors, Attitudes and Recent National Trends* (Rockville, Maryland: National Institute on Drug Abuse, 1979). 2) J.A. O'Donnell, H.L. Voss, R.R. Clayton, et al., *Young Men and Drugs—A Nationwide Survey,* NIDA Research Monograph 5 (Rockville, Maryland: National Institute on Drug Abuse, 1976).

use approximated a Gutman scale. The first was almost always cigarettes, beer, or wine: some who used these then went on to hard liquor; some who turned to hard liquor then went on to marijuana; and some who used marijuana next tried stimulants, sedatives, or tranquilizers. Finally, some in that group went on to opiates.[11]

One of the current debates about the degree to which marijuana use is dangerous grows out of this observation of successive stages of drug use: since almost all users of hard drugs have already used marijuana, the question is whether marijuana causes drug addiction. Those who say "yes" point out that little addiction to hard drugs occurs without prior marijuana use; those who say "no" point out that less than half of all marijuana users subsequently try other illicit drugs.

The first group calls marijuana a "stepping stone" to addiction. If this is so, then cigarettes and alcohol should certainly be the "stepping stones" to marijuana use, and so indirectly to the use of hard drugs. But the "stepping stone" metaphor is inappropriate: while few young people start other drugs without first trying marijuana, they do not move on to another drug as one goes from one stepping stone to the next; the pattern is one of accretion, not succession. With the exception of inhalants, the drugs of initiation are not abandoned when new drugs are tried; new drugs simply constitute an enlargement of the repertoire. The drugs tried later actually *preserve* the use of the earlier drugs. In our interviews with young black men in their thirties, only those still using marijuana had moved on to hard drugs; those who had used only marijuana had given it up in their twenties.[12]

MOTIVATIONS FOR USE

One may wonder what persuades young people to try drugs, and whether motivations vary for different types of drugs. O'Donnell found the principal motivation for use of *all* types of drugs was pleasure—achieving a "high." But pleasure is by no means the only purpose for which drugs are used illicitly. Stimulants are used to achieve alertness by youths worried about studying for examination or staying awake during long automobile drives; sedatives, alcohol, marijuana, and narcotics are all used as aids to fall asleep; marijuana, LSD, and cocaine are enjoyed because they heighten ordinary experiences such as listening to music, tasting food, and engaging in sexual activity; alcohol, marijuana, and heroin are regarded as ways to avoid boredom; sedatives and heroin are used by a few people to numb their concern about current problems; and the use of alcohol is sometimes due to social pressure rather than to a desire to enjoy its pharmacological effects.

HEAVY DRUG USE

The results we have presented so far refer to *any* use of a particular category of drugs in the adolescent age group. While the number of users of alcohol and marijuana may seem staggering, we should not infer that most young people use them frequently enough to create problems for themselves. As Figure 1 indicates, at the time of Johnston's survey only cigarettes were currently being used on a daily basis by at least one-fourth of senior high school students; some 11 percent were daily marijuana users, and almost 6 percent were daily drinkers. No other drug was being used on a daily basis by even 1 percent of these young people.

If daily use rates are low and "ever-used" rates are high, then it must be possible for many youths to use drugs occasionally, even hard drugs,

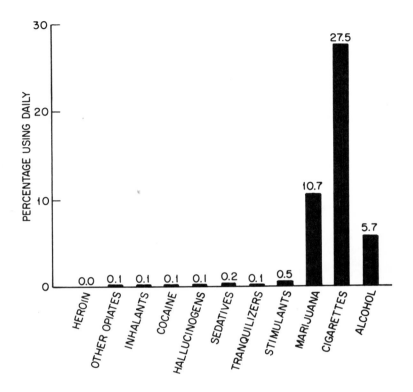

Figure 1. 1978 high school seniors: daily use of drugs in the thirty days preceding the survey. Daily use of all drugs except cigarettes is defined as use on twenty or more days during that thirty-day period. Daily use of cigarettes is defined as smoking half a pack or more a day during the same period.
SOURCE: L. Johnston, J.G. Bachman, and P.M. O'Malley, *Drugs and the Class of '78: Behaviors, Attitudes and Recent National Trends* (Rockville, Maryland: National Institute on Drug Abuse, 1979).

without becoming dependent on them. This inference illustrates one of the most important achievements of epidemiology: it dispels myths common not only among the general population but among scientists. Heroin is reputed to be a very dangerous drug, whose use was thought to lead rapidly to addiction—and addiction to heroin was thought to be well-nigh incurable. If this were actually the case most young people in the Johnston survey who reported they had used heroin should also have reported they were daily users. But heroin use by adolescents was in fact no more likely to be recent or to have progressed to daily use than was the case for any other drug (Table 3). Among high school seniors who had used heroin in the year before the interview, only 38 percent had done so during the previous month, a rate very similar to that found for users of most other drugs. Marijuana, stimulants, and alcohol were all more likely than heroin to be continued if ever used. Further, none of the seniors who had used heroin were now daily users. Thus the dangers of rapid addiction to heroin, or indeed to any hard drug, would seem to be considerably less than had been feared.

One interpretation of Johnston's findings might be that they indicate that daily use of hard drugs is incompatible with high school attendance, that is, no daily heroin users were found because they had dropped out before the survey in grade XII. Luckily we have O'Donnell's study of a general sample of young men, as well as the Vietnam veteran study. O'Donnell also found that only one-third of those who had used heroin in the previous year had used it in the last month, and less than 5 percent had used it in the last day.[13] Similarly, among veterans who had become addicted to heroin in Vietnam, only 27 percent of those who resumed use after their return became addicted during three years of follow up.[14] It is

TABLE 3. RECENT USE OF DRUGS IN THE JOHNSTON 1978 SURVEY

	Percent of Users in 1977−78 with	
Drugs in Order of Number of Users	Any Use in the Previous Month	Use on 20+ Days in the Previous Month
Alcohol	82	6
Marijuana	74	21
Stimulants	51	3
Cocaine	43	1
Sedatives	42	2
Hallucinogens	41	1
Heroin	38	0
Opiates other than heroin	35	2
Tranquilizers	34	1
Inhalants	33	2

SOURCE: L. Johnston, J.G. Bachman, and P.M. O'Malley, *Drugs and the Class of '78: Behaviors, Attitudes and Recent National Trends* (Rockville, Maryland: National Institute on Drug Abuse, 1979).

not clear why heroin has so much less addictive power in humans than one would expect on the basis of experiments in the laboratory, where animals can rapidly become addicted. Our current assumption is that the quality of heroin available on the streets of the United States is so poor and so erratic that few users get a large enough dose consistently enough to develop addiction.

TRENDS IN USAGE

The period of greatest concern over the use of drugs by young Americans was at the end of the 1960s and the beginning of the 1970s; the excitement has quieted down somewhat in the last few years, which might suggest that drug use is tapering off. There is no evidence for a tapering off, however, in Johnston's successive studies of high school seniors.[15] Marijuana use has continued to increase every year since 1975: from 47 percent of high school seniors ever having used it in 1975 to 59 percent in 1978 (Table 4); use of cocaine also increased from 9 percent to 13 percent in those four years. Other drugs did not show a similar increase in popularity; the use of

TABLE 4. HIGH SCHOOL SENIORS:
TRENDS IN LIFETIME PREVALENCE OF DRUG USE

	Percent Ever Used			
		Class of		
Usage	1975 (N = 9,400)	1976 (N = 15,400)	1977 (N = 17,100)	1978 (N = 17,800)
Increasing				
Marijuana	47	53	56	59
Cocaine	9	10	11	13
Stable				
Stimulants	22	23	23	23
Heroin	2	2	2	2
Decreasing				
Sedatives	18	18	17	16
Hallucinogens	16	15	14	14

SOURCE: L. Johnston, J.G. Bachman, and P.M. O'Malley, *Drugs and the Class of '78: Behaviors, Attitudes and Recent National Trends* (Rockville, Maryland: National Institute on Drug Abuse, 1979).

stimulants and heroin remained constant across the four years, and there was some decrease in sedative and hallucinogen use, but hardly a sufficient drop to warrant the claim that the day of LSD is over.

It is puzzling that public concern seems to be subsiding as rates of usage are increasing. The decline in concern would be justified if the rise were attributable to the spread of use to regions of the country not affected in the past, and a decline were discernible in the cities where the epidemic began. Such a pattern would probably indicate that the peak national use figure would soon be reached, to be followed shortly by an overall decline.

Surely use is spreading to new geographic areas. In the early 1960s it was chiefly a phenomenon of large coastal cities: New York probably had the highest rate in the country. The Northeast and large cities still have the highest rates of use by adolescents, but rates are now becoming remarkably uniform in all regions of the country and in cities of all sizes. Unfortunately, the spread to new areas has *not* been accompanied by a reduction in use in areas where the epidemic began. As indicated in Figure 2, while use outside major cities has been growing faster than use inside them, the trend everywhere remains upward. In 1978, 60 percent of high school seniors in large metropolitan areas had tried marijuana, as had 55 percent in smaller cities—the same rate found in large cities four years earlier.[16] Thus some illicit drug experience is clearly becoming the norm rather than the exception in the United States.

CORRELATES AND PREDICTORS OF DRUG USE

Most recent studies have demonstrated that drug use by adolescents is associated with other forms of adolescent deviance such as skipping school, drinking, early sex experience, and delinquent behavior.[17-19] As drug use becomes increasingly common one wonders whether those associations remain valid. We can examine that issue only indirectly in Johnston's study[20] as he does not provide direct evidence about deviance. He does, however, provide information about the sex distribution of users.

Sex Differences

As is true of other forms of deviance, adolescent drug use has been observed more among boys than girls. If deviance plays less of a role in drug use as it becomes more common, one might expect the gap between the sexes to

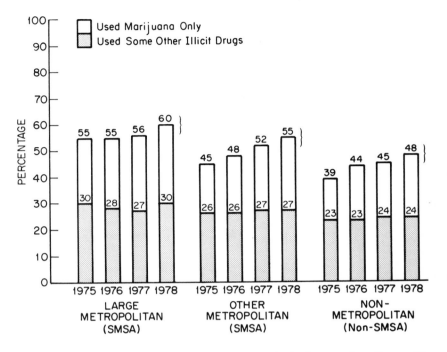

Figure 2. Small towns are catching up with large cities in the use of marijuana. The brackets near the top of the 1978 bars indicate the lower and upper limits of the 95 percent confidence interval. Use of "Some Other Illicit Drugs" includes all use of hallucinogens, cocaine, and heroin, and use of other opiates, stimulants, sedatives, and tranquilizers if not prescribed by a physician.
SOURCE: L. Johnston, J.G. Bachman and P.M. O'Malley, *Drugs and the Class of '78: Behaviors, Attitudes, and Recent National Trends* (Rockville, Maryland: National Institute on Drug Abuse, 1979).

close, but so far there is little or no evidence of this. Boys exceeded girls in the use of alcohol and marijuana by as much in 1978 as in 1975 (Figure 3). Indeed, with respect to the *daily* use of marijuana, the gap according to sex seems to be widening (Figure 4). Among girls the rise in daily use of marijuana parallels the increase in any use during the preceding year, whereas daily use of marijuana among boys seems to be increasing faster than any use. For daily cigarette use, however, rates according to sex seem to be converging; nor are boys greater users of tranquilizers or stimulants than girls.

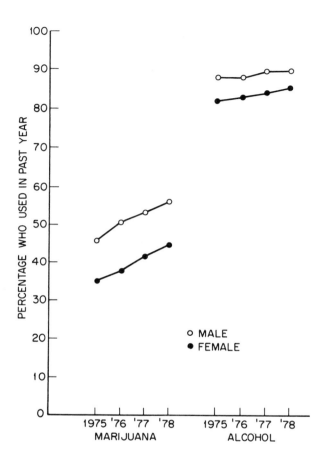

Figure 3. Four cohorts of high school senior boys and girls: use of marijuana and alcohol in the year preceding the survey.
SOURCE: L. Johnston, J.G. Bachman, and P.M. O'Malley, *Drugs and the Class of '78: Behaviors, Attitudes and Recent National Trends* (Rockville, Maryland: National Institute on Drug Abuse, 1979).

    This indirect evidence is thus not very informative. For the two most commonly used drugs, marijuana and alcohol, there is not the convergence of the sexes that one might anticipate, with redefinition of use as nondeviant; the more "deviant" drugs show more convergence.

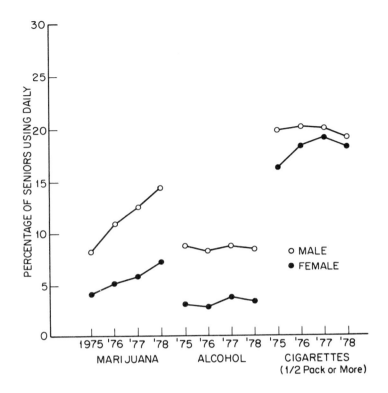

Figure 4. Four cohorts of high school senior boys and girls: daily use of drugs in the thirty days preceding the survey. Daily use of alcohol and marijuana is defined as use on twenty or more days in that thirty-day period. Daily use of cigarettes is defined as smoking half a pack or more a day during that same period.

SOURCE: L. Johnston, J.G. Bachman, and P.M. O'Malley, *Drugs and the Class of '78: Behaviors, Attitudes and Recent National Trends* (Rockville, Maryland: National Institute on Drug Abuse, 1979).

Socioeconomic Status

Another avenue of indirect evidence might be socioeconomic status, as reflected in social class and ethnic group. Serious deviance, as expressed in officially reported delinquency, is found more among the children of the poor, particularly the black urban poor. If drug use is becoming less deviant it should become less associated with these socioeconomic markers. Sure enough, in every American study blacks and Spanish Americans are shown to have high rates of drug use. It has also been the impression that drug users were predominantly of the lower class, but use has certainly spread to the white middle class over the last twenty years. If drug use is becoming less deviant, usage rates among white middle-class Americans should be approaching the rates found among the poor and minorities.

Unfortunately, measures of socioeconomic status are largely absent from large-scale surveys of young people. Johnston, for example, presents trends in prevalence by only one status indicator, college plans—a variable that may in part be affected by drug use as well as a predictor of it. In any event he found no evidence for convergence here: in the last three years rates of marijuana use have been rising for both college-degree-oriented and nondegree-oriented seniors; the difference between them is approximately constant.[21]

Other studies that present more complete socioeconomic data do not provide the necessary information about trends to establish convergence between social classes, but differences in social class are not normally found. In our study of young black men, for example, the family occupational status of young drug users was slightly higher than that of their fellow students.[22] Similarly in our study of Vietnam veterans and matched controls there was no association between low socioeconomic status and the use of illicit drugs.[23] These results may merely indicate that drugs are expensive and that the poorest adolescents cannot afford them.

In short we lack trend data that could tell us whether, as drug use becomes more common, it is losing its association with adolescent deviance.

DRUG USERS COMPARED WITH DELINQUENTS

Johnston's studies report no standards of behavior that could serve as direct measures of official or unofficial delinquency. But many other studies have found that student drug users are more delinquent than other students.[24,25] Further, like delinquents, they are less interested than other students in school achievement and religion, and less close to their parents. They differ from delinquents, however, in their identification with social protest.

Another way in which young drug users differ from delinquents is in their good peer relationships. In the early 1960s it was sometimes hypothesized that adolescent drug users were using the narcotizing effect of drugs to escape from difficult interpersonal relationships. Quite contrary results have since been found in every study of the relationships of drug users and their peers, which are usually positive and normal. Indeed the first drug used is ordinarily a gift from a friend. Without good peer relationships they would not have the opportunity to start drug use. Typical adolescent delinquents, on the other hand, are often unpopular with their contemporaries.

There are also interesting differences between drug users and delinquents in terms of IQ and early school behavior. As indicated in Table 5, drug abuse is not associated with the slightly depressed IQs common among delinquents. The upper part of the table shows the relationship between IQs and adolescent drug use, delinquency, and high school dropout in our study of young black men, who were selected for IQs of 85 and higher as measured in elementary school. At the bottom of the table the same information appears for our sample of Vietnam veterans. Lacking an elementary school IQ test, we had to use results of tests given by the army at the time of induction. It is noteworthy that in both samples drug users tend to have slightly higher IQs than average, although the differences are not great. Among young black men both dropout and delinquency are associated with low IQs; among veterans, dropout is associated with low IQ, but delinquency is not. (Of course it may be that if a young man had both a low IQ and a record of delinquency he would not have been inducted into the service.)

The black adolescents who used drugs also differed from delinquents and dropouts in *not* having had serious school problems in grades I to VIII. In our sample excessive truancy and being held back in elementary school,

TABLE 5. IQs AND THREE FORMS OF ADOLESCENT DEVIANCE:
DRUG USE, DELINQUENCY, AND SCHOOL DROPOUT

IQs	Number	Drugs	Delinquency (Percent)	Dropout
			Young Black Men	
85-89	53	22	51	55
90-99	83	15	32	33
100-109	57	26	38	39
110+	28	31	33	33
			Vietnam Veterans	
<90	136	17	26	43
90-99	103	20	24	37
100-109	97	27	35	20
110+	217	23	32	10

typically beginning in grades I and II, forecast high school dropout and delinquency, but not drug abuse (Table 6).

Once these youngsters reached adolescence, however, it became almost impossible to distinguish the behavior patterns of drug users from those of delinquents and dropouts. All did poorly in high school. Like delinquents and dropouts, drug users were typically "underachievers"—that is, they made poorer grades in high school than their IQ tests showed them to be capable of (Table 7).

The adult outcomes of adolescent drug users are as disturbed as those of dropouts and delinquents, and worse than the outcomes of children with early school problems (Table 8). For young black men the association of drug use in adolescence with later difficulties is replicated in the Vietnam

TABLE 6. DEVIANCE AMONG YOUNG BLACK MEN:
DRUG USE, DELINQUENCY, AND DROPOUT

School Problem	Number	Drugs	Delinquency (Percent)	Dropout
Both held back and truant	53	24	62	69
Held back	56	24	37	28
Truant	26	14	22	34
Neither	88	20	28	30

TABLE 7. UNDERACHIEVEMENT AND ADOLESCENT DEVIANCE
AMONG YOUNG BLACK MEN

	Achievers N = 92	(Percent)	Nonachievers N = 129
Deviance			
Drug abuse	10		30[1]
Dropout	19		54[1]
Delinquency	27		46[2]

NOTES: 1) p < .01.   2) p < .001.

TABLE 8. CHILDHOOD AND ADOLESCENT DEVIANCE AS PREDICTORS OF ADULT DEVIANCE

Proportion with Three or More Adult Deviant Behaviors

Childhood or Adolescent Deviance	Young Black Men				Vietnam Veterans			
	Present[1]		Absent[2]		Present[1]		Absent[2]	
	Number	Percent	Number	Percent	Number	Percent	Number	Percent
Drugs	48	49	175	15[3]	125	47	446	13[3]
Dropout	87	35	133	15[3]	146	42	425	14[3]
Delinquency	85	38	138	13[3]	166	28	405	18[4]
High School Underachievement	131	28	92	15[5]	Not available			
Elementary school Held back and truant	53	33	170	19[5]	Not available			

NOTES: 1) "Present": percent with adult deviant behavior computed for those *with* childhood or adolescent deviance listed in column one. 2) "Absent": percent with adult deviant behavior computed for those with no such deviance. 3) p < .001. 4) p < .01. 5) p < .05.

veteran follow up (right-hand columns of Table 8). Adult outcomes were measured with respect to eight types of problems: crime; unemployment; excessive drinking; heavy drug use; marital disruption; violence; vagrancy; and financial difficulties.

One might expect that the increased risk of adult problems among adolescent drug users required their continuing drug use. Table 9 shows there was an association between veterans' adolescent drug use and later outcomes, even for those who had used no illicit drugs in the two years before our interviews. Rates of recent problems were much lower in men who had discontinued drug use; among men who had not used drugs in the last two years, however, those who had used drugs in adolescence more often currently had at least three of the eight behavior problems—18 percent of cases as compared with 7 percent of those who had not used drugs in adolescence. Similarly, recent drug users had more current adult problems if their use had begun in adolescence that if it had begun later. As indicated in Table 9, the long-term consequences of adolescent drug use parallel the long-term consequences of juvenile delinquency. There seems

TABLE 9. Do the Long-Term Effects of Adolescent Drug Use Require Current Use by Vietnam Veterans?

| | Proportion with Three or More Adult Deviant Behaviors | | | |
| | Little or No Drug Use in Last Two Years | | Used Two or More Drugs[1] in Last Two Years | |
	Number	Percent	Number	Percent
Used drugs in adolescence	28	18[2]	97	55[3]
Did not use drugs	342	7	104	35
	No Arrests in Last Two Years		Arrested in Last Two Years	
Arrested in adolescence	124	18[3]	41	61
Not arrested	320	7	85	55

NOTES: 1) Opiates, amphetamines, barbiturates, or marijuana. 2) $p < .05$. 3) $p < .01$.

to be a continuing impact in adulthood, made worse if the adolescent behavior continues, but present even if the behavior stops.

THE SIGNIFICANCE OF RECENT DRUG TRENDS

The picture we have discovered is a troubling one. Adolescent drug use often occurs among young people whose early school records look promising; who get along well with their peers; have better-than-average IQs; are not economically disadvantaged; and are interested in social issues. Despite these advantages their adolescent and adult pictures look very much like those of typical children with conduct disorders who have slightly low IQs; come from lower status families; have problems in getting along with peers; and have experienced truancy and failure in elementary school.

One must wonder, therefore, if illicit drugs might have lasting consequences when used by immature persons. Our studies of young black men and Vietnam veterans indicated that drug use taken up after age nineteen had little significance.[26,27] Men beginning drug use late usually either did not become dependent, or did so only transiently without later adverse social effects.

We cannot, however, be so sanguine about the use of drugs and alcohol beginning at an early age. This is of special concern because drug use seems to be becoming steadily more pervasive among adolescents, and is reaching down into younger age groups. Of course it may be that the adverse adolescent and adult outcomes we have found are not the effects of drugs themselves, but of some underlying set of predispositions and attitudes not yet measured. Until we have evidence that this *is* the case, however, we can only recommend a cautious approach: that governments and families attempt to limit adolescents' access to drugs, whether licit or illicit.

NOTES

1. L. Johnston, J.G. Bachman, and P.M. O'Malley, *Drugs and the Class of '78: Behaviors, Attitudes and Recent National Trends* (Rockville, Maryland: National Institute on Drug Abuse, 1979).

2. J.A. O'Donnell, H.L. Voss, R.R. Clayton, et al., *Young Men and Drugs—A Nationwide Survey*, NIDA Research Monograph 5 (Rockville, Maryland: National Institute on Drug Abuse, 1976).

3. L.N. Robins and G.E. Murphy, "Drug Use in a Normal Population of Young Negro Men," *American Journal of Public Health* 57 (1967): 1580-96.

4. L.N. Robins, *The Vietnam Drug User Returns*, Special Action Office Monograph, Ser. A, No. 2 (Washington: U.S. Government Printing Office, 1974).

5. D. Kandel, E. Single, and R. Kessler, "The Epidemiology of Drug Use among New York State High School Students: Distribution, Trends and Change in Rates of Use," *American Journal of Public Health* 66 (1976): 43-53.

6. R. Jessor and S.L. Jessor, *Problem Behavior and Psychosocial Development—A Longitudinal Study of Youth* (New York: Academic Press, 1977).

7. G.M. Smith and C.P. Fogg, "Psychological Predictors of Eaɪ., Use, Late Use, and Non-Use of Marijuana among Teenage Students," in *Longitudinal Research on Drug Use: Empirical Findings and Methodological Issues*, ed. D. Kandel (Washington: Hemisphere-Wiley, 1978): 101-13.

8. Johnston, Bachman, and O'Malley, *Class of '78* (See note 1).

9. O'Donnell, Voss, Clayton, et al., *Men and Drugs* (See note 2).

10. L.N. Robins, "Interaction of Setting and Predisposition in Explaining Novel Behavior: Drug Initiations Before, in, and After Vietnam," in *Longitudinal Research on Drug Use; Empirical Findings and Methodological Issues*, ed. D. Kandel (Washington: Hemisphere-Wiley, 1978): 179-96.

11. D. Kandel and R. Faust, "Sequences and Stages in Patterns of Adolescent Drug Use," *Archives of General Psychiatry* 32 (1975): 923-32.

12. Robins and Murphy, "Young Negro Men" (See note 3).

13. O'Donnell, Voss, Clayton, et al., *Men and Drugs* (See note 2).

14. L.N. Robins, J.E. Helzer, E. Hesselbrock, et al., "Vietnam Veterans Three Years After Vietnam: How Our Study Changed Our View of Heroin," in *Problems of Drug Dependence: 1977* and in *Yearbook of Substance Abuse*, ed. L. Brill and C. Winick (New York: Human Sciences Press, forthcoming).

15. Johnston, Bachman, and O'Malley, *Class of '78* (See note 1).

16. Ibid.

17. Jessor and Jessor, *Problem Behavior* (see note 6).

18. L. Robins and E. Wish, "Childhood Deviance as a Developmental Process: A Study of 223 Urban Black Men from Birth to 18," *Social Forces* 56 (1977): 448-73.

19. Kandel, Single, and Kessler, "Epidemiology of Drug Use" (See note 5).

20. Johnston, Bachman, and O'Malley, *Class of '78* (See note 1).

21. Ibid.

22. Robins and Murphy, "Young Negro Men" (See note 3).

23. L.N. Robins, M. Hesselbrock, E. Wish, et al., "Polydrug and Alcohol Use by Veterans and Nonveterans," in *A Multicultural View of Drug Abuse*, ed. D.E. Smith, S.M. Anderson, M. Buxton, et al., (Cambridge, Massachusetts: Schenkman Publishing Co., 1978).

24. Jessor and Jessor, *Problem Behavior* (See note 6).

25. Robins and Wish, "Childhood Deviance" (See note 18).

26. L.N. Robins, H. Darvish, and G. Murphy, "The Long-Term Outcome for Adolescent Drug Users: A Follow-Up Study of 76 Users and 146 Non-Users," in *Psychopathology of Adolescence*, ed. J. Zubin and A. Freedman (New York: Grune & Stratton, 1970): 179-96.

27. L.N. Robins and J.E. Helzer, "Drug Use among Vietnam Veterans—Three Years Later," *Medical World News—Psychiatry* 16, no. 23 (1975): 44-49.

EPIDEMIOLOGY OF DRUG USE AND ABUSE: SOME METHODOLOGICAL ASPECTS

Olivier Jeanneret

INTRODUCTION

As a general rule the application of epidemiological concepts and methods to the study of behavioral phenomena is now accepted.[1]

Striking contrasts can be found, however, in countries on both sides of the Atlantic. Published in France in 1978, the *Report of the Study Commission on Drug Problems*, which was presented to the president of the Republic by Monique Pelletier, is known as the Pelletier report.[2] While the report never explicitly refers to epidemiological methods or data, it does, for example, call for "longitudinal research," "research on control groups," and a better "statistical appreciation of the problem," as one of two objectives for improving knowledge of the phenomena of drug use and abuse.

By contrast, in the introduction to the National Institute on Drug Abuse (NIDA) monograph, Louise G. Richards points out that: "In the government's classification of research projects, epidemiology has been singled out as a prime focus."[3]

Such a contrast is not too surprising to European epidemiologists, who are well acquainted with the difficulties inherent in obtaining accreditation for the discipline in its modern conception. Nor will they be astonished by the contrast between the sophisticated approach outlined in the preceding chapter in this volume by Lee N. Robins,[4] an internationally renowned expert in the field of epidemiological application, and the present report, which is much more schematic and didactic in purpose, by an "epidemiological generalist."

243

In the following pages, I will review from an essentially methodological perspective the various contributions epidemiology can make to applied research. The majority of sources consulted are in the English language literature, for reasons I have just mentioned.

Broadly speaking, what expectations do people have of epidemiology?

• At the national level, planners and decision makers want to know the *numbers* of persons now affected, and trends concerning these numbers in terms of time and space.

• Local authorities want to know more about local *epidemics* and how to identify "contaminators" in order to "eliminate" them.

• Clinicians want to know the medium and long-term effects of *different treatment methods*.

• "Preventionists" want to know the *risk factors* in order, if possible, to predict risk and to identify groups and individuals at high risk.

• Those responsible for health education—a special breed of "preventionists"—ask for more help in *evaluating their actions*, which are sometimes called counterproductive.*

I shall review rapidly the answers to the demands of national and local planners and decision makers, and omit the area of clinical trials.

EVALUATING NUMBERS AND TRENDS

In order to fully grasp their epidemiological dimensions, I shall deal, successively, with the indicators, obstacles, and biases encountered in using them, and, finally, with operational definitions.

Indicators

The 1979 report published by the United Nations, *Drug Abuse: Extent, Patterns and Trends*, contains information submitted by each country.[6] Table 1 shows the information on France, Switzerland, and the Netherlands contained in that report.

The report from *France* puts the number at "about 30,000 . . . who abuse very potent substances;"[7] in reality the total varies from several thousand to about 100,000, depending on the source. Successive or simultaneous use of more than one substance is emphasized. Only the statistics for infractions of the law are correctly reported.

---

* See, in particular, the elegant quasiexperimental study of Richard H. Blum in California schools.[5]

TABLE 1. REPORTS ON DRUG ABUSE RECEIVED BY THE COMMISSION ON
NARCOTIC DRUGS OF THE UNITED NATIONS ECONOMIC AND SOCIAL COUNCIL
FROM THE GOVERNMENTS OF THREE EUROPEAN COUNTRIES UP TO 15 OCTOBER 1978

FRANCE:

The authorities are very concerned about the drug abuse situation, which has
worsened. In 1977 the president of France requested a study of drug problems,
which was carried out by a multidisciplinary team over a six-month period. Its
report estimated that the drug addict population consists of about 30,000 persons
who abuse very potent substances. Most persons taking drugs are multiple drug
abusers who change from one to another or abuse several drugs simultaneously.
Some 4,315 drug abusers and intermediaries were involved in drug offences.

SWITZERLAND

Abuse of heroin is on the increase, some 1,830 persons being recorded. Heroin has
been the cause of death in some instances: 84 persons died from heroin overdose so
far in 1978. The illicit consumption of cannabis is also on the increase—5,641
persons recorded. Abuse of LSD and cocaine has leveled off, to 715 and 292,
respectively. There is also some abuse of amphetamines—318 persons. A sharp
increase in burglaries from pharmacies has been reported—35 in 1978; 181 in
1977—as well as in forged prescriptions. Persons abusing drugs are mostly males in
the 15-25 age group.

NETHERLANDS

It is estimated that approximately 10,000 persons, mostly young, are addicted to
opiates (principally heroin) and amphetamines. Abuse of legally obtained psychotropic substances is more frequently encountered among adults. So far in 1978 some
6,000 persons have been treated for heroin and amphetamine addiction in outpatient
and inpatient centers, which include crisis intervention centers, halfway houses,
therapeutic communities, and special wards in psychiatric hospitals. Many of the
young addicts are unemployed and unskilled; special aid programs are being
developed, in particular, for drug abusers belonging to ethnic minorities.

SOURCE: United Nations Economic and Social Council, *Drug Abuse: Extent, Patterns,
and Trends,* Note by the Secretary-General, Presented to the Commission on
Narcotic Drugs, Doc. E.CN 7/629 (Geneva: United Nations, February 1979).

Switzerland makes note of deaths from overdose, and of some trends concerning infractions of the law to obtain illegal drugs. Two indicators are given: burglaries from pharmacies, and mention of a particularly exposed group defined by sex and age.

The *Netherlands* report underlines the contrast between the addiction to opiates and amphetamines by young people, and the abuse of legal psychotropic substances by adults. A new source of numerical data appears: persons cared for in treatment centers either as in- or outpatients.

It is obvious that these countries are far from even dreaming of providing classical epidemiological indicators such as:

• *The prevalence rate*, defined as the number of cases reported at a given time in relation to the population generally, or to the group exposed at that time.

• *The incidence rate*, defined as the number of new cases reported over a given period of time in relation to the real or estimated population in the middle of that period.*

Only these two indicators permit:

• A description of secular trends for the same population or the same country.

• Geographic comparisons for the same period, for example, from country to country.

• True epidemiological surveillance.

It is therefore of interest to examine closely the principal *obstacles* to obtaining these rates. Only the numerator interests us; consideration of the denominator would take us too far from our main purpose.

Obstacles and Biases

As is often the case in epidemiology, the phenomenon under study can be represented by an iceberg (Figure 1). The tip is represented by deaths due to several causes; death by overdose seems to predominate. Even here, however, the quality of available epidemiological data is not guaranteed: it depends on expert reports by pathologists and toxicologists—and on their reliability.[8]

Below the tip, but still above the usual visibility level of the authorities, are two of the three "nonwatertight compartments"—the two treatment institutions, medical and penal, and, in part, the community. The first two

---

* The reader who is acquainted with modern epidemiology will pass rapidly over these elementary notions. Experience has shown, however, that in France, at least, many clinicians, even among psychiatrists, are not always familiar with them.

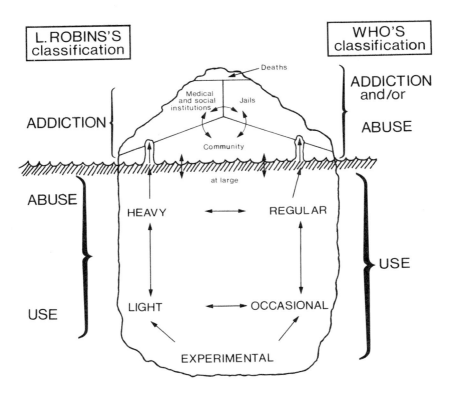

Figure 1. The iceberg of the illegal drug scene. To the left is L.N. Robins's classification and to the right the WHO classification of addiction, abuse, and use. SOURCES: Lee N. Robins, "The Natural History of Drug Abuse," (Paper presented at the Symposium on Treatment Evaluation in Drug Abuse, 19th Scandinavian Psychiatric Congress, Uppsala, 15 June 1979); *Report of the World Health Organization Committee on Drug Dependence*, Technical Report Ser. 407 (Geneva: World Health Organization, 1969): 6.

can provide data on the numbers of persons affected, although at great risk of error.

Among the *biases*, which have been well analyzed in several recent publications, the principal ones are:

• Statistics for persons imprisoned represent only a fraction of those in jail, while the latter are but a fraction of those who have actually committed crimes. Leonard Savitz reminds us it is not easy to identify these factors.[9]

• The same may be said of persons under treatment in outpatient or inpatient medical centers. Errors can be found when the reporting systems of different medical services are compared,[10] thus demonstrating the usefulness of specially designed systems.[11] Moreover, all the factors that tend to modify supply and demand for medical care render the indicator "persons under treatment" somewhat precarious.[12]

• Different medical, social, and judicial institutions run the risk of registering the same cases. Adding together the number of cases in each system, in terms of prevalence or incidence, results in a gross overestimation of the total numbers involved. Hence the utility of a single reporting form and of pooling local and regional systems, as has been done since 1974 in the Canton Vaud in Switzerland.[13]*

Finally, below the visibility level is the vast range of users who only occasionally come to the attention of the authorities, as indicated in Figure 1 by the small arrows in the larger waves. It is they, apparently, who are the subjects of the large number of cross-sectional studies[15] and surveys that have been conducted for many years, namely, primary and secondary school students, as in France,[16] and of more recent and smaller scale longitudinal or prospective studies.[17]

To the extent that cross-sectional studies are concerned primarily with determining the number of users, they are of interest to us here; when they deal with motivation, it is in terms of predictors that they will be of interest later in this paper.

Because of the sequential observation of the variables under study, only longitudinal studies are deemed capable of providing a sense of causal relationship—or, to be more precise, plausible hypotheses concerning this relationship—to the statistical correlations observed between these variables.[18]

It should be noted in passing that it is possible to give a dynamic sense to the submerged part of the iceberg, indicated by the arrows in the figure, while at the same time recognizing that a piece of ice, regardless of its size, does not represent the physical ideal of a dynamic model!

Operational Definitions

It remains now to explore the third methodological field, that of operational definitions, which conditions the quality of statistical evaluation.

To give an example of a major difference of opinion, I will begin by quoting the definitions of *use* and *abuse* employed by different authors.

---

* For the limitations of this type of reporting system for epidemiological purposes, see Irving Rootman.[14]

In Robins's view the important distinction to be made is not between use and abuse but between addiction, on the one hand, and use and abuse taken together, on the other.[19] This view is similar to that expressed by Richards:

> . . . the term "drug abuse" is employed broadly here to include all non-medical drug use, with recognition of the fact that not all use results in adverse consequences.[20]

These adverse consequences are contained in the definition of the National Clearinghouse for Drug Abuse Education in Washington, which, as applied to primary and secondary school and college students, defines abuse as "any use that interferes with . . . physical, mental, social, or academic well-being."[21]

It is possible to recognize here terms from the definition of health found in the constitution of the World Health Organization (WHO); it is the threat to personal health that specifically distinguishes abuse. The 1969 report of the WHO Expert Committee on Drug Dependence defined abuse as "excessive, persistent or sporadic use incompatible with, or without relation to, accepted medical use."[22]

But the most recent WHO expert committee report, nine years later, rallied to the support of the international convention, which defines abuse as "the use of psychotropic substances in a way that would constitute a public health and social problem."[23] As indicated to the right of our iceberg, this definition obliges us to place abuse and addiction at the visible level, and use at the invisible level. Robins's definition, to the left of the iceberg, has an advantage in that it separates abuse and addiction at the threshold of visibility, and places use at a lower level, without any clear demarcation between use and abuse. But this no longer corresponds to the different types of use indicated in the submerged part of the iceberg!

Other operational definitions can be grouped according to the usual questions raised by epidemiologists (Table 2). I will comment briefly on some of the more controversial terms.

- Is the line between *user* and *nonuser* the fact that a person may have been a user at any time, or is a current user? Can the dose limit of marijuana, for example, change with time and with the generalization of use?[24] For example, is a person who smokes a "joint" from time to time considered to be a current user or, by analogy with the classification normally used for tobacco smoking, to be a nonuser if he does not smoke at least one joint a day?

- Does the term *current use* take into consideration only the fifteen days immediately preceding data collection, or does it include the entire preced-

TABLE 2. SOME TERMS USED IN OPERATIONAL DEFINITIONS OF DRUG USERS

Who?	User, ever
	User, current
When?	Onset of use:
	Recent
	or } use
	Current
	Time interval
How much?	Frequency
	Amount
	Multiple use
How?	Methods
	Conditions } of use
	Typology
Why?	Interest in
	Trying
	Maintaining } use
	or
	Changing
Consequences?	Positive } effects
	Negative
	Pathology
	Public health } problems
	Social

SOURCES: J. Elinson, "Status of Operational Definitions," in Louise G. Richards and Louise B. Blevens, eds., *The Epidemiology of Drug Abuse: Current Issues*, National Institute on Drug Abuse Research Monograph no. 10 (Rockville, Maryland: National Institute on Drug Abuse, March 1977): 10-13; L.D. Johnston, "Surveys: Longitudinal Studies," in idem: 60-67.

ing year,[25] which evidently changes the prevalence rate of use? Or is it preferable to define current use with reference to the interval between past use and next use?[26]

• *Multiple drug use*, defined in the United States as the use of several drugs without any clear preference for one, is also understood to mean the simultaneous use of more than one drug, with the exception of heroin, at least once a month.[27]

As can be seen from these few examples, precise operational definitions are obviously indispensable from the moment an epidemiological study is conceived, as well as when the time comes to prepare questionnaires—as suggested in a recent WHO project[28]—or interview schedules, to mention only two principal working instruments.

Such definitions are in effect a necessary, although by themselves insufficient, condition for comparing the results of epidemiological studies. As Robins wisely points out, however, "just getting incidence and prevalence out of a survey of drug users is not getting very much for your money."[29]

Let us therefore go beyond this initial step, which meets the first and often only need of the authorities,[30] and examine more closely some approaches that respond to expectations mentioned at the beginning of this paper.

THE COMMUNICABLE DISEASE MODEL

I will now discuss the communicable disease model initially proposed by R. de Alarcon and coworkers[31] and developed especially by Patrick H. Hughes and colleagues.[32,33] It is based on the concept that each outbreak of a heroin epidemic depends on the concomitant existence of the following classical sequence for such an outbreak in a well-defined neighborhood of a large city: isolated case, microepidemic, macroepidemic. Using this model, intervention obviously consists of the early detection of new outbreaks and treatment of all affected persons in order to prevent the epidemic from spreading.

Although the communicable disease approach seems to have proven useful in English-speaking countries in the course of the 1960s, it is questionable if it is applicable today because of the greater rapidity in the spread of epidemics and their increasingly endemic character. This rapid spread can even give an explosive character to the epidemic, as was emphasized in the 1973 Canadian report on the nonmedical use of drugs.[34]

It is of interest that the 1977 report of the NIDA, *The Epidemiology of Heroin and Other Narcotics*, which reviews a series of methodological aspects, does not mention the communicable disease approach;[35] in fact it refers only once—in the bibliography of a single contribution[36]—to the works I have just cited. This approach could, however, be usefully applied to the study of an unexpected arrival of a new illegal drug in a community.

SURVEYS OF GENERAL POPULATIONS

Broadly, these entail:

1. Identifying the progressions and individual trajectories from one type of drug use to another.

2. Defining these types of use with greater precision.

3. Correlating independent variables (linked to persons and context) with different types of use and different trajectories.

4. Attempting to determine on the basis of the foregoing:
   - The predicting factors—and evaluating their predictive power.
   - The cause and effect relationships, taking into account
     a) the complexity of behavior; and
     b) the multifactorial character of the motivations underlying them.

Figure 2 shows diagrammatically, and with considerable simplification, the pathways and types valid for any addiction-producing drug. The first stage is *experimental use*, which results from a set of motives and factors that stimulate a desire to experiment. At this point some experimenters, influenced by a set of motives and factors that stimulate a desire or a decision to stop, will cease using drugs and become abstainers.

One group of experimenters, however, and it may be a majority or a minority, will go on to *occasional* or *recreational use*. This type of use then continues (as indicated by the horizontal arrow), or leads (the vertical arrow) to *intensive use*, influenced by motives and factors that are partly similar to and partly different from the preceding ones.

What are the outcomes of intensive drug use? Obviously the possibility of continuation exists, as does a return to occasional or recreational use, or the transition to *addiction*. This last stage is the result of a continuation of well-known factors, as, for example, the deleterious effects of the drugs or rejection of the user by society, both of which lead to changes in lifestyle. Finally, addiction can end in *death*. But, through the influence of motives and circumstances as yet poorly understood, and through the success of medical treatment, addiction can also lead to a return to intensive or

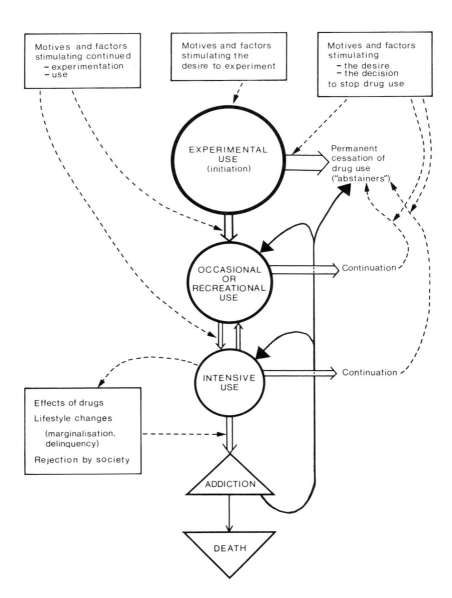

Figure 2. Types of drug use and pathways seen as parts of a dynamic system.

occasional use, and even, probably at a much more later stage, to a permanent cessation of drug use. What is obviously missing from Figure 2, therefore, is the "box" containing motives and factors to explain this move away from addiction and the gradual return to various preceding stages, including abstinence.

All the literature I have read recently on this subject insists on the need for studies similar to that of Robins, which deals with a sample of drug-using or -addicted Vietnam war veterans, most of whom completely abandoned their abuse and even their addiction on their return to the United States.[37] Such longitudinal studies, continuing on through adulthood, are still too rare.

Since Robins has already elegantly demonstrated the nature, number, and respective weights of several predicting factors, mainly through her own investigations,[38] I propose to limit myself to an outline of five particularities and difficulties related to population studies, and then to examine in more detail the question of longitudinal studies.

General Population Studies

1. *The rarer the phenomenon, the larger and less-biased must be the sample.*[39]

Let me cite by way of example the contrast between the frequency of marijuana use by primary and secondary school students and the rarity of heroin addiction in the adult population as a whole.

2. *The more marginal the phenomenon, the more difficult it is to reach the subjects.*

The contrast usually cited in this context is that between the use of illegal drugs and legal drugs such as alcohol. For so-called hard drugs, habitual household survey procedures must evidently be replaced by less conventional methods such as the nonsurvey observational technique.[40]

3. *Validity is much more difficult to test when an objective reference point is either lacking or unclear.*

Exceptions exist, nevertheless; in her study of Vietnam veterans, Robins was able to compare the subjects' interview results with their military medical records and urine tests. The results appeared valid, and she concluded that

> addicts may be more honest with interviewers who are going to go away and never come back again, than they are with the doctors they see in drug treatment programs.[41]

Robins thus draws attention to a problem that should be taken into account in a longitudinal study where there is a repeated contact between the investigator and the user of an illegal drug, who, often having become addicted, is suspicious of any follow up.

It should be noted that the validity of results is also essential in nonsystematic observation. In her presentation of the advantages and disadvantages of this technique, Gail A. Crawford compares information collected by ad hoc investigators, usually former addicts, with that obtained by the research sociologist supervisor who undertakes special surveys for this purpose.[42]

4. *The more the field investigator works with marginal groups, the more up-to-date must be her/his vocabulary.*[43]

This points up the usefulness of a continuously updated glossary, which seems to me equally valuable for investigators and educators working in the school environment.

5. *The more the investigator differs culturally from the interviewees, the more she/he risks becoming the victim of negative prejudices about them, and the more these prejudices can lead to an underestimation of the real prevalence of drug use.*[44]

This fifth difficulty requires no comment.

Longitudinal and Prospective Studies

It would be impossible here to present a complete overview of the longitudinal studies undertaken in this field; they are the subject of an entire volume.[45] I would therefore like to use a somewhat schematic approach to:

- Emphasize the advantages of such studies.
- Summarize the results obtained thus far.
- Recall some of the difficulties encountered.
- Suggest a way of mitigating some of these difficulties.

ADVANTAGES

In the preface to her book Denise Kandel recalls that longitudinal studies, in the absence of opportunities for experimentation, provide the assortment of data most useful for testing causal hypotheses.[46] Their analysis remains complex, however, and the techniques for exploiting them are still at a fairly early stage of development. This is due also to the fact that empirical use of these techniques can only be made as the studies proliferate. Peter Bentler elaborates on this point in the final chapter on methodology in Kandel's book.[47]

For Lloyd D. Johnston, longitudinal studies permit one:

• To verify whether a relationship between variables is simultaneous or sequential, which is crucial for suggesting causal hypotheses or for renouncing them at the outset.

• To estimate maturational changes, namely, in adolescents, that occur with increasing age.

• To evaluate the impact of environmental factors. Here Johnston cites Robins's experience with Vietnam veterans.

• To estimate the effects of planned interventions, whether they be preventive—for example, educational—or therapeutic; here of course one passes from the longitudinal to the experimental.[48]

A final and major advantage of these studies is that they help to dispel any misunderstanding caused by studies that concentrate only on drug addicts, notably concerning the frequency of the escalation phenomenon. In this regard, Kandel states:

> Research based on already addicted individuals precludes the investigation of many issues relevant to our understanding of drug behavior, which takes many forms other than addiction. Furthermore, although longitudinal in character, studies of this nature do not permit a clear assessment of the precursors and the consequence of drug use. Such an assessment requires contact with a population at risk for drug use and follow up over time in order to identify and to compare the characteristics of individuals who initiate the use of drugs and of individuals who do not. Continued follow up of such populations also makes it possible to identify both consquences of use and further changes over time of the variables related to use.[49]

RESULTS OBTAINED THUS FAR

In Kandel's opening chapter, in which she attempts a synthesis of the principal longitudinal studies undertaken in the United States, she highlights nineteen propositions divided into three groups:

• Types of involvement
• Antecedents to this type of use
• Consequences of this type of use[50]

We may omit here those propositions that simply confirm what we already know from cross-sectional studies, and concentrate on the most original findings resulting from longitudinal studies.

Table 3 lists the findings that seem to me to be the most interesting from the viewpoint of this conference. One may wonder if eventually they will be confirmed on this side of the Atlantic!

Psychiatrists will be interested in an example, even if only one, of concordance between the results of a cross-sectional French study by Françoise Davidson and coworkers[51] and a longitudinal American study by C.H. Haagen,[52] although the methodology used was very different.

Table 4 outlines the comparative profile of adolescents either attracted primarily to experimentation or to habitual use, thus prolonging the experimental phase, as described by Davidson.[53]

For Haagen, adolescents who describe themselves as worried, pessimistic, discontented, anxious, agitated, fickle, and in conflict with others became *habitual* marijuana users. Those who, on the contrary, rate themselves positively on the same attitude and behavior scales became *occasional* users.[54]

DIFFICULTIES

Even if difficulties are not necessarily limited to longitudinal studies of behavioral phenomena, it is worth noting their existence and nature, according to Johnston.[55]

TABLE 3. EIGHT OF NINETEEN PROPOSITIONS RELATED TO
LONGITUDINAL STUDY RESULTS IN THE UNITED STATES

---

1. The period for risk of initiation into illicit drug use is over by the mid-twenties.
3. Later age of onset is associated with lesser involvement and greater probability of stopping.
5. Addiction to heroin is not necessarily a permanent state.
6. Occasional use of heroin does not necessarily lead to addiction.
8. Personality factors, indicative of maladjustment, precede the use of marijuana and of other illicit drugs.
14. Parental behavior, parental attitudes, and parental closeness to their children have differential importance at different stages of involvement in drugs.
18. Nonaddictive illicit drug use has not been shown to lead to increased criminality.
19. Drug use has not been shown to lead to the amotivational syndrome.

SOURCE: Denise B. Kandel, "Convergencies in Perspective: Longitudinal Surveys of Drug Use in Normal Populations," in *Longitudinal Research on Drug Abuse. Empirical Findings and Methodological Issues,* ed. Denise B. Kandel (New York: Halsted Press, John Wiley, 1978): 3-38.

TABLE 4. INDIVIDUAL PSYCHOLOGICAL PROFILE OF
FRENCH ADOLESCENTS, AND TYPE OF DRUG USE

Personality Traits Predisposing Adolescents to Experimentation	Personality Traits Predisposing Adolescents to Habitual Use Following Experimentation
Expansive	Not very expansive
Active	Isolated
Unconventional	Friendless
Open to others	Ill at ease
Sociable	—with family
Opposing	—at school
	—in a group
	Marked by boredom

SOURCE: Françoise Davidson, M. Choquet, and M. Depagne, *Les Lycéens Devant la Drogue et les Autres Produits Psychotropes* (Paris: National Institute of Health and Medical Research [INSERM], 1973).

• *Anonymity.* In order to trace persons who have been interviewed previously, it is obviously necessary to identify them; this means recording their names, even if the information is subsequently kept in coded form.

• *Follow-up interviews.* These are more difficult to obtain as the time interval between them—or their frequency—increases, or when the persons interviewed are marginal and thus mobile.

• *Bias.* There is a risk of attributing to processes of individual maturation what, in reality, is a result of the evolution of practices, for example, in the form of fashions. It is therefore important to assemble information on these persons independent of the cohort being studied, although in the same temporal and spatial context.

A COMBINED STRATEGY

Among the rare research strategies capable of optimizing longitudinal studies, I should like to draw attention, without comment, to one by Johnston.[56] He suggests combining the short study of a very large sample with a longer survey of a more limited sample—of more exposed subjects, for example—proceeding later to a "recalibration" of the second on the first by means of a completely acceptable statistical technique.

CONCLUSIONS

Considering the various difficulties—particularly ethical—that epidemiological research encounters, is it reasonable to persist in advocating its use parallel to other possible approaches to the study of this phenomenon? It seems to me that one can honestly answer in the affirmative, given the remarkable results registered, especially in longitudinal studies, several of which are still in progress.

Future research will probably focus as much on the study of factors at play and of consequences as on types of use, abuse, and addiction. To this end, it should:

• Associate behavioral science specialists more closely with physicians—epidemiologists and psychiatrists, above all, although not exclusively—and with statisticians and data-processing experts.

• Open up the study of illegal drug use and abuse to include legal drugs, also, particularly medicines, as suggested in the 1973 Canadian report[57] and in the 1978 French report.[58]

• Allow, in the long run, for a broader vision of the phenomenon as a social problem.

• Continue for short and medium periods to measure the epidemiological importance of dimensions explored by workers in other disciplines.

What prevention programs aimed at adolescents could emerge from these (partly new) epidemiological research orientations?

• With regard to the use of both legal and illegal drugs, should specific preventive measures focus on the harmful effects of abuse, rather than on use itself, given the generally underestimated range of "nonharmful effects" of use, particularly on the adolescent?[59,60]

• As for the hypothesis of reciprocal maladaptation of adolescents and society, a series of generally unspecific preventive measures should be developed, such as those suggested in the Pelletier report,[61] with the far-reaching goal of improving the "functioning of society"; this should make it possible to achieve a halt in the evolution—and perhaps even a regression—of other types of behavior such as suicide or aggression against other persons.

According to some observers, "every society has a system of social expectations regarding appropriate age-behavior."[62]

To account more specifically for adolescent maturation and socialization processes, we must ask if this observation is still valid in so-called postindustrial Western society, which today most often seems to ignore not only the place and role of adolescents, but the competencies it is willing to accord them as regards certain behaviors, notably drug use.

The crucial question no longer seems to be, as it was ten years ago, whom to blame, but how to substitute for this ignorance a knowledge based on rigorous, irrefutable facts.

SUMMARY

Because drug use and abuse are anchored in the behavioral sphere, their epidemiological study presents difficulties that are important to identify and consider when choosing models and methodological approaches.

Even the enumeration of different categories of users, for example, is not as simple as one would like to believe, to say, and sometimes even to write. This is demonstrated by the comments about Table 1 and Figure 1, and by examples of obstacles to the adoption of apparently simple operational definitions.

Population studies, which fortunately are increasingly replacing studies of addicts, allow us gradually to detect, in the midst of this complex field of research, a certain number of risk factors, even though their predictive power is still weak. Undoubtedly it will be prospective longitudinal studies, of which a series is now in progress in the English-speaking countries, that will best enable us to verify these predictions. Verification is made more difficult, however, by the mobile character of the problem: this multiplies the number and variety of factors that intervene to obscure or mask medium- and long-term verification.

As for the adolescent, I admit that epidemiology aims at preparing the ground for preventive measures that take into account types of drug, forms of use and abuse, and the complex network of individual trajectories from one type of use to another. The question at the present, however, is whether—and in what instances—prevention of the harmful effects of drug use should be given priority over the prevention of drug use, up to now considered the only legitimate form of prevention.

NOTES

1. Eva J. Salber, "Epidemiology as a Technique in the Study of Drug Dependence," in *The Epidemiology of Drug Dependence* (Copenhagen: World Health Organization, Regional Office for Europe, EURO 5436 IV, 1973): 4-15.

2. Monique Pelletier, *Mission d'Étude sur l'Ensemble des Problèmes de la Drogue,* Report to the President of the Republic of France (Paris: Documentation Française, 1978).

3. Louise G. Richards, "Introduction," in *The Epidemiology of Drug Abuse: Current Issues,* ed. Louise G. Richards and Louise B. Blevens, NIDA Research Monograph no. 10 (Rockville, Maryland: National Institute on Drug Abuse, March 1977): 1-18.

4. Lee N. Robins, "Adolescent Development: Epidemiology of Drug Use and Abuse," in *Psychopathology of Children and Youth: A Cross-Cultural Perspective,* ed. Elizabeth F. Purcell (New York: Josiah Macy, Jr. Foundation, 1981).

5. Richard H. Blum, *Drug Education: Results and Recommendations* (Lexington, Massachusetts: Heath, 1976).

6. United Nations Economic and Social Council, *Drug Abuse: Extent, Patterns, and Trends,* Note by the Secretary-General, Presented to the Commission on Narcotic Drugs, Doc. E.CN. 7/629 (Geneva: United Nations, February 1979).

7. Pelletier, "Problèmes de la Drogue" (See note 2).

8. Louise A. Gottschalk, "Indicators of Drug Abuse. Drug-Involved Death," in *Epidemiology of Drug Abuse* (See note 3): 98-122.

9. Leonard Savitz, "Institutional Sources: Arrests," in *Epidemiology of Drug Abuse* (See note 3): 84-88.

10. Ira H. Cisin, "Surveys of General Populations," in *Epidemiology of Drug Abuse* (See note 3): 34-38.

11. Saul B. Sells, "Institutional Sources: Treatment," in *Epidemiology of Drug Abuse* (See note 3): 91-95.

12. Lee N. Robins, "Estimating Addiction Rates and Locating Target Populations. How Decomposition into Stages Helps," in *Epidemiology of Drug Abuse* (See note 3): 25-39.

13. Armand Delachaux, Eileen M. Brooke, and E. Haller, "Les Toxicomanies dans le Canton de Vaud," manuscript submitted for publication.

14. Irving Rootman, "Registers as Contributors to Estimation," in *The Epidemiology of Heroin and Other Narcotics,* ed. Joan Dunne Rittenhouse, NIDA Research Monograph no. 16 (Rockville, Maryland: National Institute on Drug Abuse, November 1977).

15. J.A. O'Donnell, "The Methodology of Retrospective Studies," in *Epidemiology of Drug Dependence* (See note 1): 31-34.

16. Françoise Davidson, M. Choquet, and M. Depagne, *Les Lycéens Devant la Drogue et les Autres Produits Psychotropes* (Paris: National Institute of Health and Medical Research [INSERM], 1973).

17. Lee N. Robins, "The Methodology of Prospective Studies of Drug Abuse, in *Epidemiology of Drug Dependence* (See note 1): 26-30.

18. Denise B. Kandel, "Convergencies in Prospective: Longitudinal Surveys of Drug Use in Normal Populations," in *Longitudinal Research on Drug Use. Empirical Findings and Methodological Issues,* ed. Denise B. Kandel (New York: Halsted Press, John Wiley, 1978).

19. Lee N. Robins, "The Natural History of Drug Abuse" (Paper presented at the Symposium on Treatment Evaluation in Drug Abuse, 19th Scandinavian Psychiatric Congress, Uppsala, 15 June 1979).

20. Richards, "Introduction" (See note 3).

21. National Clearinghouse for Drug Abuse Education, *Resource Book for Drug Education,* 2nd ed. (Washington: U.S. Government Printing Office, 1972).

22. *Report of the World Health Organization Committee on Drug Dependence,* Technical Report Ser. 407 (Geneva: World Health Organization, 1969): 6.

23. *Report of the World Health Organization Expert Committee on Drug Dependence,* Technical Report Ser. 618 (Geneva: World Health Organization, 1978): 8.

24. Richards, "Introduction" (See note 3).

25. Lee N. Robins, "Discussion on Status of Operational Definitions," in *Epidemiology of Drug Abuse* (See note 3).

26. Cisin, "Surveys of Populations" (See note 10).

27. James C. Sample, "Concept of Polydrug Use," in *Epidemiology of Drug Abuse* (See note 3).

28. R.G. Smart, P.H. Hughes, L. Johnston, et al., *A Methodology for Student Drug-Use Surveys*, WHO Offset Publication 50 (Geneva: World Health Organization, 1980): 1-55.

29. Lee N. Robins, "Surveys of Target Populations," in *Epidemiology of Drug Abuse* (See note 3): 39-45.

30. _____, "Brief Terms of Reference," in *The Epidemiology of Heroin and Other Narcotics*, ed. Joan Dunne Rittenhouse, NIDA Research Monograph No. 16 (Rockville, Maryland: National Institute on Drug Abuse, November 1977): 12-14.

31. R. de Alarcon and N.H. Rathod, "Prevalence and Early Detection of Heroin Abuse," *British Medical Journal* no. 2 (1968): 549-53.

32. P.H. Hughes, N.W. Barker, G.A. Crawford, et al., "The Natural History of a Heroin Epidemic," *American Journal of Public Health* 62, no. 7 (1972): 995-1001.

33. P.H. Hughes and G. A. Crawford, "A Contagious Disease Model for Researching and Intervening in Heroin Epidemics," *Archives of General Psychiatry* 27 (1972): 149-55.

34. Commission of Inquiry into the Non-Medical Use of Drugs, *Final Report* (Ottawa, Canada: Commission of Inquiry into the Non-Medical Use of Drugs, 1973).

35. Joan Dunne Rittenhouse, ed. *The Epidemiology of Heroin and Other Narcotics*, NIDA Research Monograph No. 16 (Rockville, Maryland: National Institute on Drug Abuse, November 1977).

36. Fred Goldman, "Narcotics Users, Narcotic Prices and Criminal Activity: An Economic Analysis," in *Epidemiology of Heroin* (See note 14): 130-36.

37. Robins, "Natural History of Drug Abuse" (See note 19).

38. _____, "Adolescent Drug Abuse" (See note 4).

39. _____, "Target Populations" (See note 29).

40. G.A. Crawford, "Observational Techniques," in *Epidemiology of Drug Abuse* (See note 3): 73-77.

41. Robins, "Target Populations" (See note 29).

42. Crawford, "Observational Techniques" (See note 40).

43. Robins, "Target Populations" (See note 29).

44. Ibid.

45. Kandel, "Surveys of Drug Use" (See note 18).

46. Ibid.

47. Peter M. Bentler, "The Interdependence of Theory, Methodology, and Empirical Data: Causal Modeling as an Approach to Construct Validation," in *Research on Drug Use* (See note 18): 267-302.

48. Lloyd D. Johnston, "Surveys: Longitudinal Studies," in *Epidemiology of Drug Abuse* (See note 3): 60-67.

49. Kandel, "Surveys of Drug Use" (See note 18).

50. Ibid.

51. Davidson, Choquet, and Depagne, *Lycéens Devant la Drogue* (See note 16).

52. C.H. Haagen, 1970, quoted in *Research on Drug Use* (See note 18).

53. Davidson, Choquet, and Depagne, *Lycéens Devant la Drogue* (See note 16).

54. Haagen, 1970 (See note 52).

55. Johnston, "Surveys" (See note 48).

56. Ibid.

57. Commission of Inquiry, *Final Report* (See note 34).

58. Pelletier, *Problèmes de la Drogue* (See note 2).

59. *Report of the World Health Organization Committee on Drug Dependence*, Technical Report Ser. 551 (Geneva: World Health Organization, 1974).

60. O. Jeanneret, "Prévention Primaire de l'Usage des Drogues par les Jeunes ou Prévention des Conséquences de Cet Usage" (Paper presented at the 2nd National Colloquium on Alcoholism, Lausanne, 1979).

61. Pelletier, *Problèmes de la Drogue* (See note 2).

62. B.L. Neugarten and N. Datan, "Sociological Perspectives on the Life Cycle," in *Life-Span Developmental Psychology: Personality and Socialization*, ed. P.B. Balter and K.W. Schaie (New York: Academic Press, 1973).

DISCUSSION

Predictors of Drug Use

There is data from the work of Denise Kandel and other investigators that personality maladjustment predisposes to marijuana use. The data Robins presented suggests there is no evidence for that. Was a different sampling technique used?

Robins's point was that the very early school behavior indicators that are typical of conduct disorders and predict the antisocial personality seem to be lacking. Those who have looked closely at the onset of drug use in adolescents have found a number of predictors in the immediate vicinity of the decision to use, which could be called "maladjustment."

The Jessors are perhaps the best example. They found at least four kinds of behavior—drinking, losing interest in achievement in school, losing one's virginity, and general deviance—that predicted the onset of drug use. When any of these occurred they increased the likelihood that drug use would begin within the year. They interpret this finding as indicating that onset of drug use is part of a maturational stage at which young people are freeing themselves from their parents and becoming peer-centered; the stage occurs at various ages, but the behaviors are interchangeable parts of the same phenomenon.

Progression from Marijuana Use

The only additional piece of information Kandel added is that those who moved from marijuana to a hard drug showed somewhat more depression prior to that move. She made two studies of high school students in New York State, observing what their drug use was in the fall and how it had changed by the following spring. She found that if those using marijuana in the fall were depressed they were more likely to move on to other drugs. Another possible interpretation is that they had used *more* marijuana than other students, and that heavy use had made them both depressed and more likely to use other drugs.

There is no question that highly deviant children have an increased risk of using drugs, but they do not represent the great majority of drug users; many have no prior history of deviance.

Instead of the typical pre-antisocial personality picture, Robins found that prospective drug users were early maturers who drank, stayed out late, and dated the opposite sex earlier than most. This type of deviance is called "status offense." Typically the drug-users-to-be were not violent and did not steal; although they did things considered inappropriate for their age level—at least by their parents.

Outcomes of Drug Use

Are there any data on the factors that mediate between drug outcome and drug usage—bad outcome, for example? Is there evidence that poor outcome is conditional upon continued drug usage or amount of usage? Or is it related to predisposing factors? Is the outcome worse depending on whether one lives in a small town or a large city?

The information Robins has on bad outcomes derives from a new study of young black men who were born and raised in St. Louis. If they quit drugs the rate of later problems is still above the rate for nonusers; it is intermediate between rates for those who never used drugs and those who continue to use them.

No comparable analysis has been done for the Vietnam veterans, who come from all over the country. Robins tried to find situational variables, such as city size and region of the country, that might mediate between adolescent drug use and later problems, but she found no relationship. Drugs are available everywhere in the United States; no one need be deprived.

Psychiatrists who treat heroin addicts apparently see psychopathology, which some explain as being a response to the drug and the drug culture and maintenance of the habit.

Experimental Reinforcement

Some people have carried out experimental studies. Mendelson in Boston, for example, has worked with both alcoholics and heroin addicts in an experimental unit where the subjects can self-medicate at whatever rate they choose for a period of several weeks; the drug reinforces behaviors without providing any apparent euphoria. That is, if one observes the behavior or asks about the response, the good feeling that is supposed to accompany administration of the drug is not at all evident.

The behavioral unit at Harvard has demonstrated that by modifying reinforcement conditions a monkey will give itself what appears to be a painful electric shock for no other benefit or reward than the pain. The word "pain" is used in the sense that the monkey can be conditioned to push the button to give itself an electric shock and maintain that behavior over long periods of time.

Another model relates to smoking. In one study a number of smokers reported they took up the habit initially under conditions of stress. After such dependence has occurred, however, if they do not smoke there is still enough of an effect, even with a drop in nicotine, that they continue to smoke. They appear, on observation, to be reluctant to avoid the unpleasantness of the absence of the nicotine. This raises a very important problem in methodology; the factors behind initiation may not be identical to those related to maintaining and sustaining a behavior.

Social Class and Drug Use

With regard to the new recruit to the drug abuse field, how do the figures break down in terms of social class and ethnicity? While the minority representation in the drug use or abuse arena is an important one, are the numbers of middle-class whites becoming significant? What is the overall distribution? Are we seeing any change?

In Robins's experience minorities are overrepresented among drug users, but most drug users are not minority members. In the Vietnam study, which covered quite a representative sample of the population, there was virtually no correlation with social class. The little relationship that did exist was the reverse of what one might expect—there was a slight increase of use at the highest socioeconomic level.

In a national study of high school students followed a year after graduation, Johnston found no association between social class and drug use. Drug users may have been believed to be disadvantaged because only treated cases had been studied.

Variations by Geographic Region

Is it possible that the figures in the Johnston study might be misleading with respect to local trends, which could differ from one place to another one?

Johnston does not present data town by town, but by regions of the country and by city size. Although there is variation, with the Northeast region and large cities having the highest rates of use, in none of the locales on which he focused was there a level of marijuana use below 40 percent. So although there is certainly variation, it is common everywhere.

"Recreational Use" of Drugs

Robins was asked to define "hard drugs": which drugs are considered hard? People do not agree on definitions at the present time. Often the term "hard drug" is used to refer to all illicit drugs except marijuana.

The proposals of Kandel stress that, contrary to popular belief, especially on the basis of retrospective studies, "recreational use" applies as much to heroin as to marijuana, and it does not lead necessarily to addiction or dependence. In WHO parlance, addiction is called dependence; it is not a permanent state or condition.

In other words, individuals have been observed who use heroin, but who do not look like our stereotype of the heroin addict and who do not become addicted. For a long time clinicians have known perfectly well that, perhaps more among adults than adolescents, the use of heroin is not necessarily incompatible with a normal social and professional life.

Drugs on the College Campus

One of the observations of those who work near college campuses in the United States is with respect to the use of LSD, which was the most sensational of the drugs in the late 1960s. It is clear that college students developed an underground therapeutic service from their personal experience with LSD. In a short period of time students were less frequently brought to the infirmary of the college service. The faculty began to think LSD use had diminished, when in fact what had happened was that students became used to talking a fellow student down from a trip and would stay with her/him, so the student overcame the experience with less difficulty. The students had a supply of chlorpromazine available, which they administered instead of seeking medical help. Conclusions as to the extent of the phenomenon in a community, based on observation in the medical setting, can therefore be most misleading.

VII. INNOVATIVE CARE PROGRAMS FOR ADOLESCENT DRUG USERS AND ABUSERS

DRUG USE AND ABUSE:
INNOVATIVE CARE PROGRAMS
IN THE UNITED STATES

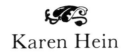

Karen Hein

I will discuss an aspect of adolescent health—or ill health—that has become a focal point of debate and discussion in America during the past decade. I am particularly pleased that a pediatrician was chosen to present the issues of innovative care for the drug-using or -abusing teenager. In the United States there is now a group of physicians, most of them pediatricians, specializing in the medical care of the adolescent, whose needs have until recently been poorly defined and largely unmet by health professionals worldwide.[1]

Whether adolescents are seen in a hospital or in a community-based educational, recreational, or social institution, health care providers are faced with the challenge of trying to offer meaningful services to those who use drugs; give advice to concerned parents and community organizations regarding the use of licit and illicit drugs; and plan programs to meet the needs of young people for whom drugs may play a minimal or maximal role in their lives.

Of the 40 million teenagers in the United States, approximately 90 percent will have used alcohol and 60 percent an illicit drug by the end of their adolescence. In this paper I will address the response to drug use by the community or health professional.

Young people who abuse drugs have a wide variety of motivations; a diversity of needs and potentials; many different patterns of abuse; and experience different consequences of drug abuse. I have therefore chosen to divide adolescent drug users and abusers into three groups. I will present two conceptual models that are used as the basis for many treatment programs, and then discuss seven approaches—two based on the first model and three on the second, and two innovative programs that have been developed on the basis of both models. Finally, I will comment briefly on the special problems of inner-city, minority group youngsters for whom the problem of drug use may be compounded by economic, legal, and social factors.

For the purpose of this discussion drug abuse is defined as

> the use of any substance in a manner which deviates from the accepted medical, social, or legal patterns within a given society. It is behavior that results from a complex interaction of an adolescent, his social and cultural environment and the pharmacology and availability of particular drugs.[2]

One might argue that in the worldwide adolescent community, and certainly in American society, there exist many subgroups in which the use of a given drug is acceptable. This is true. A discussion of innovative care must therefore begin with some agreement as to who needs the care.

THREE DRUG-USING GROUPS

Three groups of drug-using adolescents can be identified in the United States. The largest group is composed of those for whom drug use is a part of normal experimentation and exploratory behavior. Adolescence is a period of life characterized by marked changes in physical, sexual, intellectual, emotional, and social functioning. The readjustment to a new body, mental outlook, and social set results in periods of confusion and anxiety. As the young person moves from a dependent relationship toward independence, feelings of insecurity and depression are common. The awareness that she/he is expected to acquire skills necessary to function successfully as an adult is similarly anxiety producing. At this critical stage of life, drug experimentation may be viewed as a means of gaining peer acceptance, establishing a separate identity from that of the family, and satisfying the need to experience a physical or psychological lift through the anticipated "high."

Since by the end of adolescence the majority of young people have, at least once, tried smoking a cigarette, consuming alcohol, and/or using marijuana, these practices might be viewed as normal. The perceived health consequences, however, are usually thought of as sufficiently detrimental to declare such behavior a problem. In adolescence the pharmacological properties are not necessarily the most harmful aspect of drug usage; rather, the potential deleterious effect of drug-using behavior on psychosocial development should be used as a criterion for intervention. Thus innovative care for these teenagers is an attempt to curb their use of drugs through education, limiting access, or providing alternatives that offer the youngsters other means of satisfying a need to demonstrate burgeoning independence. Although this group accounts for the largest number of teenage drug users, probably close to 80 percent of all users, the other two groups receive a disproportionate amount of adverse attention.

The second group of drug-involved teenagers are those for whom drug use dominates intra- and interpersonal relationships; it becomes a means to promote socialization. Drug use is part of the fabric of the group, providing a common language and a mutuality of practice that unifies the group and gives an identity to it and to its members. Among certain groups such as some tribes of native Americans, the use of hallucinogens is recognized as an integral part of their ceremonial life; the use of peyote is legal in this instance. In the 1960s and early 1970s, however, groups of young people used similar mood-altering substances that are not condoned legally or socially, despite their insistence that the role of such drugs is not dissimilar to that of peyote for native Americans.

The response to such groups has tended to be in one of two spheres. First, the communities in which they reside often call on law enforcement agencies to monitor the activities of the members and to disperse the groups by incarcerating key members when or if an infraction of the law occurs. The second response seems to have sprung from within the groups themselves: other means of mood alteration such as meditation are viewed as a safer and equally effective means of achieving higher states of mental and physical well-being. In summary, the second group depends on drugs to ease the pangs of adolescent development, whereas the first group accomplishes this despite some drug experimentation.

The third group of drug-involved adolescents are those for whom usage is an attempt at self-medication to ameliorate severe depression or psychopathology. Such attempts usually fail, because the medications are obtained through illegal means and their continued usage usually forces the individual to resort to illegal acts to continue support of the habit, whether it is alcohol, an opiate, or a stimulant.

Attempts to mask severe signs of psychopathology are not usually successful, and the individual comes quickly to the attention of mental health, social welfare, or legal authorities. The small number of these adolescents, probably no more than 5 percent of all drug-using teenagers, has probably remained static over the past few years, but they are becoming more visible due to the recent movement toward deinstitutionalization.[3] While there is a trend toward no longer housing these young people in mental hygiene facilities, it now appears they are being incarcerated in jails or in juvenile detention or other types of residential treatment facilities. Innovative care for this group cannot be really innovative at all. Factors such as socioeconomic status and discriminatory racial practices may dictate the type of care offered.

TREATMENT PROGRAMS

I would now like to discuss briefly the rationale behind treatment or prevention programs, which can be conceptualized as being part of one of two models. The first places the emphasis on the individual drug user, based on the belief that the adolescent uses or abuses drugs because of the biological or psychological effects produced.

Chemical Substitutions

For those who adhere to the biological concept, treatment or prevention is designed to identify those who are at risk and then to change the body chemistry, physiology, or structure to correct a preexisting or induced abnormality. Methadone maintenance programs for adolescents are an example of this approach.[4] It was originally assumed that an underlying craving or an induced abnormality in a central nervous system receptor site was corrected by opiate use; by supplying a substitute the adolescent would be able to resume normal functioning. The discovery of endorphins has provided fuel to this particular fire, and has offered a physiological explanation for the observed difficulty in detoxifying opiate-addicted individuals and enabling them to remain drug free following a period of physiological addiction. A few programs specifically designed for adolescents employ methadone maintenance as the mainstay of therapy. As with adults, however, the chemical substitution alone is not adequate to correct the deficits in self-esteem and social functioning or the lack of employment opportunities for heavily drug-involved youth.

Programs that weigh personality factors as being more important than biological features have approached drug treatment through alteration of the psyche rather than the soma as the solution to the problem. Through psychotherapy, and a consequent appreciation of the subconscious underlying causality, the adolescent is able to change drug-using behavior. A body of literature describing the drug-prone personality has been developed by the proponents of this approach. Psychotherapy has not been the answer for the majority of drug-involved Americans, however, because of the high cost, limited availability, and unacceptability to many teenagers.

Self-Help Groups

The second conceptual model underlying many drug treatment programs is that of the self-help group. These programs are based on the assumption that the social environment determines whether or not, and to what degree, an adolescent will become involved with drugs. Therapeutic communities such as Phoenix House, Odyssey, and Synanon were created in an attempt to establish a subgroup that would counterbalance the detrimental effects of a hostile or exclusionary society.

These programs, although still in existence, have not been popular with most adolescents, who abhor their self-imposed isolation from the family and community; vigorous techniques for self-appraisal, including verbal encounters; and merit systems for earning privileges. Many of the programs have recently been exposed by the legal authorities and mass media as being tyrannical and dictatorial in style, and of using illegal means to restrain individuals or to obtain funds to continue operation. Most therapeutic communities are not equipped to deal with the multiple, complex problems that young people have in addition to their drug usage. The programs are not as a rule based on sufficient awareness of the developmental dimensions of adolescents, and usually require that the younger people mix with an older population of drug addicts or abusers. Participation in these residential programs calls for a commitment to a highly structured environment; most teenagers have neither the motivation for or the interest in such a commitment.

The self-help groups try to find alternatives to drugs as a means to alleviate inner tension and offer substitute means of satisfaction. One successful example of youth counseling and support is Alateen, the branch of Alcoholics Anonymous that was originally established for the teenage offspring of alcoholics. Since many of these young people themselves suffer from the social consequences of excessive alcohol intake, such groups provide an opportunity to discuss common family problems and personal and peer difficulties. Peer teaching has become recognized as an effective means of stimulating otherwise poorly motivated individuals. This model is now being tried in schools as well as in free-standing, self-help groups in the community.

Often one of the first steps the self-help groups take is to acquire age-appropriate educational materials that present the risks, benefits, and alternatives to many licit and illicit drugs.[5] The concern of the mass media about drug use has resulted in a proliferation of pamphlets, books, and audiovisual aids prepared for a variety of adolescent audiences. Some are largely pictorial or in cartoon style, while others delve extensively into research data in an attempt to provide appropriate material that will allow adolescents to make informed decisions regarding their use of drugs.

In the presence of organized, receptive groups, appropriate educational material, and a structure in which to function, peer counseling is a major innovative force in drug treatment. Originally aimed at young adults and middle adolescents, the use of peer teaching teams has now been extended to the dissemination of health information material to youngsters of elementary school age.

One particularly noteworthy program in adolescent smoking prevention was recently described by a group at Stanford University.[6] Rather than use the medical model as the basis for disease prevention, the group selected the educational model, which emphasizes the planning and implementation of organized programs of communication to guide socialization. The Stanford group reports that a more successful approach is use of an educational model of "psychological inoculation," in which the goal of prevention is to provide protection from and immunity to the pressures on young children that result in their smoking tobacco in early adolescence. Seventh-grade peer leaders are identified, trained over a period of weeks, and then return to school to conduct sessions for their classmates in which a short play is presented depicting a situation in which a young person is being pressured to smoke or drink. A contest has been devised, and a prize is awarded to the student who drafts the best plan to help an individual resist such pressures. Early data suggest that, in addition to reducing tobacco use, some decline in drug and alcohol use may be being achieved.

ALTERNATIVES TO DRUGS

The second phase of such campaigns is to provide alternatives to drugs, such as the following three programs.

The first is organized, physical risk-taking through sports and athletics. One national organization called Outward Bound uses this model to try to provide experiences replete with physical and emotional thrills and a sense of mastery and accomplishment, with minimal risk, to the adolescent participant.

The second includes yoga and meditation, which provide an alternative means of achieving a "high" and are safe ways of managing stress.

The objective of the third category is to augment the individual's self-esteem; in general, the greater the self-esteem the less likely the person is to be vulnerable to social or peer pressure or to feel the necessity to prove her-himself by risk-taking behavior.

Thus far I have described three groups of American teenagers who use drugs and two models of programs that treat them. The model that concentrates on treating the individual is most appropriate for the small percent of teenagers who fall into the third group—those with severe psychopathology. The second model, the self-help concept, is best utilized by the first and second groups of teenagers.

The Door Program

I would now like to discuss a program that uses a combination of the individual and self-help approaches. It is the finest example of innovative services that I am aware of. Because of its adaptability it is suitable for youngsters in any of the three groups mentioned. Although its reproducibility appears to be limited, this program has survived the transition from the type of services available in the 1960s to those still available at the present time.

During the 1960s innovative services were created outside the established care facilities because of the apparent inability of these traditional institutions to respond to the perceived needs of young people. Storefront clinics, ad hoc health teams at rock concert festivals, and hostels for runaways typified the early attempts to reach young people who are disenfranchised from school, family, or place of work. They were founded and maintained by the voluntary efforts of dedicated physicians, nurses, social workers, and street workers. The immediate need they served and their initial success resulted in a proliferation of similar programs throughout the United States. Attempts to translate these temporary crises-oriented programs into viable permanent ones with financial backing met with little success, however. Those programs that did survive beyond the initial phase, which was supported by the zeal of volunteer professionals, have been able to obtain small grants from a variety of sources to piece together a program that offers comprehensive services to young people.

This is the story of The Door, A Center of Alternatives, a New York City community-based, comprehensive, multiservice center for youths between age twelve and twenty-one. Programs and activities are provided free of charge, no parental consent is required, and confidentiality is assured. Professional services include general medical care, psychiatric and social services, nutritional, educational, vocational, and legal guidance, counseling in family planning, and sex education, as well as recreational sports activities such as instruction in Eastern martial arts. By placing these services in one facility it is feasible to integrate them and to offer continuity of care. The Door has approximately sixty-five full-time clinical staff members; fifty-five students from the various professional disciplines in field placements; and approximately fifty professional volunteers.

All the services and activities at The Door function as points of entry into the drug and alcohol treatment programs. Those young people who are not willing to identify themselves as drug abusers or to admit that their drug use is having a detrimental effect on their lives can enroll in the Crisis Intervention and Short-Term Treatment Program. The help they receive in resolving acute problems is important in preventing them from becoming increasingly reliant on drugs. The emphasis is on the resolution of problems and conflicts and on involvement in alternatives before abuse becomes a central life focus.

For those who acknowledge the deleterious effect of drugs on their lives and are motivated to reduce or discontinue drug use, the Intensive Treatment Program provides structured, long-term support. Following an initial period of orientation, an individualized treatment program is developed that includes the definition of specific treatment goals. The program focuses on group psychotherapy, family counseling, comprehensive medical care, "community" meetings, life education workshops, and classes of the person's selection; the participant may also join physically related activities such as sports, martial arts, or dance. The therapeutic milieu of the program provides a sense of belonging that is often absent in the lives of many of these young people.

The duration of the Intensive Treatment Program is approximately two years and consists of four phases:

In *Phase I* (Life Stabilization) the client deals with the realities of her/his present life structure and is introduced to the therapeutic process. This phase takes about three months.

Phase II (Confrontation and Therapy) is of approximately ten months' duration. It helps the young person develop a greater awareness of her/his feelings, conflicts, and patterns of behavior.

Phase III (Reintegration and Exploration of Alternatives) usually lasts for eight months and consists of engaging the client in a search for a meaningful, alternative lifestyle, an exploration of new values, and the development of a new and positive attitude toward life.

Phase IV (Autonomy), the final element of the program, taking about three months, focuses on termination of treatment and complete reintegration within the community. At the end of this period the young person may graduate from the program if she/he has successfully given up drugs, established a constructive and satisfying lifestyle, and demonstrated a high degree of responsibility and autonomy.

Those graduates who have shown themselves to have special therapeutic capabilities are employed as receptionists, youth workers, counselors-in-training, medical or laboratory assistants, or workshop instructors. Those who do not continue to participate in The Door's activities are followed up over a two-year period; contact is made monthly for the first three months, then once at intervals of six months, one year, and two years after termination.

This innovative program has all the elements required for a successful outcome. The services are comprehensive, yet developed exclusively for teenagers. The program is individualized, so that the time course and content are not beyond the control of the adolescent. The Door is able to accommodate 350-400 young people a day, approximately 200 of whom enter the program each month. About 10 percent are appropriate candidates for enrollment in the Drug Treatment Program.

Although The Door is a nationally recognized model program for teenage drug users and other troubled youngsters, its funding problems have not eased over the past few years. Despite acknowledgment by federal and local agencies that the majority of drug-involved adolescents require comprehensive services, The Door is still struggling for survival by piecing its budget together with small grants from multiple sources. The time, energy, and uncertainty inherent in this effort have resulted in a decline in the number of groups attempting to provide this sort of innovative care outside the traditional agencies.

TRAINING PROGRAM FOR PROFESSIONALS

I would now like to describe another approach to drug use that emphasizes innovative training of health professionals in drug use issues, rather than provision of innovative services to teenagers.

For the past twelve years the Division of Adolescent Medicine of the Albert Einstein College of Medicine at Montefiore Hospital has been participating in one such training program in the only secure detention facility for juvenile delinquents in New York City.[7] In the process of providing health care for incarcerated youth, medical students and house

officers learn about the special aspects of adolescent growth and development and the impact of drug use and institutionalization on young people.
The trainees are taught to include a confidential drug history in their initial
assessment and to recognize the clinical expressions of drug abuse during
the physical examination. The appropriate use of laboratory screening tests
in the evaluation of somatic consequences of drug abuse is demonstrated,
and emphasis is placed on the importance of being aware of current trends
in drug usage in the adolescent community.

During the past decade care has been offered to 17,945 drug-using
adolescents. Thirty-seven percent of those tested were found to have
abnormal liver function, but the majority were unaware of a history of
hepatitis. Pediatric house officers have been given an opportunity to observe
the complex interrelationship between drugs and the maturing adolescent
patient.[8]

The trainees are also counseled to be more discriminating in their
analyses of data on the impact of legal intervention in drug abuse. A
superficial review of the effects of the harsh 1973 "Rockefeller drug laws"
in New York, for example, might lead one to believe the use of opiates
declined dramatically after these statutes were enforced. An examination of
the epidemiological patterns of use at the detention center from the late
1960s through the 1970s, however, revealed that the decline preceded these
laws by several years.[9,10]

The detention house setting affords an opportunity to demonstrate the
ethical and legal dilemmas inherent in caring for the drug-using adolescent,
including issues of confidentiality; consent for release of records; and the
role of the health professional in including health needs among the list of
priorities of youngsters with pressing personal, family, and societal conflicts. Thus far approximately 80,000 young people and 400 pediatric
trainees have rotated through the detention center; it is hoped that both
groups have come away with a better sense of the role licit and illicit drugs
play in the life of youngsters identified by legal authorities as being in
trouble.

SOCIAL CONSEQUENCES OF DRUG USE

The last two programs described, The Door, A Center of Alternatives, and
the detention center training program, primarily serve youths who are
disenfranchised from family, school, or work. Many other programs are
geared to the needs and practices of middle-class youngsters. Additional
subgroups, however, require special consideration. Female drug abusers,
for example, have different issues to face than their male counterparts when

confronted with options for care. The intake process, goals, methods of treatment, and outcomes of programs such as methadone maintenance are often heavily weighted toward what is most acceptable to their male clientele.[11] Similarly, the plight of the drug-involved rural youth or minority group member is quite different from that of white middle-class Americans.

Even if the pattern of drug usage were similar among groups of adolescents, the social consequences may differ dramatically. It has been said that the war declared on drug abuse might more accurately be described as a war on the drug abuser. Inner-city minority group adolescents are frequently arrested on suspicion of having committed a crime related to obtaining or using a drug: nine out of ten urban black youths will be arrested on suspicion of some criminal offense during their lifetimes.[12]

Given that the 1979 unemployment rate of urban blacks age sixteen to nineteen is 30 to 35 percent,[13] the combination of unemployment and high rates of arrest for suspected drug-related crimes makes the future of large numbers of American youth appear bleak indeed. In the National Council on Crime and Delinquency survey of employers, 88 percent said they would not consider hiring anyone who had been arrested, even if the person had been acquitted. These data demonstrate the multiplier effect of drug use by inner-city minority youths, where legal involvement and subsequent limited employment opportunities have a far worse effect than the damaging pharmacological properties of the drugs alone.

ESSENTIALS FOR INNOVATIVE CARE

As we now approach the end of the 1970s I would like to reiterate those elements I consider essential for truly innovative care of the drug-involved adolescent.

First must be the recognition that there are distinct subgroups of adolescents who take drugs with a variety of motivations and with very different personal, legal, and social consequences. Most of these individuals use drugs as part of a temporary stage of exploratory behavior that appears to be a normal phase of adolescent development. Innovative care for them should consist of increasing their awareness of their needs as adolescents living in an adult community, and providing acceptable alternatives when necessary.

For the second group of drug-involved adolescents the most successful innovative attempts are those that turn the locus of responsibility back to the teenager or peer group. Health professionals can become advocates for those programs that create a nurturing, safe, supportive background for personal growth and expression without dependence on drugs.

For the third group, traditional structured programs that often seem to restrict rather than to enhance personal freedom and choice, although not innovative, continue to be the mainstay of therapy. Since this group is so small in relation to the others, the emphasis on community care should probably be shifted toward the larger number of drug-involved teenagers in the first two groups.

The challenge for all of us here and for those youngsters and their concerned parents, teachers, and health providers in our respective communities is to recognize the three groups of drug-using adolescents and to design innovative programs for each group. Care should be provided in a manner consistent with our own national traditions, but clearly recognize the unique features of adolescent development that are common to teenagers of all nations.

NOTES

1. World Health Organization Expert Committee, *Health Needs of Adolescents*, Technical Report Ser. 609 (Geneva: World Health Organization, 1977).

2. R.B. Millman, "Drug and Alcohol Abuse," in *Handbook of Treatment of Mental Disorders in Childhood and Adolescence*, ed. B. Wolman, J. Egan, and A. Ross (Englewood Cliffs, New Jersey: Prentice-Hall, 1978): 238-67.

3. M. Kramer, *Psychiatric Services and the Changing Institutional Scene, 1950-1985*, DHEW Publication No. (ADM) 77-433 (Washington: U.S. Government Printing Office, 1977).

4. B. Kissin, J.H. Lowinson, and R.B. Millman, eds., "Recent Developments in Chemotherapy of Narcotic Addiction," *Annals of the New York Academy of Sciences* 311 (1978): 1-313.

5. "Student Association for the Study of Hallucinogens," Educational Offprint Series, *Journal of Psychedelic Drugs* (Madison, Wisconsin: Stash Press, 1979).

6. A.L. McAlister, C. Perry, and N. Maccoby, "Adolescent Smoking: Onset and Prevention," *Pediatrics* 63 (1979): 650-58.

7. K. Hein, M.I. Cohen, I.F. Litt, et al., "Juvenile Detention: Another Boundary Issue for Physicians," *Pediatrics*, in press.

8. I.F. Litt and M.I. Cohen, "The Drug-Using Adolescent as a Pediatric Patient," *Journal of Pediatrics* 77 (1970): 195-202.

9. K. Hein, M.I. Cohen, and I.F. Litt, "Illicit Drug Use among Urban Adolescents: A Decade in Retrospect," *American Journal of Diseases of Children* 133 (1979): 38-40.

10. Joint Committee on New York Drug Law Evaluation, *The Nation's Toughest Drug Law: Evaluating the New York Experience* (Washington: Drug Abuse Council, Inc., 1977).

11. W. Cuskey, L. Berger, and J. Densen-Gerber, "Issues in the Treatment of Female Addiction: A Review and Critique of the Literature," *Contemporary Drug Problems* (1977): 307-71.

12. C.M. Bryan and P. Crawshaw, "Law and Social Policy," in *Core Knowledge in the Drug Field*, ed. L. Philips, G. Ramsey, L. Blumental, et al., National Planning Committee on Training of the Federal Provincial Working Group on Alcohol Problems (Ottawa, Canada: Ministry of Supply and Services, 1978).

13. "Hard Core Jobless Count Politically, Economically," *New York Times* (9 September 1979).

DRUG USE AND ABUSE: INNOVATIVE CARE PROGRAMS IN EUROPE

Claude Olivienstein*

It is difficult to separate the institutional admission and treatment of teen-age drug addicts from the admission and treatment of all drug addicts. Some experts believe that addicts should be placed in facilities with a general patient population consisting, for example, of psychotics and social deviates—marginal elements, delinquents, and sexual deviates. They consider this approach to be an "innovation," in that the addicts are not locked into a hermetically sealed world consisting only of others like themselves; it also creates potential areas of difference that can be useful in the context of the therapy given to drug addicts and to other deviates.

We do not agree with this approach. Aside from certain problems peculiar to members of minority groups and to adults who became addicted in the course of an illness, drug addicts in the Western nations also have problems that are peculiar to, and originate within the limits of, their adolescent years.

Involved here are special relationships with time, especially with time lived, and with space. What is needed is an approach to these specific relationships with time and space and a new concept of therapeutic time

* In preparation for the conference the author consulted the following specialists: Jean Bergeret, professor at the National Center for Defence against Tuberculosis, Lyon; Professor Aldo Calenca of the Hospital Sery in Lausanne, Switzerland; Dr. Nicole Friedrich, Department of Education of UNESCO, Paris; Dr. Rodolphe Ingold, working on a grant with Professor Daniel X. Freedman in Chicago; Professor Henri Loo, Clinic for Mental Diseases, Paris; Professor Madeddu of Milan, Italy; and Professor Pierre Rey, Centre du Levant, Switzerland.

and therapeutic space, the fundamental aspect of which is the institutional setting. We believe this is an innovative concept; it does not vulgarize what drug addiction signifies: the adolescent's search for identity and, alternatively, extremely rapid and infinitely slow flights into contradictory entities.

The completion of the therapeutic circle thus requires us to take this specific nature into consideration so it can be eliminated, not on the grounds of morality or standards of behavior, but because the adolescent is suffering.

We should first like to point out that, contrary to ideas advanced by certain fashionable pragmatists, the adolescent, perhaps more than any other human being, is entitled to an ethical approach to his self and to his suffering. Moreover the end must never justify the means.

THEORIES OF INSTITUTIONALIZATION

Among the dominant theories about the institutionalization of drug addicts, that of Jean Bergeret of Lyon distinguishes three principal methods of operating clinics for addicts:*

• "Fusion" systems treat psychotic or prepsychotic adolescents, or those perceived as such. In such systems the therapist maintains a positive, fusional relationship with the latter's inner "I."

• "Anaclinical" (narcissistic) systems are directed at subjects with depressive tendencies. The technique consists of the therapist's orthopedic reinforcement from outside; the therapist and the institution act as "strong" partners vis-à-vis the "weak" patient in a passive, receptive position.

• In "objective" systems the therapist voluntarily helps the personality to regain its coherence and independence. In centers of this type the guiding personnel are often accused of being "cruel."

The second and third systems operate effectively in what are known as "therapeutic communities."

Each of these systems tends to assume that it has "the" solution. The fact is, we are beginning to realize that each may have good and bad features, and that the failures of a given system result more from its totalitarian dogmatism than from its nature, and from the fact that each is integrated into a polyvalent whole.

We are also beginning to perceive that another source of their failure is their unduly close connection with a psychopathological or sociopathological concept of drug usage, which implies a normative and curative

---

* Jean Bergeret, 1979; personal communication.

connotation. In our opinion their failure can be attributed more to a lack of a harmonious development than to the addict's continued use of toxic substances.

An "innovative" approach to the care of adolescent drug addicts must pay more heed to the dynamic lived experience and to the ludicrous imaginary world of the adolescent than to the similarities to psychotic, depressive, and other structures—similarities that block the adolescent and eliminate the possibility of change.

Experiments are now moving more toward a flexible, polyvalent, and competitive concept of institutions for the treatment of addicts. This concept takes into consideration both the specific nature of drug addiction and the time lived by the adolescent. As the sphere of reflection and action, it introduces the kinetic idea: the rate of growth; the rapidity of the effects—and cessation of the effects—of the drug; the rate at which emotional relationships are established; and the speed of the addict's personality changes, particularly from the nonpathological to the pathological, and vice versa.

The polyvalence and competition among institutions go hand in hand with a range of biomedical, psychotherapeutic, and sociotherapeutic methods. In recent years these methods have produced some successful results—the success rate in terms of serious addiction has risen from 5 percent in 1969 to 30 percent at the present time.

In the following pages we shall limit our consideration essentially to adolescents addicted to so-called "hard" drugs: opiates, amphetamines, barbiturates, and organic solvents.

Obviously, however, there is a preliminary procedure that consists of offering an indiscriminate welcome into a formal structure to any adolescent who is having problems with the use of legal or illegal toxic substances. Such front-line structures play a basic role in guiding the addict toward a given method of acceptance and treatment. At this stage it would be dangerous and unwarranted to specify the type of acceptance and to segregate the adolescent drug user. The screen should be a two-way street, because it is extremely important that the adolescent not feel, or be, trapped.

THERAPEUTIC MEASURES

This does not concern our topic, however; our purpose is to discuss the adolescent who is a permanent and continuous user of hard drugs, which modifies time lived and space. Before analyzing the therapeutic measures, we must show clearly that these relationships are altered in the direction of excess and megalomania.

What makes this particularly important is the fact that adolescence is already a time of searching for an identity model and of rejecting the total illusion of the law of the parents, who are embodied, symbolically, in the leaders of the therapeutic communities. When drugs are consumed this search is completely altered by dazzling trips: the addict feels as though he were God, and when you are God you cannot have a father. But when the effects of the drug wear off, the victim feels worthless and falls into a complete state of melancholia. Thus the alternative is God or nothing. These problems are classic in adolescence, but with drugs they oscillate between vertiginous precipices, added to the continually repeated possibility (denied to the normal adolescent) of becoming God twice, three times, or n times.

Another example is esthetics and the body. When he is "up," the male adolescent may feel as beautiful as Apollo; when he is "down," he may regard his genital organs as ridiculously small, which may lead him to attempt suicide, with the same hypertrophy of values as in the previous example. The addict's relationship with pleasure—a pleasure that is repetitive, quasi-organic, and in all cases nonphantasmic—is unequaled by any other, and only the addicted adolescent enjoys it.

So, because the adolescent does not have the reference points provided by lived experience and the equalizing corrective factor of the years, the frustrations, which are unbearable in comparison with the pleasure and its dazzling modifications, create the outrageous disturbances in behavior and the explosions that are well known to therapists and treatment centers. (It should be noted in passing that force is helpless against memory, which is why imprisonment fails.)

We now understand why only a thorough knowledge of these phenomena, and particularly of the changes in the content of the imaginary world of the addicted adolescent, can enable us to adopt a coherent therapeutic attitude, that is, an attitude that has both an identity and its opposite—ambiguity.

This means the therapeutic attitude must permit flexible transitions from one structure to another and from one attitude to another, provided each of them is identifiable, has a law, and is nondemagogic, that is, it does not replace one dependence with another dependence.

For example, if there is someone the adolescent sees as a father image it is absolutely necessary that the image be destroyed and that there be a period of mourning for his all-powerful image, a process made difficult because it wounds the narcissism of the therapist, who initially is gratified that his strong image is being substituted for that of a parent who is more often perceived as absent than as in conflict.

Parental void; Oedipal archaisms; sharp changes in the psyche, the libido, and the body; pregenital regressions and astonishing trips into an imaginary trans-sideral world; absence of identification; and multiple and bizarre identities—these are the problems we are dealing with, and these are what the treatment must handle.

BIOMEDICAL METHODS

Let us first consider, under these conditions, the contributions of biomedical methods.

Here again things are not simple, for a contradiction is involved: we must first eliminate terrorism, with its dehumanizing aspect, from the medical system; but we must know how to utilize the reassuring points of reference offered to the child by pediatrics.

Any acceptance into a treatment program must include, preferably at the start, a thorough medical examination, if only to reassure the adolescent that he is normal. But we must not ignore the image roles played by the doctor and nurse, and we must learn to utilize them judiciously. We have to recognize the limits of this approach, however: the adolescent drug addict is not a sick person, and we must let him know this.

Moreover, the addict and his family must be warned that there is no vaccination against drug addiction; the problem is a behavioral one, a transgression, and while it represents a refuge from anxiety it is also a search for pleasure. We repeat: it is the recollection of this pleasure that is the principal obstacle to the end of the addiction—and medicine, like prison, is helpless against the memory of pleasure. Medicine occupies a fundamental position, however, that tends to be minimized unduly in the withdrawal stage.

Withdrawal is a period during which the addict expects to suffer, but it is also a time when he is shown it is possible to gain ascendancy over suffering; during this process it is important for the addict to learn how to handle drugs. If the doctor has the capacity to communicate this power and demonstrates its effectiveness, the adolescent will suspend his distrust and accept the fact that the doctor can help him overcome the addiction.

Except for the opinions of certain sadistic behaviorists, the general consensus at this time seems to be that moralistic, punitive techniques must never be employed. Suffering, which for a long time was believed to be unavoidable in withdrawal syndromes, is being increasingly eliminated, either by degressive treatment with morphine-like substances, or by antihypertension drugs that are still in the experimental stage. These products have an advantage: they are not mood elevators. The requirement that the subject be comfortable during the withdrawal period is a most important innovation. Antihypertension drugs have an enormous theoretical advantage, and their significance and practical application should be explored further.

For the first time drugs other than morphine products can block the feeling of a lack without causing the user to regress to the euphoria and the memory, if dimmed, of pleasure. The subjects are precipitated into a feeling of existentialist uncertainty that bears no relation to their previous experience. They can no longer make comparisons, and they have no reference point for the effect of the medication. When it is better understood, this new "space," which is unknown to both the patient and the therapist, can be used for a new psychotherapeutic approach.

Up to the present time maintenance programs have been based on morphine-type substances such as methadone or long-acting methadone, which transform an illegal drug addict into a legal medical patient. For an adolescent who is seeking an identity, however, this status is unacceptable. Maintaining him in the condition of a lifelong drug addict thwarts his chances of "escape," confines him to a specialized institution, and binds him in a collusive position with drugs.

With antihypertension drugs, and in cases where the relationship with drugs is such that the addict's frustration can be alleviated only by using chemical shock absorbers of this type, there is hope of removing the subject from the specialized field by making the drug a routine for him. Prescriptions for these remedies by the family doctor are, at worst, a means of treating a health problem.

We are not yet at this stage; this method offers only the prospect of an initial reaction against the hyperspecialization that is necessary at the present time. In the meantime therapists are aware of the need to provide medical treatment for insomnia, depression, and inability to function, disturbances that for too long have been neglected by psycho- and sociotherapists, and that often lead to a relapse.

We should mention here that epidemiological and anthropological surveys are contributing to our understanding and treatment of adolescent drug addicts. Follow-up studies, unfortunately still fragmentary, are making it possible to recognize that there are two major types of adolescent drug addicts:

• Those who were at high risk from childhood: insomniacs; children who had nightmares; school dropouts; unstable children; runaways; and those from broken homes. Such youngsters, who should be identified before they reach the drug-addict stage, are filling the jails and the special institutions. These are the unfortunate ones whose treatment at the drug-addict level has to oscillate between two contradictory requirements: they must be overprotected and controlled throughout their lives, and the break with their condition as perpetual welfare cases must be organized without precipitating a catastrophe—the only way to free them from their addiction. For this category of addict, the biomedical methods may perhaps offer a guarantee, and a protection against lifelong deviance.

• For well-integrated adolescent addicts, to whom drugs represent a hedonistic encounter at a time when they are having problems recognizing their own sexuality, medical treatment should be very short and rapid; institutional treatment should lead them to find physical satisfaction apart from the autosexuality that drug addiction represents. The largest percentage of therapeutic successes have occurred with this category of addict.

On the level of medical treatment we should stress the training that must be given to pediatricians and general practitioners in order to put an end to the excessive sedation of infants and children that is often discovered in the background of adolescent addicts—just as we too often find that at least one parent takes too many sedatives. The time will come when psychotherapists will have to clash with some elements of the pharmaceutical industry.

To conclude the medical aspects of the treatment of adolescent drug addicts, we should state that theoretical research on a therapy specific to an endogenous and organic cause of drug addiction has not yet discovered a satisfactory practical application. In particular, studies of the brain and knowledge of specific receptors has not led to practical applications. If such an outlet should be found it would be a serious error to ignore the conflicting data on drug addiction, even in an adolescent who has an innate or acquired biological disorder.

OTHER APPROACHES

Specialists are becoming increasingly aware that a multidisciplinary approach has to be taken to this problem. Thus the role of the various types of psychotherapists continues to be one of the essential components in accompanying the adolescent drug addict along the road to a level of maturity at which he can begin to accept a certain degree of frustration.

The nature of the psychotherapies to be selected presents a problem. Psychoanalysts are familiar with Bergeret's story of the "leopard with the helmet": the recommendation was to "remove his helmet and treat him as you would an ordinary leopard." This demand for orthodoxy would seem, at least initially, to be inapplicable. The speed of an analytical cure is incompatible with the speed of the "vibrations" experienced by the drug addict.

Here again empiricism points in the direction of a combination of group and individual techniques. Some replace orthopedics, while others act to increase awareness of the psychic and relational mechanisms that led the drug addict into this particular lifestyle.

As for group techniques, we are familiar with the essential role of games, but greater emphasis is now being placed on the ludicrous aspect that should characterize some games. To achieve this it is necessary to have the use of audiovisual taping equipment, for example, with the participants themselves doing the filming; the tapes should subsequently be shown during criticism sessions.

The use of music is equally important. We refer not to passive listening, but to the formation of musical groups led by a musician-psychologist who guides the participation of each addict in accordance with his personality, and who, working through musical criticism, makes it possible to approach certain personal problems less explosively.

These techniques with increasing frequency involve bodily participation: body expression, acting, massage, acupuncture—all these are being used with a view to, and oriented toward, a method of approach and of contact, to the point where the adolescent describes his symptom: addiction involves a body, a body that moves. The needle is pushed into a selected vein and it changes the body and its reaction just as it changes the imaginary world and the fantasy. In using any of these techniques it must be remembered that they act on two levels.

Individual psychotherapy, however, continues to be the preferred treatment for the adolescent drug addict, who, unlike other adolescents, is incapable of enduring frustration in order to cope with his failings. The therapist must take this into account when organizing the program; he cannot close himself off in temporal and spatial dogmatism; from the outset he must *entice*, just as the flash of drugs entices the addict. He must design the therapeutic program in a flexible manner, without unduly restrictive obligations in terms of time and place—sometimes it may be necessary to go into the field—and also without demagogy. At all times the therapist must affirm his position, so that his relationship with the adolescent will start out by being fusional, gradually become increasingly orthodox, and lead to the patient's acceptance of the frustrations and the indispensable compromises that mark the transition to adulthood.

The concern of the authorities and of members of the addict's family, who may also need to be treated, is understandable in face of the scope of the task and the quasi-elitist nature of this approach. Psychotherapy is often a torment for the family, for it frequently brings to light a swamp of corruption and even intrafamily and intrasocial perversions. Confronted with this prospect, a permanent, healthy alliance should be formed to explore the causes of the disturbances of adolescence.

EFFECTIVENESS OF TECHNIQUES

The paternalistic behavior practiced in some therapeutic communities seems dated; it is gradually being replaced by behavior that is more moderate, less solicitous, and more dehumanized—but also more scientific. With increasing frequency it is relegating dependence on a charismatic personality or a miracle institution to the background by stating it is attacking only the symptom that causes the suffering. The problem is that on the drug addiction scene the family suffers as much as the subject. The current normative view of behaviorism in relation to the state and its powers, whether it be the Soviet or the American model, raises serious ethical problems.

As regards effectiveness, with all the precautions taken these techniques can be viewed only as additions, for by their very nature they ignore the kinetic data characteristic of the adventure of adolescence—biological, sexual, emotional dimensional, and other changes. In the absence of a comprehensive view of the hypertrophied and megalomaniac factors of adolescence, amplified by drugs, the best these techniques can do is make it possible to shift the symptom, replacing the taking of drugs with other transgressions, or, if that is not possible, transferring to serious and repeated depressive disturbances.

Institutional methods represent the most important advance. As mentioned earlier, they take into consideration two basic theoretical factors:

• The idea that time and space for any adolescent vary in accordance with his state of maturation.

• The idea that the time and space of an adolescent who takes drugs have specific and variable meanings.

THE THERAPEUTIC CHAIN

To meet these specific problems it seems essential to avoid focusing the treatment of the adolescent drug addict on a single place and a single time. Here the idea of the "therapeutic chain" becomes extremely important.

Therapeutic chain refers to a group of persons and places that are interrelated, that exchange information, and that come to an agreement as to the end point of the action, but that have different theoretical positions and offer specific places. This chain extends from the indiscriminate acceptance to "specific centers" of any adolescent with problems. These centers can be medical treatment centers; psychoanalytic-type centers; shelters; surrogate families; long- or medium-term residence facilities; therapeutic apartments; marginal communities; ideological communities; or production cooperatives.

Here again we must stress an aspect that is contradictory, but indispensable: each place and each person must have its own characteristic and function. In contrast, the adolescent must, in the event of conflict or distress over a place or a person, and even if he is punished—and punishment is indispensable in relation to the law of acceptance—know there is another place or other persons who can meet his needs.

This does not mean that the aid-and-assistance system is completely linked to the interchanging whims of an adolescent who is "king," and who may indulge in all sorts of errors or transgressions; on the contrary, it means he will be able to choose from among a variety of laws. He will thus have to serve an apprenticeship in various institutions, which, regardless of where it takes place, will teach him that law is necessary to collective and individual survival.

We have learned that if law is present only in the form of a "punishment-cure" the adolescent will become either a lifelong welfare case and a broken human being or a perpetual rebel and delinquent living on the fringes of society. In contrast, if he can see that acceptable laws are embodied in persons who are contradictory, and even in conflict, he will be able to find his place among them and become once again a part of the clan or the tribe, and this will enable him to find his identity.

The diversity of the centers or types of acceptance does not mean that one can do everything, or that optimal standards are the result of the experience. For example, for a center with walls that serves as a long-term residence, it seems necessary to establish in advance a date for release—the idea of a contract made between acceptors and acceptees is basic for these centers, as indeed it is for the addict. The advantage of this system is that it helps the adolescent to realize he has a future for which he must prepare.

To take another example, experience has taught us that both residence centers and treatment centers should have no more than five to twenty adolescents in treatment. When there are fewer than five the result is anxiety and depression or plots; when there are more than twenty the result is anonymity and a return to the world of prison. Finally, all the centers agree that the construction and furnishing of the residence where the adolescent will live is an essential element of the treatment.

In this conception, the gradual change in the adolescent's room is surprising. At the beginning of his residence he removes the furnishings; later he creates a dream world, with posters, an enclosed bed, a Lilliputian atmosphere, and so on; if the treatment is a success, there is a gradual scaling down of the room. Therapists realize the meaning of this remodeling of the addict's room.

We could cite innumerable examples of the little things that have to be done which, when combined, make it possible to create a smooth merger of the many elements that constitute a successful treatment.

The most important factor is that the therapeutic chain be a coherent whole, with different places and personnel, where all the foregoing methods are practiced. The maturing of the adolescent, who at first is incapable of enduring frustration and to whom a certain type of enticement is offered, and who is then forced to grow up, must have as its counterpart a maturing of the offerings: an exploded time and space to begin with, then a more limited space and a limited time at the end of the stretch. The stated goal, which must be a real goal in the minds of the treating personnel, must be the autonomy of the patient. We find it inconceivable that treatment ideology should be pessimistic by nature and consist of maintaining the adolescent in a state of suffering in one way or another until his age and his condition permit him to be channeled toward the medical and criminal assistance of the adult world. The aim of the therapeutic chain, the total action of which now takes place within a two-year period, is the independence of the young person.

In setting up a treatment plan for drug addicts it is completely wrong to show preference for a given method of relational operation, or to establish a hierarchy of methods, assigning a noble activity to one aspect and a lesser role to another. The essential thing is to understand that in a given transition of a single adolescent, or of two adolescents whose cases are identical, a given option may be catastrophic at one point and beneficial at another. Here is where prime importance is attached to the coherence of the entire therapeutic chain, and particularly of its leaders, who must submit to checks and criticism.

The concept described here makes it possible to achieve a 30 percent rate of positive results. In a follow-up study by the French National Institute of Health and Medical Research (INSERM) at the end of a two-year period, 17 percent of the subjects were completely free of trouble and could be considered balanced; 14 percent were off drugs but still had many personal problems. Nevertheless, a 30 percent success rate means a 70 percent failure rate, which in turn means that prevention continues to be the main problem. There are two aspects to prevention:

• First, health education for young people in the context of a genuine policy on youth. Three interesting experiments have been carried out in Canada, Switzerland, and France, using as a test group a number of preadolescents who are given information and perform practical studies on the problems of ecology, alcohol, tobacco, and drugs.

• The detection of children and families who are at risk. This raises the fundamental ethical problem, which cannot be neglected, of the risk of labeling families, particularly the most disadvantaged families.

A combination of these preventive methods and treatment methods, however, is now making it possible to achieve a noticeable improvement in the problem of drug addiction among young people.

DISCUSSION

Separate Services for Drug Abusers

Should services focus on the issue of drug use, or should there be separate services for that problem as opposed to other adolescent concerns? In the British setting, as part of the solution there is a procedure that separates services thought to restrict the contagion of drug use. It sounds as though it is too late for any such system in the United States.

Are the errors of the temperance movement being repeated, in that the focus is on toxicology rather than on graver social ills? And does this mean that access to services is undesirably concentrated on the fact of drug use?

The style in America, at least, is to identify a small part of one problem and to try to solve it, rather than to recognize the unique qualities of the adolescent. First the problem of adolescent drug use was addressed, and then "the problem of adolescent pregnancy." There is a flood of associated establishments running after the tip of the iceberg, which is not the way to go about it. It would make much more sense to provide comprehensive, long-term services for all adolescents rather than to identify one problem or another.

Once one is involved in so-called innovative services, whether a group treatment center or something similar, the usual pattern in America is that the youngsters leave the program whether or not the treatment succeeds; so the end point is always departure. One major emphasis in the creation of an innovative service, whether for the healthy, the emotionally deviant, or the drug-involved adolescent, should be to ensure that it guides them through adolescence, whether they are doing well or not.

Detoxification Process

Hein was asked if a selection procedure is employed, in terms of excluding some adolescents from treatment. Are neuroleptics used? The Door program receives clients of any kind; if they need detoxification that is done in a nearby inpatient unit.

The detention center is rather like the tail end of a Gaussian curve for almost all the patients who are sent there; they usually have no identified family support and are actually placed there by the legal authorities. No self-selection is involved; most of the youngsters do not want to be there. But they are given good medical care during their stay at the detention center, which is, on an average, about two weeks.

As for the pharmacological agents employed, Valium is given. Originally it was given because the detention center was not licensed to give methadone to this younger age group when it opened thirteen years ago. The drug is apparently a safe and quick form of covering the patient during the detoxification period. For opiates this usually takes forty-eight to seventy-two hours, for methadone, five to seven days; for the barbituate addict, phenobarbital is used and detoxification takes about ten days to two weeks. The trouble with giving Valium to an addict, however, is that there is a danger of becoming addicted to the tranquilizer later.

What about hard core dealers? Some centers have had trouble with them. The detention center deals with adolescents up to age sixteen. The population includes relatively few successful pushers and many unsuccessful junkies.

European Programs

A survey has been made of innovative services in eleven European countries under the leadership of the World Health Organization (WHO) Regional Office in Copenhagen. The investigators were impressed by how often these services are either discontinued or change a lot in terms of objectives, clientele, and so on; a follow-up study is therefore being made.

Peer counseling does not seem to be employed often in Western Europe, except, perhaps in England. The Pelletier Report tried to introduce to French schools what were called *Club Chateau la Vie* to improve communication among young people, and especially to prevent deviance. But according to a recent report it seems that this movement has not been very successful.

Leaders of Self-Help Program

One participant was struck by the frequency with which therapeutic leaders are at risk in new drug programs, at least in the United States. Some impressive solutions to the problem are offered by such programs as Odyssey House and Synanon, which depend on a charismatic leader. But often the movement grows and the leader gets richer and richer and more and more important, and then one learns the operation has been corrupt or fascistic.

The second level at which the problem occurs in America is in the self-help groups run by former addicts under the guise of therapeutic programs. It often turns out that some leaders are in fact maintaining their own habit; some are even pushing drugs. Perhaps it is inevitable, for the drugs represent a hazard for both therapists and patients, and some people are lost along the way. But despite the fact the there are some crooks in the machinery, on an overall basis the programs do more good than harm.

In France, also, one has this phenomenon of dependence on the charismatic leader and the many abuses that arise as a consequence. The problem can even be encountered in the scientific community. To combat this, the authorities have tried to create plural institutions, so that one idea never dominates. Control is in the hands of governmental authorities, and special inspectors of health deal with the problem. There are also associations of therapists that meet annually and criticize the people whose programs are not conducted properly. In that respect the media sometimes play an ambivalent role by excessively evaluating one category of therapist, and, at the same time, trying to destroy certain others. But on the whole their influence is for the good.

In the New York detention center program, what is called the third group—the hardcore addicts—is so down-and-out in terms of personality, economic disadvantage, self-esteem, and a support system that it is certainly open to deviant leadership. But the problem is somewhat more widespread than that of one or two crazies leading a group of urban nomads nowhere. There has been a shift from racial discrimination toward fear and hatred of delinquents, which in many ways is just a masked form of racial discrimination because so many of the youngsters are minority group members. The solution does not lie in trying to identify better leadership for these groups: they are down-and-out, and they will remain so as long as our society has a need to identify a scapegoat group.

Use of Community Resources

Hein was asked to what degree, in dealing with adolescents, particularly younger adolescents, community resources and the community itself are involved—mention was made of clubs, neighborhood units, churches, and other groups. Second, what attempts are made to work with the families of the adolescents, who are also at risk?

For the younger population, particularly, the approach should be toward the community, which has resources that could be mobilized and harnessed for such programs. The community agencies in the New York City area, for example, certainly are extensively organized, with various clubs and neighborhood organizations, including black and Hispanic church groups.

Attitude of Professionals

If one looks back to the early 1960s when the addiction rate first started to rise in the United States, followed several years later in Europe, the professionals, by and large, avoided this field; it was considered dirty work, and the few who were involved tended to be scorned by their colleagues—it was not nice clean work like dealing with schizophrenics. Many of the self-help groups started at that same time because nobody else was doing anything.

It was not until the problem became enormous and the federal government started putting a lot of money into rehabilitation programs that a number of professionals and others saw the opportunities.

There is a not too dissimilar history in the United States in regard to the care of the mentally retarded. The approach was not how these individuals could be helped, but how to keep them out of institutions and clinics because they were difficult to treat and they did not respond.

Once the shift occurred to look for solutions to drug addiction following the medical model, and to have doctors become involved, it soon became apparent that this was not going to be the answer. That is why there is now a shift back toward educational and other models for prevention and treatment.

Drugs as Big Business

No one at this meeting has looked at the phenomenon in another way: in the United States drugs represent a very sizable business. The people who peddle drugs are happy to see therapeutic and detoxification centers set up because they preserve their customers; moreover they make only marginal dents in the size of the market. Whoever comes up with a really effective antiheroin agent that threatens to cut into that market had better surround himself with armed guards because he will be in mortal peril.

Crime in America is a big business that compares favorably in size with a number of large industrial enterprises, and it obviously has a receptive field of customers. So, in addition to all the aspects of the addict's side of the picture, what about the question of the drug industry and its potential to maintain itself? If one were to make a study of automobiles and accident prevention one would not do so without considering the market for automobiles. What about the drug industry, the "General Motors of heroin?"

Fred Goldman in New York has written extensively about the economics of the drug industry. He not only makes the point that it is big business and that an enormous amount of money is involved, but that it is a very important industry for professionals, many of whom would be without jobs were it not for the existence of drug addicts.

Drug Addiction versus Emotional Disturbances

The trouble with creating drug treatment services is that they have a way of making the problem look much larger than it really is. One Vietnam veteran became addicted while he was there, but by the time he came back to the United States he was completely off drugs. He later got into trouble with the law and decided that the solution was to shoot up with heroin so he could get certified as an addict and go into a treatment program, rather than to jail. He did just that, and it did keep him out of jail.

People who work in adolescent drug programs find that many youngsters present themselves as addicts because the program exists, but drugs are not their real problem. Robins, when interviewing a veteran in a VA hospital drug program, was trying out a new technique. When she came to a question about depression, his mouth dropped open and he said: "What kind of a doctor are you?"; he felt she was reading his mind because he had been in the program for months, but had never been asked about his depressive symptoms.

That is essentially what happens in a VA drug program, which is usually operated by one doctor and a large staff of counselors. The doctor almost never sees the patients, and no one ever asks them about symptoms. They are treated as drug patients. That is very unrepresentative of what the problems really are. In interviews with Vietnam veterans, when they were asked about the drugs with which they had problems they had many more with amphetamines and with alcohol than they had with heroin. The programs do not meet the need.

The issue is not that we should not have drug programs, but that they should be different—they should be viewed as an opportunity. To underscore the point Hein made, we need more comprehensive services and more awareness of the intercorrelated other behaviors.

TEENAGERS AS PARENTS: DEVELOPMENTAL ISSUES IN SCHOOL-AGE PREGNANCY

Beatrix A. Hamburg

In October 1978 the 95th Congress of the United States passed Senate Bill 2910, the "Adolescent Health Services and Pregnancy Prevention and Care Act of 1978." The bill describes the findings of Congress regarding "the high risk of unwanted pregnancies among adolescents, the severe adverse health, social and economic consequences of adolescent pregnancy and parenthood, and the lack of availability of services to assist these adolescents." Although the bill provides for the care of young women up to age twenty-one, a major impetus for the legislation is a national concern about the trend toward increasing numbers of very young adolescents, age fifteen and under, who are becoming pregnant, carrying the pregnancy to term, and keeping the babies. The depth of congressional concern about these problems is reflected in the fact that the bill authorized appropriations of $60 million for fiscal year 1979, $70 million for 1980, and $80 million for 1981. Despite this dramatic legislation, however, by the end of 1979 only $1 million had been spent on new programs to meet these needs.

Teenage pregnancy is a highly visible issue that is viewed with great alarm; it has even been called a national epidemic.[1] The reasons for these recent high levels and rising rates of early adolescent sexual activity and fertility are not clearly understood. Systematic research on the antecedents and consequences of adolescent parenthood was virtually nonexistent prior to 1976; since then there has been a steep rise in research attention to selected dimensions of the problem. Some of the major findings will be reviewed briefly. For the most part they describe the perinatal outcomes for mother and child and the long-term economic consequences for the mother.

The focus of this paper is on early adolescence. Reasons are given for delineating early adolescence as a distinct life stage, and the developmental characteristics of this period are described in detail. The match of these characteristics with parenting roles and developmental tasks is discussed, as are typical social, psychological, educational, and economic outcomes for the young mother. Some physical, cognitive, and psychological outcomes for the child are also given. These discussions are placed in a lifespan context in which the implications of the asynchronous timing of events in the life cycle can help explain the altered maternal life course and the role confusion for the child, teenage mother, and maternal grandmother. Finally, there is some discussion of probable future trends with and without specific interventions.

DEFINITIONS

The tasks of trying to marshal data, sort out significant issues, and plan meaningful interventions have been complicated by semantic confusion. In the area of teenage pregnancy there is a lack of consensus within the ranks of medical professionals and social scientists on the meaning of most of the commonly used terms. My definitions and use of terms in this paper will be specified for the sake of clarity.

Early adolescence covers the ages of twelve to fifteen. In the United States this coincides roughly with attendance at junior high school. The unitary construct of adolescence should be further divided into a middle adolescent period—sixteen to eighteen—which coincides with high school attendance. In the United States high school is usually completed by age eighteen. Late adolescence is also a distinctive phase and should refer to individuals age eighteen and older who are still in transition to adult roles.

School-age pregnancy appears to be a preferable term to teenage pregnancy. The occurrence of pregnancy in a school-age girl poses high risk in the multiple ways that will be elaborated in this paper. The same issues do not apply to post-high school eighteen- and nineteen-year-old mothers. In conventional usage adolescent or teenage populations usually include persons through the age of nineteen. It is misleading to group the data for all teenage pregnancy and childbearing because the significant differences between early and late adolescence are obscured. Fertility rates and birth trends vary for the different teenage cohorts. Rates of childbearing for the oldest teenagers have shown a decline in recent years, whereas rates for early adolescents are rising. The lumping of data does occur, however, and some of them can be usefully reported. In these instances *teenager* will be used, and should signify that the term includes eighteen- and nineteen-year-olds in addition to the younger age groups.

Inappropriate pregnancy. This term is chosen instead of unwanted pregnancy to reflect the fact that, particularly among younger adolescents, many of the pregnancies are desired even though they are not planned. After the birth, however, the responsibility for the baby may be unwanted. These are issues that will be discussed more fully later in this paper.

Families. In this usage the term will be broadened beyond the immediate unit of the school-age mother and her child. Family will be used in the standard Census Bureau definition of members related by blood, marriage, or adoption who live together in one household; beyond that it is also useful to include the wider family kinship network of persons not living in the household. Finally, the family of the teenage father should be included as a third relevant family sector.[2]

SCOPE OF THE PROBLEM

The nature and extent of the problem is fairly well documented. The childbearing rate of American teenagers is among the highest in the industrial world. Of twenty-two industrial countries studied, the United States ranks nineteenth in the number of births to females between age fifteen and nineteen: 58 per 1,000. The range is from 5 per 1,000 in Japan to 72 in East Germany and Bulgaria. The same study reports that approximately 600,000 American teenagers give birth each year.[3]

In the past decade overall fertility rates have declined sharply in the United States. Birth rates among very young teenagers are increasing, however, while the rates for all other age groups are declining. Because of this differential in fertility rates, births to teenage mothers are now a higher percentage of all births—up from 14 percent of the total births in 1960 to almost 20 percent in 1974.[4]

Table 1 shows the number of births and percent changes for American teenagers between 1961 and 1977. This clearly underscores the fact of differential fertility rates: there has been a 17.8 percent decline in births for eighteen- to nineteen-year-olds. School-age adolescents show a rising trend, with an increase of 54.8 percent for girls under age fifteen.

For reasons chiefly related to ignorance, early adolescents use virtually no birth control methods other than abortion. Typical reasons reported by girls for failure to use contraceptives are: "wrong time of the month," 39.7 percent; "low risk of pregnancy," 30.9 percent; contraceptive unavailable,

TABLE 1. NUMBER AND PERCENTAGE OF BIRTHS TO AMERICAN TEENAGERS,
1961 AND 1977

Age (Years)	1961	1977	Percent Change
Under 15	7,400	11,455	+54.8
15-17	178,000	213,788	+20.1
18-19	424,000	348,366	−17.8

SOURCES: National Center for Health Statistics, unpublished tabulations. U.S. Congress, Senate, Human Resources Committee, statement prepared by Wendy Baldwin, Ph.D., Center for Population Research, National Institute of Child Health and Human Development, 14 June 1978.

30.5 percent; and interfere with pleasure, 23.7 percent; only 6.5 percent reported wanting a baby as the reason.[5,6]

Figure 1 shows that the rate of abortion for the under fifteen age group is far higher than for any other age group. Nonetheless about 50 percent of school-age pregnant girls decide to carry the pregnancy to term, and over 95 percent elect to keep the baby.[7]

Early and out-of-wedlock childbearing tend to be linked. Table 2 indicates that 85 percent of births to mothers under age fifteen are out of wedlock. Early pregnancy, married or not, usually means the end of formal schooling for the girl.

SOCIAL CHANGE AND ADOLESCENT
SEXUAL PATTERNS

There seems very little doubt that there has been a significant recent rise in the amount of sexual activity among adolescents and a trend toward increasingly younger ages of initiation. It seems unlikely that the downward trend in age of initiation and the increase in the overall level of adolescent sexual activity can be largely attributable to biological changes leading to earlier maturation. The secular trend toward earlier menarche has generally been accepted as only three months per decade. Furthermore, in the more affluent and healthy sectors of the world, secular declines appear to have leveled off.[8] In any event the sharp rises in sexual activity of adolescents have far outstripped the rates of biological change: there has

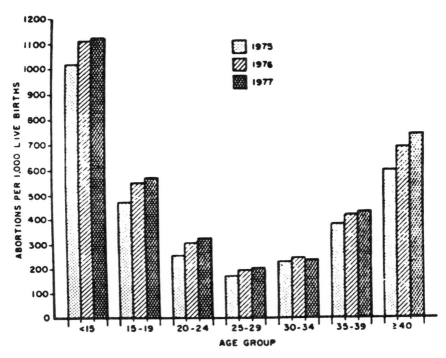

Figure 1. Legal abortion ratios, by age, the United States, 1975-77.
SOURCE: National Center for Health Statistics, *Abortion Surveillance Reports for 1975, 1976, and 1977* (Washington: U.S. Government Printing Office, 1977): Table 6. Based on all states with data available: 34 in 1975; 36 in 1976; and 37 in 1977.

been at least a doubling of rates of sexual activity in recent decades. This can be illustrated using the example of data on fifteen-year-old girls: in 1953 A. Kinsey reported a sexual activity rate of 3 percent;[9] A. Lake reported a rate of 6 percent in 1966;[10] for 1971 and 1976 J.F. Kantner and M. Zelnick reported rates of 13.8 and 18 percent, respectively.[11] When H. Presser studied age at menarche, sociosexual behavior, and fertility, she found that age of menarche was not a good predictor of the timing of the first birth—age at first intercourse was the best predictor, and this in turn was strongly related to age at first dating experience.[12]

The United States has had a long history of a double standard regarding sexual activity. There is evidence, however, that females are now beginning to narrow the traditional gap between the sexes in terms of rates

TABLE 2. PERCENT OF OUT-OF-WEDLOCK BIRTHS TO AMERICAN TEENAGE GIRLS,
1960 AND 1974

Age (Years)	1960	1974
	(Percent)	
Under 15	68	85
15-17	24	48
18-19	11	27
All under 20	15	36

SOURCES: National Center for Health Statistics, *Trends in Illegitimacy, United States, 1940-1965*, Vital and Health Statistics Series 21, no. 15 (Washington: U.S. Government Printing Office, February 1968): Table 9. National Center for Health Statistics, "Advance Natality Statistics 1974," *Monthly Vital Statistics Report*, 24, no. 11, suppl. 2 (13 February 1976): Table 11.

of sexual activity. This trend is also true for smoking and alcohol and drug use, where current female rates have risen over the past decade and are now nearly comparable to those of males.

It would appear that a confluence of social factors has independently and collectively shaped an enduring change in the societal stance toward approval of increased sexual freedom for both married and unmarried persons.[13] Since 1960 there have been significant developments in birth control technology; the legalization of abortion; a sharp rise in the number of working women; and liberalized perceptions of women's roles. Moreover, the youth of the nation has been influenced considerably by the rise of the counterculture in the middle and late 1960s, with its emphasis on hedonism and the linking of drugs, free sex, and rock music as a youthful lifestyle. Most recently the media and movies have glamorized the sexiness of early adolescents, portraying them in roles of explicit sexuality. *Time* magazine referred to "Hollywood's Whiz Kids" in a recent admiring cover story.[14]

There appears to be a very recent upsurge in motivated pregnancies.[15,16] There are disquieting reports in the press that indeed there is a burgeoning fad of "baby chic," whereby pregnancy is perceived as giving higher status to schoolgirls.[17] One hopes this is a passing fad, but it is disturbing to read that at the end of the first month of the 1979 school year some high schools report that the number of pregnant girls equals the total for the entire 1978 school year.

The recent congressional tendency to limit access to abortions paid for by public funds may be significant. If the trend toward an increase in sexual activity in early adolescence and resistance to the use of contraception by this age group is coupled with sharp restrictions on access to abortion it seems likely that school-age parenthood could continue to rise even more sharply. In an article that projects trends from existing demographic data, C. Tietze predicts a substantial increase in out-of-wedlock births for early adolescents unless protective interventions are introduced.[18]

PARENTING ROLES AND DEVELOPMENTAL CHARACTERISTICS OF EARLY ADOLESCENCE

Early adolescence as a distinctive developmental period has received sparse attention until recently because of the pervasive tendency to view adolescence as a unitary period of development. As a result the specific and relevant issues of this period are poorly understood by those who deal with early adolescents.

Since this group represents a sizable and expanding proportion of teenage parents, it is worth examining the fit between their normative attributes and abilities and the tasks of parenthood. For the school-age parents this "goodness-of-fit" has serious implications for the course of the adolescents' own growth and development and for the future of the children to be nurtured by them. This is a neglected area of research, but an analysis must be done in order to target effective preventive, supportive, and remedial services to these very young parents. Lacking the benefit of a consistent, informed approach, many efforts so far have been disappointing and have failed to reverse the disturbing trends of high birth rate and poor outcome for both mother and child.

DEVELOPMENTAL TASKS OF EARLY ADOLESCENCE

Three sets of novel preemptive challenges inevitably confront the early adolescent. The first set relates to the multiple impacts of the biological changes of puberty; the second derives from entry into the new environment of junior high school; the third reflects the problems of sudden entry into the new role status of adolescence that is conferred by virtue of entering junior high school. These new role expectations are poorly defined for both the young persons and the adults who deal with them, and thus the ambiguity concerning early adolescent role behaviors becomes a stress in its own right.

For early adolescents there is the sharpest possible discontinuity with past situations. Their novel problems often defy familiar ways of behaving, and it is not possible to draw on analogous past experience as a source of relevant information to guide their actions. At this critical time the previously dependable sources of parental and school support are often weakened or withdrawn. The special adaptive challenge posed by confronting three superimposed developmental tasks is often underestimated. Anticipatory coping is not used, and networks of familial and other social supports that might serve to attenuate, regulate, or otherwise modify the stressful impacts are not provided because of the general lack of awareness of the predictable tasks and challenges of the period.[19]

BIOLOGICAL CHANGES OF PUBERTY

J.M. Tanner has stated that

> for the majority of young persons, the years from 12 to 16 are the most eventful ones of their lives so far as their growth and development is concerned. Admittedly during fetal life and the first year or two after birth development occurred still faster . . . but the subject himself was not the fascinated, charmed, or horrified spectator that watches the developments, or lack of developments, of adolescence.[20]

This quotation underscores the psychological impact of pubertal events, but it also reminds us that puberty is more than a time of sexual changes—it is a time of general growth spurt; changes in facial contours; in fat distribution; in psychological functions; in pelvic proportions; and in muscular strength and development. These are at least as important as the changes in genitalia and secondary sex characteristics, and they function independently in shaping the course of development.

Furthermore, the changing gonadal hormones may have direct effects on emotional lability, moods, and behaviors of the young adolescent. Typical ages are generally given for the timing of these pubertal events: for example, menarche at age twelve and a half. Comparable midpubertal events for males usually lag roughly two years behind the female. The range for the occurrence of pubertal change is very great, however: the normal range of ages for onset of pubertal changes in girls is from eight and a half to thirteen;[21] the same investigators found the range for boys to be from ten to fifteen.[22]

It has been established that the timing of puberty—early versus late maturation—has significant and differential behavioral consequences for boys and girls.[23-25] Parents, teachers, health providers, and adolescents themselves are not acquainted with these or other facts of normal pubertal development that might spare much needless worry. National surveys, both public and private, have consistently shown over several decades that there is a steep upsurge in bodily concerns between the ages of twelve and fifteen.[26-28]

SEX EDUCATION

Given the recent national trend toward heightened early adolescent sexual activity and the rising rates of school-age pregnancies, there is research interest in learning about the extent, sources, quality, and effectiveness of sex information and preparation for sexual activity that teenagers are receiving. Data are still rather sparse, but the accumulated evidence indicates there is very little communication about sex in the home.[29-33] These studies demonstrate that parents are never cited by adolescents as their first or major source of sex instruction. It is typical to find that 20 percent of mothers of seventh grade girls have never told them about menstruation; 50 percent have not discussed the male role in reproduction; and 68 percent have not discussed any aspect of birth control.[34] When literature is offered, or when sexual matters are discussed in the family, the mother is the usual agent. It has also been noted, however, that the impact of parental communication about sex is significant. Available research indicates that even minimal attempts at sex education are associated with postponement of the age of sexual activity; when daughters are already sexually active, parental discussions seem to be related to the most effective use of contraception.[35,36] Unfortunately, methods to enhance parental involvement in sex instruction are not considered an important ingredient of family planning services for teenagers. On the contrary, there is an erroneous belief that adolescents benefit from disengagement from parents, particularly in sexual discussions and decisions.

Neither are schools a major source of sex information. Many schools avoid the topic because of parental and political pressures based on the conviction that presenting the issue leads to promiscuity. When material is offered in schools it is often highly anatomical, overly didactic, and of little practical use. Early adolescents are for the most part dependent on haphazard and often distorted information derived from their peers and from the media. Physicians are viewed by adolescents as a potentially good source of information,[37] but they seldom visit physicians.

The biology of pregnancy, medical aspects of childbirth, and facts of child development have, if possible, received even less attention in the

education of early adolescents. Again this ignorance has serious consequences for both parents and child. Even at the high school level most
adolescents are unaware of the early pregnancy risks for mother and fetus.
They do not, for example, know about the hazards to the fetus of smoking
or alcohol consumption; such ignorance may contribute to their failure to
seek early or regular prenatal care.

Early adolescents also display very unrealistic and highly precocial
expectations for the timing of developmental milestones of infants and
children. They expect and want infants who are capable of a high degree of
independent activity from the time of birth.[38] The same study revealed that
very young mothers report they are often intolerant of crying and tend to
use physical punishment when babies cry or do not meet their unrealisti-
cally high expectations. Early adolescent mothers are clearly unprepared
for a small, often sickly baby who will have a prolonged period of
helplessness and dependence. The mother's immaturity, impulsiveness, and
low frustration tolerance add to the risk of abuse of the child as well as to a
sense of personal failure and unhappiness.

CHALLENGES OF JUNIOR HIGH SCHOOL

The drastic change in school format from the self-contained classroom of a
small elementary school to the rotating classes of a very large junior high
school represents one of the most abrupt and demanding transitions of the
educational career. Elements that contribute to the high rate of distress
are: 1) a general sense of confusion about the bigness and complexity of the
new school format; 2) insecurity about inability to cope with the interpersonal demand of having to relate to a different teacher and a different group
of students on an hourly basis; 3) concern about the ability to make and
hold friends; 4) ignorance about role expectations now that they are
considered to be adolescents; and 5) fear of academic failure.

A great many students have deep-seated fears of academic inadequacy
and failure. One important issue for early adolescents is their perception of
the sharp escalation in academic demands, both in terms of expected output
and complexity of tasks; evidence tends to confirm that such fears may be
well-founded. Studies in the 1960s demonstrated a startling drop in school
performance associated with entrance to junior high school;[39] in a study by
C. Armstrong in New York, 45 percent of the boys and girls with good
elementary school records performed at a poor level in junior high school.[40]
The author further noted that whereas grades in elementary school were
closely related to intelligence, intelligence was largely unrelated to the
changes in performance at the junior high level.

Despite the fact that *intelligence* per se is not an issue in the school performance of early adolescents, it is worth reexamining their style of cognitive functioning. By and large it has been assumed that early adolescents move to logical operations and abstract thinking,[41] but several lines of evidence suggest this is not generally true. First, teachers of high school students invariably report they are unable to succeed with the same approach in junior high school. E.C. Martin states that

> when I moved from high school to junior high school teaching I was an experienced teacher with a reputation for good performance. I went to my class of eighth graders with confidence. After forty-five minutes, I knew I had entered a different world and would have to begin learning about teaching again. . . . These were people who were different from the fifteen- to eighteen-year-olds I had been teaching.[42]

Teachers are frustrated unless they revise their presentations from the predominantly logical and abstract to a more concrete approach.

Recent research indicates that the junior high school student is deficient in the ability to make valid generalizations, use symbols, and process information with objectivity. Data indicate that although some formal operational abilities begin to emerge during the early adolescent period, abilities such as "controlling variables"—the strategy of holding other things constant while exploring the effect of one variable on an outcome—may be atypical among early adolescents. The results of R. Karplus and colleagues suggest that performance of these tasks may benefit from instruction.[43] Further research is required, however, to establish the degree to which these skills are teachable to modal individuals at the early adolescent cognitive level. The National Science Foundation has reviewed cognitive issues with emphasis on the implications for teaching science to early adolescents.[44] Such research is also applicable to devising an appropriate junior high school curriculum for the teaching of social skills, interpersonal relationships, and decision-making processes.

Investigations in other areas of reasoning are relevant to early adolescents. A. Tversky and D. Kahneman have shown that some adults consistently tend to regard samples as overly representative of the populations from which they are drawn.[45] The prevalence and significance of logical errors and biases of this kind in early adolescents should be investigated. Results from survey data show that early adolescents systematically overestimate the prevalence of certain peer behaviors. For example, when the actual baseline rate of smoking in a school was 15 percent, most students estimated the level of smokers to be over 80 percent.[46] Similarly, F. Furstenberg, Jr. reports that, when asked about the prevalence of sexual activity, early adolescents report with evident sincerity that "everybody is doing it.''[47] A consistent tendency to errors due to overgeneralizations could help explain the exaggerated impact of peer and media influences on early adolescents.

D. Elkind has described the egocentrism of adolescents as showing its peak in the ages that correspond to early adolescence—twelve to fifteen.[48] One aspect of their egocentrism may be a belief in personal uniqueness, which Elkind calls "personal fable." This cognitive stance may underlie a "here and now" time perspective in which long-term consequences and future happenings do not have salience. It may also explain ideas of invulnerability that allow early adolescents to persuade themselves that they can safely take a known risk. When this immediate time perspective and the sense of invulnerability are coupled with failure to comprehend laws of probability, young adolescents may be especially prone to engage in unprotected sexual encounters with a false sense of confidence. Disbelief and denial that she can actually be pregnant also tend to lead an early adolescent girl to a pattern of delayed obstetrical attention. At times this delay may result in a pregnancy that has progressed beyond the point when an abortion can be done with safety. Similar denials about the health and well-being of the infant could compromise its health care.

Middle and junior high school teachers need to be made aware of the diversity in cognitive abilities that characterize early adolescents. A significant amount of information has been collected on the range of individual differences in their logic and reasoning skills.[49] Discrepancies in rates of cognitive development parallel the early versus late maturation in physical development in early adolescence. Further research is needed to establish the synchrony, if any, between the timing of physical and cognitive maturity. In any event, it is known that even when more mature levels of cognitive functioning are attained there is a strong tendency for reversion to concrete information processing at times of stress and anxiety. It is important to realize that most early adolescents are highly unlikely to be successful at improvising or at making balanced, effective decisions when confronted with the novelty and anxieties that may arise in parenting situations.

SELF-ESTEEM IN EARLY ADOLESCENTS

In large-scale studies in Baltimore and Milwaukee schools, R. Simmons and coworkers found that self-esteem typically drops when students enter junior high school.[50,51] Young adolescent white girls in the sixth and seventh grades showed the lowest self-esteem of the students tested. When a matched group of early-maturing girls in the sixth and seventh grades of an elementary school was compared with sixth and seventh grade junior high school girls, the former did not show a comparable fall in self-esteem. It was postulated that the girls in elementary school were shielded from the added social and sexual pressures that characterized the junior high school experience. In earlier studies of youth self-esteem, M. Rosenberg found that low self-esteem correlates with characteristic attitudes and responses. The individual is more vulnerable in interpersonal relations: is deeply hurt by criticism, for example; is relatively awkward with others; finds it hard to make conversation or to initiate contacts; assumes that others think poorly of or do not particularly like her/him; tends to put up a "front" with people; feels relatively isolated and lonely; and has low faith in people. Rosenberg states that:

> Low self-esteem makes them relatively submissive or unassertive in their dealings with others. . . . It is thus apparent that the individual's self-conception is not only associated with attitudes towards other people, it is also associated with his actions in social life and the position he comes to occupy in his high school peer groups.[52]

The attributes associated with low self-esteem represent attitudes and behaviors that diminish coping potential, heighten stress, and accentuate any preexisting tendencies to resort to maladaptive solutions.

ADOPTION OF ADOLESCENT ROLE

Entry into junior high school means leaving behind the familiar world of childhood—it defines entry into the status of adolescence. For some major role transitions such as marriage or entering the work force there are well-defined expectations for behaviors, and often a period of preparation. Early adolescents are catapulted into their new role status with no preparation and with very vague conceptions about the attitudes, behaviors, prescriptions, and prohibitions appropriate to that role. Unfortunately there is a comparable ambiguity on the part of the adults who surround them.

In the early history of the United States the cognitive, physical, and temperamental changes associated with puberty occurred in a context in which the postpubertal individual was immediately inducted into needed adult roles for which the biosocial changes were well suited. Modern postindustrial society accentuates the discrepancy between the biological proclivities and potentialities of the young person and the demands of the culture and its social institutions.

The newly labeled adolescent feels an immediate need for a new set of behaviors, values, and reference persons. She/he is aware that significant adults relating to her/him often have a reciprocal expectation that they will, in turn, now have different standards and new ways of relating to the early adolescent. The uninitiated person aspiring to a new status often tends to respond to the most conspicuous and stereotyped features of the new role. The adolescent may assume postures of exaggerated independence, often accompanied by derisive and rebellious attitudes toward parents, in particular, and perhaps toward adults in general. In response to the stereotype of emancipation, the early adolescent may also slavishly adopt styles of hair, clothing, and behaviors identified as characteristic of the youth culture. Sexual activity is a visible vehicle for testing new role behaviors.

The bulk of literature on adolescence actually derives from descriptions of the late adolescent phase. Unfortunately they are applied indiscriminately to all adolescents. Parents, in seeking guidelines for appropriate behavior in relation to their child's transition, find an emphasis on the adolescent's need for independent decision making and the development of autonomy. When taken literally this can lead to a significant renunciation of parental prerogatives and support, which may in turn lead to heightened distress on the part of the early adolescent. The result is that, in a time of major discontinuity, accustomed parental guidance is withdrawn and the young person is thrust towards uncriticial acceptance of the peer group as a model and as a major coping resource. While this uncritical allegiance to the peer group may be useful in allaying immediate anxieties, it has serious limitations: the peer group at this stage is usually too shallow and too limited to afford the necessary resources for growth and development. J. Loevinger finds that typical junior high school students are at "Stage 2" of ego development, which is characterized by impulsiveness and exploitation. When the peer group is organized around alcohol, hard drugs, and/or acting-out behaviors there is potential for considerable damage.[53]

Before junior high schools existed, a child advanced to eighth grade in an elementary school setting and premature issues of autonomy rarely occurred. As the junior high school student is usually between age twelve and fourteen, there is still four to six years before the issue of separation from the home and the parents will become real. A strong posture of independence at this early stage is not linked with a valid developmental transition. It is therefore inappropriate to convey to early adolescents and to their parents the idea that the emphasis should be on the achievement of independence; instead it should be on parental stability and guidance at a time of major superimposed biological, educational, and social discontinuity. The early adolescent cannot possess the competence and mastery needed for full independence. The early and mid-adolescent phases represent the necessary training ground and biological preparation for the achievement of autonomy by late adolescence. The success with which these earlier phases are negotiated will of course affect the final outcome of adolescent development.

TIMING OF EVENTS, AGE, AND LIFE COURSE

As individuals move through the lifespan their careers reflect a succession of culturally defined roles, which to a very great extent are age linked. Rather explicit age norms exist for the such major transitions as leaving home, getting married, having children, assuming adult work roles, and retiring. B. Neugarten has discussed the adverse consequences that can flow from pronounced deviations from the culturally approved time schedule, whether the "off-time" is too early or too late.[54]

In the usual course of events, pregnancy is expected to occur in an adult who has completed schooling and has experienced a period of adjustment to the demands of marriage. Too early timing of the first birth, whether it occurs in or out of wedlock, has profound negative implications for the subsequent life course of the mother.

The correlates of early parenthood, married or not, are:

• Dropping out before finishing high school. This is a result of the pregnancy, and not vice versa. When variables such as race, socioeconomic status, academic ability, and expectations regarding college are controlled, the adolescent childbearers do not complete high school, and matched controls graduate at a significantly higher rate.[55-58]

• Unemployment or menial jobs at low pay as both a short- and long-term consequence of a limited education.[59-61].

• High probability of welfare or aid for dependent children (AFDC) status: among AFDC recipients 61 percent are mothers who started families as teenagers; $4.6 billion was spent on such families in 1975.[62-64]

• Marital instability: 72 percent of teenage marriages break up; high probability of numerous changes in marital status; considerable time as a single parent and female family head.[65,66]

• High likelihood of a second pregnancy within two years of the first birth.[67]

• High subsequent lifetime fertility. Women age seventeen or younger average five children; close spacing; more children than desired. Comparable women over age twenty at the time of first birth average three children over a lifetime—other factors held constant.[68,69]

• Social isolation: no dependable reference group of peers or family relationships as a network of social support.[70]

• Negative effects on the physical, cognitive, and emotional development of the child.[71,72]

A perspective of sociohistorical context interacting with life stage can help us understand the current crisis of teenage parenthood. Individuals born since 1960 have moved through their developmental stages in a time of rapid social change that has had an effect on societal values and institutions. These young people have felt the continuing impact of significant developments such as changes in the traditional roles of women; advances in the technology and availability of contraception; legalization of abortion; more openness about and media emphasis on sexuality; and a decline in the stigma once attached to out-of-wedlock pregnancy.

Individuals who attained adolescence in the early 1970s are reported to engage in more sexual activity; tend not to use contraceptives; become pregnant at a greater rate; and become parents at an early age.

Women who were young adults and those who were approaching middle age reacted to the same events with a sharp decline in pregnancy and birth rates; they were knowledgeable and conscientious users of contraceptives. Further, for more mature women there was a heightened emphasis on jobs and careers: the number of working women has increased dramatically in recent years. The women of this generation are the mothers of the adolescents just described. Their daughters' pregnancies, school dropouts, and the restrictions on their future job/career opportunities come as a bitter disappointment to many of these women, regardless of their socioeconomic status. Their resulting anger and frustration over the changed life prospects is one source of the intergenerational conflict between mothers and pregnant teenage girls. Thus differential effects of sociohistorical events have been felt by women, depending on the life stage of the individual at the time of the experience. As has been noted, adult women moving through these years of change have responded in quite different ways than have adolescents during the same years.

A lifespan approach underscores the normative sequencing of stages in the life course. During the lengthy adolescent period, modal individuals come to terms with their changed body image; develop interpersonal skills; achieve cognitive competencies; experiment with roles and relationships; prepare for work roles; and make a commitment to an intimate enduring relationship. By late adolescence a substantial basis for self-esteem and independent functioning is established. The school setting provides preparation for the world of work as well as a locus for social interactions with peers.

These tasks normally are completed by adolescents before they confront the adult challenges of marriage, parenthood, and the world of work. The contemporary trend toward delay in marriage and fewer children has resulted in a further sequencing, in which adaptations to job and career often precede marriage. Parenthood is becoming a relatively late event in the life course of a substantial number of young persons in the United States. In terms of the larger society, teenage parenthood therefore becomes more discrepant and less socially acceptable as it becomes more prominent.

For reasons described, the early adolescent is singularly unprepared for parenthood. Very few or none of the normative tasks of any of the stages of adolescence have been completed. Furthermore, the preemptive demands of parenthood prevent the young mothers, and sometimes the fathers, from access to the growth experiences required to continue personal development or to achieve the necessary skills for parenting or for the world of work. These problems are compounded by the poverty that is a frequent correlate of early parenthood.

For many very young mothers pregnancy is sought to achieve peer approval. Inexperience and immature cognition, however, lead to notions of parenthood that are unrealistic. Parenthood is not another transient experiment with role taking—it is the most permanent commitment that can be made. The early adolescent also discovers that the birth of a baby is a very abrupt transition to the highly demanding task of parenthood. A new mother starts out immediately with total responsibility on a twenty-four-hour basis for an infant who may be unusually small and seem fragile. Most school-age parents have not yet resolved their own dependency needs, and they experience great difficulties with the pervasive, compelling dependence of the baby. These mothers need a great deal of practical and emotional support. Child abuse is too often the last resort of a confused and overwhelmed young parent.

When the literature on child abuse is reviewed and the variables that correlate with the probability of child abuse are sorted out, almost all of them apply to the school-age mother (Table 3).

Social isolation deserves some special mention. Almost 50 percent of school-age mothers live alone, often on welfare, as female heads of household; very few of them marry. Almost half live at home with their families. But even when a young mother stays with her family, social isolation is still an important factor. Early adolescents find that school peers often lose interest after the first flurry of visits to the new baby. The parties and peer activities that were possible during pregnancy are now

TABLE 3. SUMMARY OF RISK FACTORS ASSOCIATED WITH CHILD ABUSE

SOCIOENVIRONMENTAL FACTORS
>   Social isolation
>   Close succession of children
>   Large family size
>   Poverty
>   Unemployment
>   Poor housing

PARENTAL FACTORS
>   Unwanted pregnancy or child
>   Lack of parenting skills
>   >   a) Poor reading of child's signals
>   >   b) Lack of age-appropriate expectations
>   >   c) Lack of child-rearing skills
>   >   d) Inability to empathize with child
>   Difficult pregnancy and childbirth; sickly baby
>   History of abuse or violence in home of parents

CHILD FACTORS
>   Low birth weight
>   Physical handicap; poor health
>   Difficult temperament

SOURCES: R.E. Helfer and C.H. Kempe, eds., *The Battered Child* (Chicago: University of Chicago Press, 1968). R.D. Parke and C.W. Collmer, "Child Abuse: An Interdisciplinary Analysis," in *Review of Child Development Research*, vol. 5, ed. E. Mavis Hetherington (Chicago: University of Chicago Press, 1975): 509-90. J.J. Spinetta and D. Risler, "The Child-Abusing Parent: A Psychological Review," *Psychological Bulletin* 77 (1972): 296-304. *Annual Review of Child Abuse and Neglect Research* (Bethesda, Maryland: Department of Health, Education, and Welfare, 1978).

precluded. After a while a school-age mother may actively discourage visits of her peers because of inappropriate behavior such as their wanting to teach swear words and obscene gestures to a toddler "as a fun thing to do." There may be tension between her and her own mother over the care of the baby. The child-care routines, although demanding, are often considered as very boring by adolescent mothers. Often they have no one with whom they can discuss these issues.

Substantial research attention has been given to the birth and perinatal attributes of the baby. In addition, a few studies have been made of the later outcomes of these infants. The dismal picture of infant mortality and perinatal morbidity among offspring of early adolescents has been well described. The data show that for mothers under sixteen there is a strong likelihood that the baby will show impaired cognitive development. Table 4 indicates that in the studies done by J.B. Hardy and coworkers this relationship is strongest for some black mothers. The same group has, however, shown that the babies of other young black mothers with comparable birth weight show a superior outcome.[73] This is an area that deserves further study. More needs to be known about the factors influencing the very good and very poor outcomes in IQ status. The variables that mediate the black/white differences are not known. In addition to IQ, other kinds of emotional behavioral outcomes should be systematically studied as these offspring grow and develop.

PROSPECTS FOR THE FUTURE

A concerted effort should be made to work with the school-age mother who is having her first child. There are clear goals. There is a national concern.

From the moment the infant is born the school-age mother experiences great stress and many problems. Furthermore, the likely aspect of a dismal

TABLE 4. DISTRIBUTION OF LOW AND HIGH STANFORD BINET IQ SCORES
AT AGE FOUR BY MATERNAL AGE AT BIRTH OF CHILD

	Age of Mother (Years)					
	16	17-19	20-24	25-29	30-34	35
	Percent of Children with IQs 79 and Below at Age Four					
White	2	3.5	3	2.8	2.8	2
Black	25	14	15	11.5	11.1	13
	Percent of Children with IQs 110 and Over at Age Four					
White	1.3	4.1	5	5	2.5	4
Black	4	3.9	7.5	10.2	12.3	13

SOURCE: J.B. Hardy, D.W. Welcher, Jay Stanley, et al., "Long-Range Outcome of Adolescent Pregnancy," *Clinical Obstetrics and Gynecology* 21 (1978): 1215-32.

future life course with lost opportunities for mother and child has been well documented. These school-age mothers offer a challenging opportunity to intervene in ways that will prevent or break cycles of intergenerational poverty, misery, and high fertility. There is beginning to be sufficient developmental knowledge and a base of empirical evidence on which to mount programs to meet their needs.[74-76]

A primary aim should be to enable the mother to at least complete high school. Fortunately, laws no longer prohibit school attendance during pregnancy, but schools now need to develop alternatives that will meet the special health needs that characterize the later stages of pregnancy, and thus make regular school attendance feasible.

After the child is born, school attendance for these young mothers may hinge on the availability of transportation. There is also a need for dependable infant and child care services so the young mothers may have blocks of time for their schooling.

The poignant situation of these young mothers highlights the fact that schools can do more for all students by teaching basic practical skills. The curriculum should include instruction in child development, with practical experience in nursery schools; fundamentals of nutrition; basic cooking and housekeeping skills; budgeting; and economic uses of food, energy, and other goods and services. For teenage parents this kind of curriculum is essential.

Family health care services are also of crucial importance and should be another key aspect of services. The medical care system is likely to be the first contact of the pregnant school-age girl, and continuing contact could be a reliable vehicle for reaching mothers and their children over several years for other needed services. The teaching of parental skills could be incorporated in these services. Emphasis should be placed on long-term follow up of mothers and children to monitor their physical and behavioral outcomes over several years.

Contraceptive counseling and services should be readily available to these teenage mothers. For those who are inclined toward a deferral of pregnancy, emphasis on preventing a second prematurely timed pregnancy requires knowledge and skills. These can be taught, and the timing of this medical contact offers a critical opportunity that may have lifelong consequences.

The problem of the social isolation of these mothers will be countered in part by school attendance. Other supportive services should, however, be offered, such as self-help groups, subsidized telephone services, and drop-in centers. These services are particularly important for the teenage mother who lives alone as a single head of the household.

Poverty is a pervasive problem. Provision for the basic necessities of food, clothing, and adequate housing must not be overlooked, for teenage mothers usually need help in learning how to find and utilize community resources.

When the parents are married, vocational and job placement services for the father are generally required, for he usually drops out of school to try to earn a living for the family.

There is an urgent need to move ahead with implementation of sensible programs, and careful evaluation over time so that appropriate adaptations can be made as we learn to be increasingly effective in enabling these young people to rejoin the mainstream and lead fulfilling productive lives both personally and as parents.

NOTES

1. Alan Guttmacher Institute, *11 Million Teenagers: What Can Be Done about the Epidemic of Adolescent Pregnancies in the United States* (New York: Planned Parenthood Federation of America, 1976).

2. *Teenage Pregnancy and Family Impact: New Perspectives on Policy, A Preliminary Report* (Washington: George Washington University, Family Impact Seminar, June 1979).

3. Guttmacher, *11 Million Teenagers* (See note 1).

4. W. Baldwin, *Population Bulletin* 31 (1976): 496-1174.

5. C. Lindemann, *Birth Control and Unmarried Women* (New York: Springer-Verlag, 1974).

6. F. Furstenberg, Jr., "The Social Consequences of Teenage Parenthood," *Family Planning Perspectives* 8 (1976): 148-64.

7. Guttmacher, *11 Million Teenagers* (See note 1).

8. *Population Reports, Series J: Family Planning Programs*, no. 10, pt. 1 (Washington: George Washington University Medical Center, Department of Medical and Public Affairs, July 1976).

9. A. Kinsey, W. Pomeroy, and P.H. Gebhard, *Sexual Behavior in the Human Female* (Philadelphia: W.B. Saunders, 1953).

10. A. Lake, "Teenagers and Sex: A Student Report," *Seventeen* 26 (1967): 88-131.

11. M. Zelnick and J.F. Kantner, "Sexual and Contraceptive Experience of Young Unmarried Women in the United States, 1976 and 1971," *Family Planning Perspectives* 9 (1977): 55-78.

12. H. Presser, "Age at Menarche, Socio-Sexual Behavior and Fertility," *Social Biology* 25 (1978): 94-101.

13. B.A. Hamburg, "Social Change and the Problems of Youth," in *American Handbook of Psychiatry*, 2nd ed., vol. 6, ed. D. Hamburg and H.K.H Brodie (New York: Basic Books, 1975): 385-408.

14. J. Skow, "Hollywood's Whiz Kids," *Time* (13 August 1979): 64-70.

15. S. Panzarine, J. Kabis, A. Elster, et al., "Motivated Adolescent Pregnancies," *Journal of Current Adolescent Medicine* 1 (1979): 57-59.

16. N. Brozan, "Single Mothers Sharing a Difficult Time," *New York Times* (14 May 1979): A16.

17. " 'Baby Chic': No Stigma to Pregnancy," *Washington Post* (23 October 1979): 1.

18. C. Tietze, "Teenage Pregnancies: Looking Ahead to 1984," *Family Planning Perspectives* 10, no. 4 (1978): 205-07.

19. B.A. Hamburg, "Coping in Early Adolescence: The Special Challenges of the Junior High School Period," in *American Handbook of Psychiatry*, 2nd ed., vol. 2, ed. G. Caplan (New York: Basic Books, 1974): 385-97.

20. J.M. Tanner, "Sequence, Tempo and Individual Variation in the Growth and Development of Boys and Girls Aged Twelve to Sixteen," *Daedalus* (Fall 1971): 907-30.

21. E.L. Reynolds and J.V. Wines, "Individual Differences in Physical Changes Associated with Adolescence in Girls," *American Journal of Diseases of Children* 75 (1948): 329-50.

22. _____, "Physical Changes Associated with Adolescence in Boys," *American Journal of Diseases of Children* 82 (1951): 529-47.

23. P.H. Mussen and M.C. Jones, "Self-Conceptions, Motivations, and Interpersonal Attitudes of Late- and Early-Maturing Boys," *Child Development* 28 (1957): 243-56.

24. M.C. Jones, "Psychological Correlates of Somatic Development," *Child Development* 36 (1965): 899-911.

25. J. Clausen, "The Social Meaning of Differential Physical and Sexual Maturation," in *Adolescence and the Life Cycle*, ed. S. Dragastin and G.H. Elder, Jr. (New York: John Wiley, 1975).

26. A Frazier and L.K. Lisonbee, "Adolescent Concerns with Physique," *School Review* 58 (1950): 397-405.

27. A.T. Jersild, *In Search of Self* (New York: Columbia University Press, 1952).

28. *Examination and Health History Findings among Children and Youths, 6-17 Years*, DHEW publ. no. (HRS) 74-164, ser. 11, no. 129 (Bethesda, Maryland: Department of Health, Education, and Welfare, 1974).

29. D. Bloch, "Sex Education Practices of Mothers," *Journal of Sex Education and Therapy* 7 (1972): 1-18.

30. C. Pode, "Contraception and the Adolescent Female," *Journal of School Health* XIVI (1976): 475-79.

31. P.B. Rothenberg, "Mother-Child Communication about Sex and Birth Control" (Paper presented at a meeting of the Population Association of America, Atlanta, Georgia, 1978).

32. G.L. Fox, "The Family's Influence on Adolescent Sexual Behavior," *Children Today* (May-June 1979): 21-36.

33. Ibid.

34. Bloch, "Practices of Mothers" (See note 29).

35. Fox, "Family's Influence" (See note 32).

36. Furstenberg, "Social Consequences" (See note 6).

37. Yankelovich, Skelly, and White, Inc., *The General Mills American Family Report, 1978-79: Family Health in an Era of Stress* (Minneapolis: General Mills, Inc., 1979).

38. V. Delissovoy, "Child Care by Adolescent Parents," *Children Today* (July-August 1973).

39. J. Finger and M. Silverman, "Changes in Academic Performance in Junior High School," *Personnel and Guidance Journal* 45 (1966): 157-64.

40. C. Armstrong, *Patterns of Achievement in Selected New York State Schools*, mimeographed (Albany, New York: State Education Department, 1964).

41. B. Inhelder and J. Piaget, *The Growth of Logical Thinking from Childhood to Adolescence: An Essay on the Construction of Formal Operating Structures* (New York: Basic Books, 1958).

42. E.C. Martin, "Reflections on the Early Adolescent in School," *Daedalus* (Fall 1971): 1087-1103.

43. R. Karplus, E. Karplus, M. Formisano, et al., *Proportional Reasoning and Control of Variables in Seven Countries: Advancing Education through Science-Oriented Programs*, Report 10-25 (Berkeley, California: Lawrence Hall of Science, 1975).

44. P.D. Hurd, *Early Adolescence: Perspectives and Recommendations to the National Science Foundation* (Washington: U.S. Superintendent of Documents, Stock no. 038-000-00390-9, 1978).

45. A. Tversky and D. Kahneman, "Belief in the Law of Small Numbers," *Psychological Bulletin* 76 (1971): 105-10.

46. M. Fishbein, "Consumer Beliefs and Behavior with Respect to Cigarette Smoking: A Critical Analysis of the Public Literature," in Federal Trade Commission, *Report to Congress: Pursuant to the Public Health Smoking Act for the Year 1976* (Washington: U.S. Government Printing Office, May 1977).

47. Furstenberg, "Social Consequences" (See note 6).

48. D. Elkind, "Egocentrism in Adolescence," *Child Development* 4 (1967): 1025-34.

49. Hurd, *Early Adolescence* (See note 44).

50. R. Simmons, F. Rosenberg, and M. Rosenberg, "Disturbance in the Self-Image at Adolescence," *American Sociological Review* 38 (1973): 553-68.

51. R. Simmons, R. Bulcroft, D. Blyth, et al., "The Vulnerable Adolescent: School Context and Self-Esteem" (Paper presented at a meeting of the Society for Research in Child Development, San Francisco, 1979).

52. M. Rosenberg, *Society and the Adolescent Self-Image* (Princeton: Princeton University Press, 1965): 205.

53. J. Loevinger and R. Wessler, *Measuring Ego Development* (San Francisco: Jossey-Bass, 1970).

54. B. Neugarten, "Time, Age and the Life Cycle," *American Journal of Psychiatry* 135 (1979): 887-94.

55. Furstenberg, "Social Consequences" (See note 6).

56. J.J. Card and L.L. Wise, "Teenage Mothers and Teenage Fathers: The Image of Early Childbearing on the Parents' Personal and Professional Lives," *Family Planning Perspectives* 10 (1978): 199-205.

57. K.A. Moore, S.L. Hofferth, and R. Wertheimer, II, "Teenage Motherhood: Its Social and Economic Costs," *Children Today* 8 (1979): 12-16.

58. Baldwin, *Population Bulletin* (See note 4).

59. T.J. Trussell, "Economic Consequences of Teenage Childbearing," *Family Planning Perspectives* 8 (1976): 184-90.

60. Moore, Hofferth, and Wertheimer, "Teenage Motherhood" (See note 57).

61. Baldwin, *Population Bulletin* (See note 4).

62. U.S. Congress, House, Select Committee on Population, *The Economic Consequences of Teenage Childbearing*, testimony given by K.A. Moore, 28 February 1978.

63. Guttmacher, *11 Million Teenagers* (See note 1).

64. K.A. Moore, "Teenage Childbirth and Welfare Dependency," *Family Planning Perspectives* 10 (1978): 233-35.

65. J.B. Hardy, D.W. Welcher, Jay Stanley, et al., "Long-Range Outcome of Adolescent Pregnancy," *Clinical Obstetrics and Gynecology* 21 (1978): 1215-32.

66. Guttmacher, *11 Million Teenagers* (See note 1).

67. T.J. Trussel and J. Menkin, "Early Childbearing and Subsequent Fertility," *Family Planning Perspectives* 10 (1978): 209-18.

68. Ibid.

69. Card and Wise, "Teenage Mothers and Fathers" (See note 56).

70. *Teenage Pregnancy* (See note 2).

71. Hardy, Welcher, Stanley, et al., "Adolescent Pregnancy" (See note 65).

72. Baldwin, *Population Bulletin* (See note 4).

73. Hardy, Welcher, Stanley, et al., "Adolescent Pregnancy" (See note 65).

74. Furstenberg, "Social Consequences" (See note 6).

75. L. Klein, "Models of Comprehensive Service: Regular-School Based," *Journal of School Health* 45 (1975): 271-78.

76. L. Klerman and J. Jekel, *School-Age Mother: Problems, Programs and Policy* (Hamden, Connecticut: Linnet Books, 1973).

DISCUSSION

Adolescent Population

The question often arises of whether the large number of adolescent pregnancies currently reported does not simply reflect the fact that there has been a sharp rise in the absolute number of adolescents since 1950. In response it should be stated that while demographic factors do play some role, they are only a partial explanation. Data show that in 1950 the ten- to nineteen-year-old population in the United States was some 22 million, or 14 percent of the total population; in 1976 the same age group numbered 41 million, or 19 percent of the population. It has already been emphasized, however, that there has also been an absolute increase in overall adolescent fertility during the same period.

Rise in Fertility Rate

Furthermore, the rise in fertility has not been uniform across the various subsets of adolescents. Early adolescents have consistently shown the most striking increase in fertility rates: during the past decade births to girls under age fifteen increased by 55 percent, whereas births to those age eighteen or nineteen declined by nearly 18 percent. It is this differential in fertility rates has aroused concern for the early adolescent. Failure to differentiate early, middle, and late adolescence obscures the patterns that exist. Only recently has the unitary concept of adolescence begun to be questioned.

Prevalence of Early Adolescent Pregnancy

In the United States, early adolescent pregnancy is becoming more prevalent; it is also becoming fashionable—a source of prestige among the girls' peers.

This trend may be reinforced by the fact that the American culture reflects a strong emphasis on sexual permissiveness. The media and movies present attractive models of women who are having babies and keeping them without benefit of marriage. Present evidence suggests that early adolescents are especially sensitive to the social environment and are highly vulnerable targets for media messages.

In France the situation is somewhat different. Unmarried girls are not so proud of having babies, and they do not gain the admiration of their friends. It has also been observed that many young girls experience a narcissistic pleasure in anticipation of motherhood. The baby is viewed as an extension of the self, and, in fantasy, can be endowed with many highly positive attributes. There are other significant aspects to this situation. Very often these young girls are in conflict with their families. For them, having a child is a kind of competition with the mother—competing with her on her own ground as a mother. The adolescent mother may be proud that she, herself, will take care of the baby.

Parenthood as a Permanent Commitment

In any case, and regardless of country of origin, most very young adolescent girls share immaturity and limitations of cognitive development that predispose them to impulsiveness and poor judgment in making decisions about parenthood. This is a period characterized by many role explorations. Young adolescents do not understand that the most permanent commitment one ever makes is parenthood. Today marriage and career often are not permanent; one can get a divorce or change jobs, but one does not ever become an "unparent." So in an attempt at role experimentation with parenthood the young person finds herself with a permanent commitment.

Role of the Father

The role of the father in adolescent parenthood has received little attention. The best evidence is that even when there is a sense of commitment and an ensuing marriage, the father's role and involvement is usually temporary. Teenage marriages are usually prone to end in early divorce, but it is not only emotional immaturity and lack of parenting skills that threaten these marriages. Most young fathers drop out of school to try to support the family, but they find they have no marketable skills and are rarely successful in obtaining a job that will enable them to maintain a stable home. Young fathers are in great need of vocational training and skilled help in seeking and holding a job. When the marriage fails, a pattern often develops in which the mother has unstable liaisons with a number of different men, none of whom take real responsibility as a parent.

Prevailing Social Milieu

Meeting the many needs of these adolescents can be an especially challenging task. For some, the only acceptable services are those that are age-relevant and geared to meet their immediate, specific needs and interests. Some facilities that cater exclusively to adolescents may further isolate them from the larger society and preclude the acquisition of knowledge and skills required to achieve long-term and personal career goals.

A more complete understanding of the challenges and roles of adolescents may also require an examination of the prevailing social contexts. Some social observers feel there is virtually no place for adolescents in modern societies. They are concerned that social organization in industrial countries places constraints on the roles and options that are permitted to adolescents. They also feel there is a tendency to blame the victim and rationalize the fact that the social organization deskills adolescents, fails to provide them with interesting and productive work, and restricts their opportunities for stable relationships.

There is a prevalent and deeply held belief that adolescents must move into a separate peer culture, and that they have a developmental need to assert their independence of parents and other adults. Insofar as this is true, it is applicable to older adolescents who are in actual transition to adult roles, not to early adolescents age ten to fifteen. This is another misunderstanding that derives from the unitary concept of adolescence in which the modal adolescent is based on a prototype of the late adolescent male on the threshold of adulthood.

Different Stages of Development

The emphasis on the need to differentiate among the periods of adolescent development strikes a responsive chord. Early adolescents especially are in need of parental support and guidance as they abruptly leave the world of childhood. The prescription to distance themselves from parents and other adults has probably been very harmful to many young adolescents. Even the peer counseling projects that have been most successful in various areas of need have worked best when there is adult support and leadership.

There is evidence that, when parents maintain ties and discuss sexual matters with early adolescents, initiation of sexual activity is postponed to a later age; if the talks occur when the young person is already sexually active, there is a more responsible use of contraception. In general, there is an urgent need to provide more adult guidance to early adolescents.

CHILDREN AND ADOLESCENTS IN A CHANGING WORLD

Leon Eisenberg

The title of this presentation, for which I am unable to deny responsibility, might well have led to prosecution under truth-in-advertising legislation were symposia governed by such statutes. My defense would have been that surely so knowledgeable a group of colleagues would have understood me to mean "aspects of" or "an introduction to" or "a preliminary essay on," rather than as stated: "Children and Adolescents in a Changing World." It is not merely that I lack the competence—and the time—for such an all-encompassing survey, but that it bears upon each of the major issues the other speakers have addressed: epidemiological definitions of "caseness" in relation to cultural expectations; the parceling out of exogenous and endogenous determinants of behavior; the shaping of response to war and migration as stressors; the variability of cultural criteria for substance abuse; the factors that mold parenting behaviors; and so on. What I will attempt, therefore, is to highlight a few facets of the topic in the belief that adaptation to change is what child development is about, and that the consequences of social change can illuminate theory as well as practice in psychiatry.

In sequence I propose to consider social change and population genetics; changes in reproductive behavior; the demographic revolution and its psychiatric consequences; women, work, and child care; and, finally, mobility and social ties. In my view the commanding imperatives of technology have altered not only our culture and our social responsibilities, but human biology itself.

327

SOCIAL CHANGE AND POPULATION GENETICS

Let me begin with what may seem the most outlandish of the propositions set forth, namely, the impact of sociotechnical change on human biology. This is not a new phenomenon. Where human beings live, how many of them there are, and the way they live have always had profound effects on both the evolution of the species and the development of the individual.

Diseases such as measles and poliomyelitis could not become endemic in human populations until the agricultural revolution permitted people to aggregate in numbers sufficient to provide a host reservoir for the virus to recycle itself.[1] The penetration of the virus into a hunter-gatherer community of several hundred behaves today as it did in neolithic times; it rapidly kills or immunizes so high a proportion of the total population that the virus is unable to continue to propagate. Thus human culture created, albeit unwittingly, the conditions necessary for infectious disease to exert evolutionary selective pressures on the biology of modern man, a process limited to the past 500 generations.[2]

The sickle-cell gene, rare in other populations, reached an equilibrium frequency of 10 percent among West African blacks because the heterozygote (hemoglobin AS) is less vulnerable to falciparium malaria, even though the abnormal homozygote (hemoglobin SS) has almost no reproductive fitness. Sicklemia persists as an adaptation to a malaria-infested environment, as do thalassemia and glucose-6-phosphate dehydrogenase (G6PD) deficiencies. With the migration of populations to malaria-free zones, or with effective malaria eradication, the prevalence of the now entirely disadvantageous allele decreases.[3]

An example of another type of human adaptation is provided by the antigens of Duffy blood group system which, although otherwise innocuous, in contrast to the sickle gene, appear to act as "receptors" for the vivax malaria plasmodium at the surface of red cells. The recessive phenotype, Duffy negative, confers resistance to vivax malaria, and thus the frequency for the Fy^0 allele approximates 100 percent among Central African blacks; it approaches zero among Caucasians.[4] So much, then, for the antiquity of the process.

Genotypic change continues into the modern era, as advances in medical care permit the survival to reproductive life of persons with such diseases as galactosemia, congenital hypothyroidism, and phenylketonuria. Insofar as the deleterious effects of the double dose of the gene can be largely mitigated or entirely neutralized by medical intervention, no human loss (other than medical costs) is involved. In the instance of phenylketonuria, however, a new biological problem has arisen: pregnancy in the otherwise healthy, treated phenlketonuric female can lead to the birth of a defective infant because of in utero exposure of the fetus to toxic levels of blood phenylalanine.[5] Prenatal detection of Mendelian, chromosomal, or other congenital disease, followed by abortion of the affected fetus, does not influence gene distribution in and of itself, as the individual whose birth was avoided would not have been reproductively effective. In the past, many parents who knew themselves to be carriers would have foregone childbearing for fear of having an affected infant. The relative security now provided by amniocentesis enables such parents to give birth to phenotypically normal children, some of whom will be carriers and thus add to the genetic load of future generations. Nonetheless, since these diseases are fortunately rare, the net effect on the human gene pool need provide no reason for concern. Moreover, offsetting eugenic effects can be expected from public health measures; the eradication of malaria by eliminating the heterozygote advantage should lead to the gradual reduction of genes for thalassemia, sicklemia, and G6PD deficiency.

The genetic burden in the population with respect to the psychoses is more complex. Based upon a comparison of the frequency of schizophrenia in the biological and the adoptive parents of children who develop schizophrenia, strong evidence now exists that there is a strong genetic component in the disorder.[6] Manifestations of the clinical syndrome may well depend on environmental precipitation, but a genetic diathesis appears to be a necessary precondition.[7] The likelihood of bearing a schizophrenic offspring is approximately 10 percent when one parent is affected, and 40 percent when both parents have a history of schizophrenia. Yet only some 4 percent of schizophrenics report having had a schizophrenic parent. Thus genetic counseling can make little contribution as a public health measure. The decision not to have children, even if made voluntarily by all such individuals, would have only a marginal impact, particularly since only a fraction of such persons have their first such episode before childbearing occurs.

On the other hand, there is reason to believe that current policies favoring brief hospitalization and community care, though undoubtedly important advances for patients, are increasing the chances for fertility in schizophrenic parents and thus contributing to an additional genetic load[8] and to a stressful environment for the offspring.[9] In the case of infant psychosis, although the twin study of S. Folstein and M. Rutter has demonstrated a major heritable component,[10] the disorder is so uncommon, and so few of the afflicted youngsters go on to marriage and childbearing, that genetic issues have little public health importance.

Even if genetic counseling for the individual family is ineffective as a public health measure in schizophrenia, does it make sense as a clinical procedure? Parents must weigh the risk of having one offspring in ten manifest the disease over a lifetime—with no way of predicting whether it will be mild or severe, a single episode or recurrent, episodic or chronic— against the satisfaction of nine children who can be expected to live a normal life. There is no justification for proposals for the "prophylactic" use of phenothiazines by children in such families, despite its efficacy as a therapeutic measure, because of the high ratio of normal to affected offspring and the hazards of the long-term use of a powerful agent during the time of maximal growth and development of the central nervous system.[11]

More appropriate and ethically justified are efforts to buffer the child of schizophrenic parents against the vicissitudes of familial stress. These measures include the systematic provision of contraceptive services to schizophrenic women to limit the burden of family size;[12] day nursery and after-school programs; homemakers and social services during episodes of parental incapacitation;[13] and supportive psychiatric intervention for children in such families.[14] While there is as yet no evidence that these efforts will "prevent" the onset of schizophrenia in these children, they can contribute substantially to the relief of distress and the promotion of healthy personality development.

One striking effect of modern society has been to diminish selection pressure. Well over 95 percent of infants born alive in Western countries survive to the age of reproduction; postreproductive mortality has no selective power. Variance in the number of children born per woman does provide an opportunity for selection by differential fertility, but there is some evidence that birth control is reducing the variation in size of families. If we ever achieved a state in which each couple had only two children there would be no room left for natural selection; any subsequent evolutionary changes would be due to mutation and to genetic drift. Mutation may be on the increase as the result of man-made radiation and the introduction of chemical mutagens in the environment, but these represent challenges to the development of effective methods of public health control rather than inevitable events.

SOCIAL CHANGE AND REPRODUCTIVE BEHAVIOR

The most marked impact of social change on human biology has been on the phenotype rather than on the genotype. In all Western nations there has been a steady increase in the mean stature attained by successive generations as a result of improvements in nutrition and in the control of infection. Just as striking has been the lowering of the age of onset of puberty; it now begins some four years earlier than a century ago.[15] Although fertility occurs later than menarche, because the early menstrual cycles are anovulatory there has been an inevitable parallel net reduction in the age at which fertility can begin. This sociobiological change, that is, a change in biology resulting from socially produced alterations in health conditions, has complex consequences. When the biological phenomenon of early puberty is associated, as it is in the United States, with an increase in the frequency of adolescent sexual activity because of changes in sexual mores, unwanted pregnancy is an all too common side effect, to the detriment of both mother and infant.

In 1976 about 1.2 million abortions were performed in the United States;[16] of the women aborted, one-third were under age nineteen; two-thirds were unmarried; and one-half were nulliparous.[17] Depending on the age of the mother, maternal mortality from pregnancy and childbirth is from twice to eight times higher than from legal abortions.[18] Delays in seeking an abortion, stemming from financial or other barriers to access, guarantee additional deaths: there is a fifty-fold greater mortality from abortion after the sixteenth week than before the ninth week of pregnancy.[19] These data refer to legal abortions; the mortality from illegal abortions is conservatively estimated by C. Tietze as 100-fold greater than early legal abortion.[20] The death toll from unwanted pregnancies carried to term is highest among teenagers because of the higher rates of toxemia, abnormalities of labor, postpartum infection, and hemorrhage among this age group.

And what of the infants? Maternal immaturity is associated with a much higher rate of low-birth-weight infants.[21] Low birth weight in turn is associated not only with a much greater perinatal mortality, but with a disproportionate number of developmentally impaired children.[22] Nonetheless, despite the increased risk of low birth weight, some 80 to 90 percent of infants born to teenagers are of normal weight; of those who weigh less than 2,500 g. the majority are biologically intact when they leave hospital.

The problems these children face are social: the complex of adversity that stems from being born unwanted into a family ill-prepared or unable to provide proper care. Studies of children born to mothers who applied for and were refused abortion have been carried out in Sweden[23] and in Czechoslovakia.[24] Psychological profiles and educational accomplishments of these unwanted children were compared with a set of control children. In both studies, although many of the families did manage to cope and to love them, the children were at greater risk of developmental failure. Unwanted offspring are more often the target of child abuse.[25] All too many are abandoned to foster care and to state institutions, and it is these who suffer a heavy toll of psychiatric disorder, educational retardation, and vocational failure.[26]

The impact on the mother can be equally devastating. In a study of the social consequences of teenage parenthood, F. Furstenberg, Jr. has documented the marital instability, school disruption, economic problems, difficulties in regulating family size, and problems in childrearing among adolescent mothers compared with classmates who did not become pregnant premaritally.[27]

What of the hazards of abortion itself? As noted, maternal mortality rates for all ages are higher from pregnancy and childbirth than they are from legal abortion. In a careful analysis of the subsequent pregnancy experience of women who have had abortions, J.R. Daling and I. Emanuel have demonstrated no adverse effects on pregnancy outcome in comparison with a matched control group who have not had abortions.[28,29] As for the repeated contention that abortion presents psychiatric hazards, available data demonstrate that postabortion psychosis is less than one-fifth as common as postpartum psychosis.[30] Moreover, in a study of women who underwent first trimester abortions, H.S. Greer and coworkers found their psychosocial adjustment to be considerably better eighteen months later than it had been before the procedure.[31]

The point of this analysis is not to suggest that abortion should be regarded as a preferred method of contraception, but that it is an indispensable backup in family planning services. How long we shall have to continue to rely on abortion will be determined by our success in developing more effective and safer contraceptives; in making them universally available; and in persuading those who do not wish to have children to use them. Given the relative failure rates of the available methods[32] and the growing public concern about the hazards of the pill, if all married users of the pill under age forty were to substitute the diaphragm or other traditional measures, the additional contraceptive failures would lead to a demand for 1 million more abortions than there were in 1976.[33]

THE DEMOGRAPHIC REVOLUTION AND ITS PSYCHIATRIC CONSEQUENCES

Because of the large group still in the fertile period, at the present birth rate the population of the United States will continue to increase until the year 2040. In this respect events in Western Europe have outrun us: birth rates in France and West Germany have fallen below replacement values and the population decline has begun. The economic effects of this demographic reversal are already manifest: for the past fifteen years social security contributions have jumped by 8 percent a year in Western Europe—about twice the annual economic growth rate.[34] Whether national incentives and sanctions can smooth out the boom-and-bust cycles in fertility remain questions for the future, but it has become abundantly clear that natal policy is a major issue the world over.[35]

At the other end of the life cycle there has been a steady increase in longevity. There are in the United States more than 23 million persons over age sixty-five: there will be 30 million by the turn of the century and 50 million by 2030, even with no further increase in longevity.[36] The growing proportion of the elderly in the population is no purely American phenomenon: it is occurring in all Western European countries, particularly in Sweden.

Consider the contrast between the United States as the prototype of an industrialized society and Mexico as the prototype of a developing country. In 1976 the ratio in the United States of children under age fifteen to persons from fifteen to sixty-four was 0.377; the ratio in Mexico was 0.991, almost three times higher. Conversely, the ratio of American adults age sixty-five and over to persons from age fifteen to sixty-four was 0.165, whereas in Mexico it was 0.068, less than half as large.[37] These ratios have a great bearing on the likelihood of job opportunities for the young and on the size of the dependency burden on the working population. Such demographic data explicate the powerful thrust behind the very considerable unregistered migration from Mexico to the United States of people seeking to escape from poverty.

From the standpoint of psychiatric epidemiology, the growing proportion of the elderly inevitably predicts a larger number of individuals with senile dementia. This increase is likely to be larger than simply proportionate because of the success of antibiotics in prolonging the lives of those with senile brain disease.[38] For child psychiatrists the dependent elderly portend greater stress on the family and hence on children in the family. Moreover, these demographic changes are resulting in postponement of the age of retirement, thus slowing down vocational turnover, which creates a problem for adolescents seeking entry to job opportunities. This has serious implications for our system of higher education.

Whereas at the turn of the century no more than an elite 4 percent of eighteen- to twenty-one-year-olds in the United States went on to college, by 1979 about 50 percent were enrolled. If personal development were the primary motivation for education the social investment might be well worthwhile, but a major thrust has been for economic gain. Until recently a college degree ensured a higher income; this is no longer so clearly the case.[39] In Italy, France, and other Western European countries—and even in India[40]—university degrees are "fast becoming tickets to nowhere," according to a report from the International Labor Office in Geneva.[41] University students are ambivalent: on the one hand, they protest the irrelevance of their education to their economic future; on the other, they resist efforts to redirect the university curriculum along vocational lines. Rising expectations conjoined with diminished opportunities create the seedbed for political turmoil among disaffected adolescents and young adults.

WOMEN, WORK, AND CHILD CARE

The increase in women's longevity coupled with the decision to have fewer children—and the contraceptive technology to make that possible—has radically transformed their lives; childbearing and childrearing now occupy far fewer years of a woman's life. Two centuries ago less than half the children born survived until age ten, a statistic that still obtains in the developing world. With decreases in infant and child mortality, fewer pregnancies became necessary to assure the same family size. Moreover, social security measures diminished the reliance of elderly parents on the financial support of their children. The simultaneous demands of an industrial society required the incorporation of women into the work force; working, in turn, influenced decisions about preferred family size.[42–44]

What the sociologists refer to as a "tipping point" has been reached in the United States: today the majority of married women are in the labor force. The woman who does not work rather than the one who does now feels the necessity to justify a socially deviant role. It is clearly an extension of human freedom that women seek, and can often achieve, a wide range of life roles. In my opinion it is no mere coincidence that child development researchers and clinicians have become preoccupied with the issues of early bonding and attachment behavior at a time when women in Western society are in the process of changing their traditional roles. For if women can be persuaded that their children will suffer if they are away at work, many may be expected to alter their lifestyles accordingly.

I do not contend that investigators falsify their results because of political preconceptions, or even that conscious design is at work; that may be true for a few, but not for most. What is germane is that social problems define the relevance of research and influence the kinds of research supported by public agencies. Moreover developmentalists are influenced by their own history: the *Zeitgeist* shapes the way problems are formulated, data are collected, and findings are interpreted. Even when research findings are expressed with appropriate cautions against overgeneralization, there is a public avid to use tentative results to justify long-held biases. As Gunnar Myrdal put it so plainly:

> A "disinterested" social science is . . . pure nonsense. It never existed and it will never exist. We can make our thinking strictly rational in spite of this, but only by facing the valuations, not by evading them.[45]

An immediate example of the use and the abuse of child development data in the political arena is given by the recent history of day care legislation in the United States. During World War II, when the war effort demanded womanpower in industry, the government subsidized day care. Studies of child development had immediate utility, and the public was reassured to learn that systematic research revealed no deleterious effects.[46] With the war over, it was essential to find jobs for men and to ease women out of the labor market; not only did child development become less interesting to policy makers but the old myths about the importance of childrearing in the home flowered once again, in total disregard of the evidence. Indeed, when President Richard M. Nixon vetoed the Comprehensive Child Development Bill on 9 December 1971 he spoke of it as committing the "vast moral authority of the National Government to the side of communal approaches to child rearing over against the family centered approach"[47]—much as the Prussian police had closed Friedrich Froebel's "Gardens of Children" on the charge that they were hotbeds of atheism and socialism.[48]

Today the focus has shifted to the earliest days of the infant's life. What matters in development, we are told, is bonding, a more sophisticated version of the ethologists' theory of imprinting. B. Lozoff and G. Brittenham stress the sharp differences in maternal behavior between women in hunter-gatherer societies and in modern America.[49] As they point out, among !Kung bushmen, in the first three months of life the infant is held in close physical contact with the mother 90 percent of the time, in contrast to a figure of 30 percent in America. By the ninth month the !Kung mother is carrying her baby more than half the time, whereas her American counterpart does so less than one-sixth of the time. Further, almost all !Kung infants are breast-fed on demand until age three; only 6 percent of American infants are breast-fed for as long as six months.

Given that the social patterns of the !Kung and other hunter-gatherers typify the characteristics of infant development for the greater part of the history of our species, Lozoff and Brittenham, after a concession to the fact that a behavior pattern adaptive at one epoch need not continue to be so, go on to comment that

> the remarkable transformations in the pattern of infant care which have occurred in the last few hundred years may have had a profound impact on normal infant development and normal maternal involvement.[50]

Do I overread these authors as implying that current patterns of infant care, consequent upon new roles for women, may be harmful to both infants and mothers?

I do not for a moment suggest that these changes are unimportant for developmental outcomes. But I would argue that the developmental consequences of the kind and amount of physical intimacy between mother and infant are inseparable from the entire web of childrearing practices and related culture traits that contribute to, or militate against, adaptation to an ecological setting. Infants are not endlessly malleable: they have essential needs for affectional and cognitive intake. But just as the constituents of a diet must be in appropriate balance for adequate growth to occur, so must the social aliments an infant needs be viewed in relation to one another.

The emphasis on bonding as a crucial process has been furthered by the discovery of primate models. Removing a monkey infant from its mother leads to a phase labeled "protest" behavior, followed by one labeled "despair" and depression."[51] More accurately, this sequence occurs in *some* monkey species. There are notable differences between the behaviors of separated pigtail and bonnet macaque infant-mother pairs. A pigtail mother in a cage with other adults will not permit them to interact with her infant, and sharply limits movements of her infant away from her vicinity; a bonnet mother allows conspecifics to explore and groom her infant and restrains its departures much less often. These differences in maternal behavior are correlated with much less display of distress in the bonnet than in the pigtail infant when the mother is removed from the colony.[52]

P. Dolhinow reports that infant langurs will initiate their own "adoption" by another adult female when the mother is removed from the group. As the infant succeeds in obtaining a caretaker, symptoms are quickly reduced; indeed after most experimental separations the infant elects to remain with its adoptive caretaker even after its biological mother is returned.[53] Dolinhow concludes that:

> There are ranges of reaction to mother loss typical of every species, rather than a single, stereotyped set of responses. Reactions to mother loss presumably depend upon a number of factors involving adults as well as the immature. The langur presents a very useful contrast to the macaque, probably because of the multiple caretaking pattern, infant initiative and adult acceptance.[54]

Even among primates, "culture" appears to be a determinant of parenting behavior. Sara B. Hrdy has reported infanticide among Indian langurs. If a strange male takes over a female nursing an infant, the new consort is likely to kill the infant. This behavior makes sense to the sociobiologist because the killing of the infant terminates its mother's lactation, leads to the earlier resumption of estrus, and permits the new male to impregnate the female; thus he assures that his parental investment contributes to the survival of his genes rather than to those of the earlier partner.[55]

Yet R. Curtin and Dolinhow note that infanticide is rare or nonexistent among langurs living in "natural" conditions in the wild. They point out that the langurs studied by Hrdy were living in and around Indian villages and were undergoing major changes in patterns of foraging and colony behavior.[56] Thus, even within the same species of primate, patterns of infant-mother and infant-father relationships are influenced by ecological context. Comparitive psychology can illuminate our understanding of human behavior, but it can only do so if the analysis is sensitive to species differences, to the influence of context, and to differences in the mechanisms that may yield similar behaviors.

Early experiences may have different enduring effects, but they are less pervasive than bonding theory predicts. Barbara Tizard has demonstrated that children reared in institutions from infancy show more disturbed social behavior at school than those reared in ordinary families.[57] How far can adoption after the early years of life make up for initial deficits? She compared a group of children who had remained in institutions, or who had returned to a deprived home environment, with children who had been adopted. The great majority of adopted children were able to form close ties with their adoptive parents and showed no more behavior problems *at home* than did the controls. On the other hand, their teachers reported high rates of socially disruptive behavior among both the adopted and the institution-alized children.[58]

The results suggest that whereas late adoption helps greatly, it does not make up entirely for the lack of opportunity for early bonding. The events of the first year of life set the stage for those of the second, and events of the second year for those of the third, and so on. The outcome years later is determined by intervening experience, as well as that of the first year, despite its salience.[59]

Just how potent later experience can be is evident from the follow up into young adulthood of the children Sophie Dann and Anna Freud described after they had been rescued from Theresienstadt at the end of World War II. Shortly after the birth of these children their mothers had been killed by the Nazis and they were cared for in the concentration camp by a succession of women who were severely harassed and under the constant threat of death. None, in fact, survived. The children, when rescued at age three, were strongly attached to each other but indifferent to adults. Following a period of therapeutic residential care, all were placed in foster homes or adopted.[60]

An unpublished report of their status as young adults is extraordinary in demonstrating that they have performed remarkably well. They may still be at risk of psychiatric disorder, but none of us would have predicted so successful a life trajectory as they have exhibited up to the present time. We will never know how far they "mothered" each other; how far polymatric caretaking met their needs; how much Anna Freud's therapeutic interventions contributed; or to what extent their adoptive homes were the effective agents. But the clinical outcome provides a necessary corrective to the prevalent pessimism about the irreversibility of early deficits.

MOBILITY AND SOCIAL TIES

An industrial society demands a mobile work force. The consolidation of farming into an agribusiness diminishes the need for agricultural manpower. Increasing proportions of the population concentrate in metropolitan areas. Urbanization is a worldwide phenomenon; its effects are the more devastating in the developing world, where *barrios* and *favelas* of grinding poverty surround cities whose population growth threatens their survival.[61] People move because they despair of satisfaction in their present environments and they perceive greater opportunity as lying elsewhere. The message is clear: without the investment of national resources to improve conditions in the countryside, population movement will continue, to the detriment of both rural and urban areas.

Americans seem to be in perpetual motion: one in five families moves every year. This means fresh starts, less parochialism, and more opportunities for young couples to develop free of parental coercion. It also means loss of support of extended families, fewer ties to the community, and a sense of rootlessness and alienation. Mobility disrupts social networks.

The medical implications of mobility stem from the force of the data indicating that social ties are important determinants of mental and physical health. George Brown and his colleagues have studied the prevalence of depression among women in urban and rural settings in the United Kingdom. In London the most potent protective factor against depression proved to be an intimate and confiding relationship with a husband or a boyfriend;[62] in rural Scotland, those women least integrated into village life had the highest rates of depression. S. Henderson and his group surveyed a large random sample of the general population of Canberra, Australia, employing standardized interview schedules to assess levels of neurotic symptoms, extent of life stress, and strength of social ties. They found, as have others, that the greater the life stress, the higher the symptom score. In the presence of stress, social ties provided significant protection against the likelihood of experiencing symptoms.[63] Furthermore a large number of studies have demonstrated an excess of morbidity and mortality among the widowed during the year after bereavement.[64]

The most impressive findings of all have recently been reported by L.F. Berkman and S.L. Symes, who studied the mortality experience of a community sample of almost 5,000 men and women between age thirty and fifty-nine over a nine-year period. At the time of enrollment in the study each individual was asked about four sources of social contact: marriage; visits to and from close friends and relatives; frequency of church attendance; and level of activity in group associations. When the four ratings were combined into a Social Network Index, it proved to be a powerful predictor of life expectancy. For the succeeding nine years the age- and sex-specific death rate was more than *twice* as high for those who were the most isolated compared with those who were the most connected. The Social Network Index was found to be associated not only with overall mortality, but with four separate causes of death: heart disease, cancer, cerebrovascular disease, and circulatory disease.[65]

Family studies demonstrate the impact of interpersonal relationships on the health of both children and adults. In a study of 100 persons in sixteen families who had throat cultures taken every three weeks, as well as at times when they were ill, R.J. Meyer and R.J. Haggerty found beta-hemolytic streptococci in 20 percent of some 1,600 throat cultures; more than half of all positive cultures were not associated with detectable illness, however. The most powerful predictor of the likehood of either colonization by the bacteria, or colonization plus illness, was the stress family members had experienced in the several weeks before the cultures were taken.[66]

In a subsequent study, K.J. Roghmann and Haggerty monitored the relationship between family life crises and illness by means of a daily diary kept by 500 families. On the first day of a stress episode, illness was 2.5 times more likely than would be expected by chance. If illness was not present, stress increased the utilization of medical services; equally interesting was the finding that stress *decreased* the likelihood that a mother would seek medical care *for herself* if she was ill, but *increased* the likelihood of consulting a doctor if her child was ill.[67] In such studies the parent-child relationship is taken as the mediating variable between stress as provocation and social ties as support acting on the child.

What of the effect of social networks on child development per se? U. Bronfenbrenner, in his formulation of an "ecology" of human development, has called for the inclusion of social networks as important components of the setting that determines the behavior of children.[68] M.M. Cochran and J.A. Brassard have attempted a theoretical formulation of the relationship between personal social networks and child development. They emphasize networks as sources of cognitive and social stimulation; as direct support for the child through the provision of care when parents are absent or incapacitated; as supplying observational models for varying adult roles; and as providing opportunities for active participation in adult networks during which the child develops its own concepts of human exchange networks.[69]

It is my expectation that this level of analysis will yield evidence of effects directly on the child, as well as mediated through the parents, in promoting or retarding healthy development.

CODA

The pace of social change in the past several decades is without parallel in human history. For the greatest part of the 50,000 to 100,000 years modern man (homo sapiens) has been on earth, men and women lived in hunter-gatherer tribes of some fifty to 150 members. Apart from natural catastrophes, the day-to-day life of early human tribes changed hardly at all over the millennia. To become a competent adult, a child had only to acquire the collective wisdom of its elders. Today conventional wisdom based on the past has become anachronistic as a guide to the future.

Some suggest that the rapidity of contemporary social change driven by an expanding technology may have outpaced the capacity of the human organism to adapt to it. This view embodies a nostalgic misconception of the past and a romantic yearning to return to it because of present difficulties. It underestimates the very real benefits that have come with change and that have yet to be shared by the greater part of the world's population; their today is our yesterday. That yesterday is not only impossible to resurrect, but not worth its reincarnation. Glorification of its stability ignores the very real costs that went with it: wretched health, vulnerability to natural catastrophe; and sharply restricted opportunities for personal development, available only to the privileged few.

The task for behavioral science is to help shape social institutions to supplement the family and community networks that provided support and gave meaning to life in the past. Western society has had the ingenuity to develop social legislation to provide a floor under states of financial dependency: unemployment compensation, social welfare laws, pension plans, and the like. What has been neglected is the need for new social structures to enable the family, still the mediator between society and the child, to carry out its functions at a time when it is being buffeted by social forces beyond its means to manage. Those of us in developmental medicine and psychology must join in this effort.

What we discover in our clinical practices with children who are the casualties of social chaos, and from our systematic testing of hypotheses about the conditions necessary for human growth, can contribute to the design of public policy for a more humane world. In that task it is essential that our horizons extend beyond parochial observations in our own societies to encompass cross-cultural perspectives. We will not be able to understand children in our own corner of the world, let alone those in others, unless we attend with equal eye to all.

Social evolution must now become self-conscious: our children must be helped to understand the constraints that limit choices, as well as the options for a more fully human existence. Either we have a future in which we acknowledge each other as members of a single species, in which human differences become a cause for celebration rather than oppression, and in which fostering human development over a lifetime is the overriding concern of society, or there will be no future at all.

NOTES

1. F.L. Black, "Infectious Diseases in Primitive Societies," *Science* 187 (1975): 515-18.

2. J.B.S. Haldane, "Natural Selection in Man," *Acta Genetica Statistica Medica* 6 (1956/1957): 321-32.

3. L.L. Cavalli-Sforza and W.F. Bodmer, *The Genetics of Human Populations* (San Francisco: W.H. Freeman and Co., 1971).

4. Ibid.

5. H. Hansen, "Variability of Reproductive Casualty in Maternal Phenylketonuria," *Early Human Development* 2 (1978): 51-71.

6. S.S. Kety, "Studies Designed to Disentangle Genetic and Environmental Variables in Schizophrenia," *American Journal of Psychiatry* 133 (1976): 1134-37.

7. D.D. Rosenthal, *Genetic Theory and Schizophrenia* (New York: McGraw Hill Book Publishing Co., 1970).

8. L. Erlenmeyer-Kimling, S. Nicol, J.D. Rainer, et al., "Changes in Fertility Rates of Schizophrenic Patients in New York State," *American Journal of Psychiatry* 125 (1969): 916-27.

9. M. Rutter, *Children of Sick Parents: An Environmental and Psychiatric Study* (London: Oxford University Press, 1966).

10. S. Folstein and M. Rutter, "Infantile Autism: A Genetic Study of 21 Twin Pairs," *Journal of Child Psychology and Psychiatry* 18 (1977): 297-322.

11. L. Eisenberg, "Principles of Drug Therapy in Child Psychiatry," *American Journal of Orthopsychiatry* 41 (1971): 371-79.

12. V. Abernathy and H. Grunebaum, "Toward a Family Planning Program in Psychiatric Hospitals," *American Journal of Public Health* 62 (1972): 1638-46.

13. E.P. Rice, M.C. Ekdahl, and L. Miller, *Children of Mentally Ill Parents: Problems in Child Care* (New York: Behavioral Publications, 1971).

14. E.J. Anthony, "A Risk-Vulnerability Intervention Model for Children of Psychotic Parents," in *The Child and His Family: Children at Psychiatric Risk,* ed. E.J. Anthony and C. Koupernik (New York: John Wiley and Sons, 1974).

15. J.M. Tanner, *Growth at Adolescence,* 2nd ed. (Oxford: Blackwell Scientific Publications, 1962).

16. J.D. Forrest, "Abortion in the United States, 1976–1977," *Family Planning Perspectives* 10 (1978): 271-79.

17. Center for Disease Control, "Abortion Surveillance—United States 1975," *Morbidity and Mortality Weekly Report* 26 (1977): 241.

18. W. Cates and C. Tietze, "Standardized Mortality Rates Associated with Legal Abortion: United States, 1972-1975," *Family Planning Perspectives* 10 (1978): 109-12.

19. W. Cates, D.A. Grimes, J.C. Smith, et al., "Legal Abortion Mortality in the United States: Epidemiologic Surveillance, 1972–1974," *Journal of the American Medical Association* 237 (1977): 452-55.

20. C. Tietze, "The Effect of Legalization of Abortion on Population Growth and Public Health," *Family Planning Perspectives* 7 (1975): 123-27.

21. S.J. Ventura, "Teenage Child Bearing: United States 1966–1975," *Monthly Vital Statistics Reports* 26 (1977): 1-15.

22. J.B. Hardy, "Birth Weight and Subsequent Physical and Intellectual Development," *New England Journal of Medicine* 289 (1973): 973-74.

23. H. Forssman and I. Thuwe, "120 Children Born after Application for Therapeutic Abortion Was Refused," *Acta Psychiatrica Scandinavica* 42 (1966): 71-88.

24. Z. Matejeck, Z. Dytrych, and V. Schuller, "Children from Unwanted Pregnancies," *Acta Psychiatrica Scandinavica* 57 (1978): 67-90.

25. B. Lauer, E. Ten Broeck, and M. Grossman, "Battered Child Syndrome: Review of 130 Patients with Controls," *Pediatrics* 54 (1974): 67-70.

26. L. Eisenberg, "The Sins of the Fathers: Urban Decay and Social Pathology," *American Journal of Orthopsychiatry* 32 (1962): 5-17.

27. F. Furstenberg, Jr., "The Social Consequences of Teenage Parenthood," *Family Planning Perspectives* 8 (1976): 148-64.

28. J.R. Daling and I. Emanuel, "Induced Abortion and Subsequent Outcome of Pregnancy in a Series of American Women," *New England Journal of Medicine* 297 (1977): 1241-45.

29. _____, "Induced Abortion and Subsequent Outcome of Pregnancy: A Matched Cohort Study," *Lancet* 2 (1975): 170-73.

30. C. Brewer, "Incidence of Post-Abortion Psychosis: A Prospective Study," *British Medical Journal* 1 (1977): 476-77.

31. H.S. Greer, S. Lao, S.C. Lewis, et al., "Psychosocial Consequences of Therapeutic Abortion: King's Therapeutic Study III," *British Journal of Psychiatry* 128 (1976): 74-79.

32. N.B. Ryder, "Contraceptive Failure in the United States," *Family Planning Perspectives* 5 (1973): 133-42.

33. F.S. Jaffe, "The Pill: A Perspective for Assessing Risks and Benefits," *New England Journal of Medicine* 297 (1977): 612-14.

34. J. Kandell, "Former French Premier Seeks to Spur Lagging Birth Rates," *New York Times* (6 June 1978).

35. R. Parke, "Population Changes That Affect Federal Policy: Some Suggestions for Research," *Social Science Research Council Items* 33 (1979): 3-8.

36. Bureau of the Census, "Demographic Aspects of Aging and the Older Population in the United States," *Current Population Reports. Special Studies* Ser. D-23, no. 59 (1976).

37. *Health: The United States, 1978,* DHEW Publication 78-1232 (Washington: U.S. Department of Health, Education, and Welfare, December 1978).

CHILDREN IN A CHANGING WORLD 343

38. E. Gruenberg, "The Failures of Success," *Milbank Memorial Fund Quarterly* 53 (1977): 3-24.

39. R.B. Freeman, *The Overeducated American* (New York: Academic Press, 1976).

40. W. Borders, "Joblessness Plagues India's Educated Elite," *New York Times* (28 May 1978).

41. M.G. Scully, "Youth Employment Stirs International Concerns," *Chronicle of Higher Education* (22 May 1978).

42. H. Kahne and A.I. Kohen, "Economic Perspectives on the Roles of Women in the American Economy," *Journal of Economic Literature* 13 (1975): 1249-92.

43. V.K. Oppenheimer, "The Life-Cycle Squeeze: The Interaction of Men's Occupational and Family Life Cycles," *Demography* 11 (1974): 227-45.

44. Z. Luria, "Recent Women College Graduates: A Study of Rising Expectations," *American Journal of Orthopsychiatry* 44 (1974): 312-26.

45. G. Myrdal, *An American Dilemma* (New York: Harper & Row, 1944): 1064.

46. L.M. Stolz, "Effects of Maternal Employment on Children: Evidence from Research," *Child Development* 31 (1960): 749-82.

47. M.W. Edelman, "A Political-Legislative Overview of Federal Child Care Proposals," in *Raising Children in America: Problems and Prospective Solutions*, ed. N.B. Talbot (Boston: Little, Brown and Company, 1974): 304-18.

48. L. Kanner, *A History of the Care and Study of the Mentally Retarded* (Springfield, Illinois: C.C Thomas, 1964): 119.

49. B. Lozoff and G. Brittenham, "Infant Care: Cache or Carry," *Journal of Pediatrics* 95 (1979): 478-83.

50. Ibid.

51. R.A. Hinde and L. McGinnis, "Some Factors Influencing the Effects of Temporary Mother-Infant Separation," *Psychological Medicine* 7 (1977): 197-212.

52. L.A. Rosenblum and I.C. Kaufman, "Variations in Infant Development and Response to Maternal Loss in Monkeys," *American Journal of Orthopsychiatry* 38 (1968): 418-26.

53. P. Dolhinow, "Commentary on Infantile Attachment Theory," *Behavioral and Brain Sciences* 3 (1978): 433-44.

54. Ibid.

55. S.B. Hrdy, "Infanticide as a Primate Reproductive Strategy," *American Scientist* 65 (1977): 40-49.

56. R. Curtin and P. Dolhinow, "Primate Social Behavior in a Changing World," *American Scientist* 66 (1978): 468-75.

57. B. Tizard and J. Rees, "The Effect of Early Institutional Rearing on the Behavior Problems and Affectional Relationships of Four-Year-Old Children," *Journal of Child Psychology and Psychiatry* 16 (1975): 61-73.

58. B. Tizard and J. Hodges, "The Effect of Early Institutional Rearing on the Development of Eight-Year-Old Children," *Journal of Child Psychology and Psychiatry* 19 (1978): 99-118.

59. L. Eisenberg, "The *Human* Nature of Human Nature," *Science* 176 (1972): 123-28.

60. A. Freud and S. Dann, "An Experiment in Group Upbringing," *Psychoanalytic Study of the Child* 6 (1951): 127-68.

61. F.C. Turner, "La Estampida Hacia las Ciudades en Latino America," *Intersciencia* 2 (1977): 31-41.

62. G.W. Brown and T. Harris, *Social Origins of Depression: A Study of Psychiatric Disorder in Women* (New York: Free Press, 1978).

63. S. Henderson, P. Duncan-Jones, D.G. Byrne, et al., "Social Bonds, Adversity and Neurosis," *British Journal of Psychiatry*, in press.

64. G.L. Klerman and J.E. Izen, "The Effects of Bereavement and Grief on Physical Health and Well-Being," *Advances in Psychosomatic Medicine* 9 (1977): 63-104.

65. L.F. Berkman and S.L. Syme, "Social Networks, Host Resistance and Mortality," *American Journal of Epidemiology* 109 (1979): 186-204.

66. R.J. Meyer and R.J. Haggerty, "Streptococcal Infections in Families: Factors Altering Individual Susceptibility," *Pediatrics* 29 (1962): 539-49.

67. K.J. Roghmann and R.J. Haggerty, "Daily Stress, Illness and Use of Health Services in Young Families," *Pediatric Research* 7 (1973): 520-26.

68. U. Bronfenbrenner, "Toward an Experimental Ecology of Human Development," *American Psychologist* 32 (1977): 513-31.

69. M.M. Cochran and J.A. Brassard, "Child Development and Personal Social Networks," *Child Development* 50 (1979): 601-16.

DISCUSSION

Rooming In

Improving the interaction between the mother and the infant is to the good of both. The highly artificial practice in some modern hospitals focuses on infection and technical problems, rather than on psychological development, and separates the infant from its mother in the maternity service. The practice of rooming in, with the baby living in the same room as the mother so she is able to care for it is desirable in so far as possible.

Whether the benefits are as great as the proponents of this practice in the United States insist, however, still has to be determined.

Breast-Feeding versus Formulas

One matter of concern is that when pediatricians in the 1920s designed infant formulas and developed safe methods for their preparation it became more "scientific" to raise a baby on an artificial formula than on mother's milk because the formula was "scientific." This interrupted a practice that had gone on perfectly well since the establishment of the human species.

What we would like to see is not a return to a requirement for breast-feeding, so that the mother who does not want to or cannot breast-feed is made to feel guilty, but choices—that is, women who want to ought to be encouraged to breast-feed, and those who do not should also be supported.

The infant who is forced on its mother might have a more difficult time than if it were raised on a bottle.

It is this kind of variation that should be stressed. A return to breast-feeding and to early infant care is probably still desirable, but people in the United States, at least, are subject to waves of enthusiasm; some are now arguing that early breast-feeding will prevent drug dependence. That remains to be demonstrated.

Mother-Infant Bonding

Bonding has become quite fashionable in the United States, and a great deal of research is being done on the subject. Data on bonding describe the abnormality of the premature infant who has been isolated from the mother for the first six, eight, or twelve weeks of life, and who has missed a valuable developmental experience. When the mother is finally given custody of the infant, about whom she has been worried and whom she has only seen through a glass partition, she is nervous and apprehensive and handles it as though it were very fragile.

In contrast, when the mother is introduced to the newborn's nursery, has access to the child, and is given systematic instruction on how to manage it, the child does much better.

The alternative is to separate the infant from the mother and put it in a crib in a typical overcrowded newborn nursery. Under those circumstances there is the danger of the spread of infection; it is also impossible to maintain adequate nutritional standards. The amount of care given to the child is such that the infant fares far better in bed with its mother.

Unfortunately, pediatric investigators have been disproportionately impressed by bonding models that work well for some species of birds and some ungulates. For most animals, however, it is not so much the first ten hours of experience that count, but repeated experiences over the developmental cycle. There is no evidence that bonding takes place in primates in that short period of time, and it is certainly not true that the experience is irreversible.

Not only is it good for a mother to have access to her infant soon after birth, but birthing rooms in hospitals where the father is also present, when they both want it that way, are also commendable. What is distressing is the enthusiastic wave sweeping over the United States urging that all babies be born in a birthing room, on the one hand, or, on the other, that fetal instrumentation be used by which the monitors keep producing "noise" which the doctor mistakes for data.

Changing Roles of Males and Females

With regard to children and adolescents in the future world, what role will fathers play in terms of family structure? One of the very serious problems ahead is the likelihood that women will become more like men, rather than men acquiring some of the good traits of women. Women, for example, are taking up the habits of men: smoking among adolescent females has risen to the level of adolescent males, and more women are now dying of lung cancer.

The *New York Times* reported a single case, a prototype of the problem, of a woman who fought in the courts to be given the right to become a miner and was killed in a mine disaster. That is death that would not have occurred as long as mining was a sex-linked occupation. We have to make it less necessary for men to do the kind of jobs and lead the kind of lives that carry with them extra biological hazards.

Thus one of the challenges is to begin to think of changing the value system in order to allow men to give, to feel, to acknowledge feeling, to be concerned with closeness, to be sentimental—whatever words one wishes to use—in the way that women have been socialized by tradition to do.

There ought to be social legislation that would include, as for example in Sweden, leave for fathers as well as mothers after a child is born. Sweden has also moved away from a lifelong obligation of parenting. It now has legislation that permits children to "divorce" their parents; some parents want legislation to enable them to divorce their children.

With regard to the establishment of day care centers in the schools in order to teach parenting skills, boys should also have this kind of experience. Where systematic studies have been done, their interest, their ability, and their real concerns are evident, but their opportunities have been restricted.

Changing Social Universe

There is another phenomenon about which several speakers have expressed their views: not only is psychiatry changing, which is to be welcomed, but our social universe is changing. Who knows what the outcome will be? Who could have predicted twenty-five years ago the importance of two of the phenomena we have been discussing? First, the use and abuse of drugs by individuals at younger and younger ages, and, second, the flood of early pregnancies, despite the parallel development and exploitation of adequate means of contraception.

Plight of Disadvantaged Children

There are other more important phenomena than those, however. There is a world different from our own, a world in which our concerns and our difficulties may seem absolutely trivial. Refugee children are drowning in the China Sea; others are dying of hunger in Cambodia; and still others are being shot to death in Southeast Asia or tortured by tyrants in front of their parents, or are watching their parents being tortured. We cannot close our eyes to such events in countries other than our own—which perhaps may even happen in our own countries. Child psychiatry must be a discipline attentive to all the children of the world, attentive to other disciplines, and attentive also to political matters. Child psychiatry must realize that eventually it must mobilize its resources and do all it can to save who can be saved of all those troubled children.

Two points of view were offered: one, if we have any humanitarian impulse at all we have to be concerned about the special problems of the children in parts of the world where conditions of health are similar to those of the West 200 years ago. These problems are not the inevitable results of biological barriers, but are due to the failure to apply available social technology to their solution.

Another reason for drawing attention to children in Saharan Africa and Cambodia, for example, is to help us have a better understanding of children in America and Europe; that is, all of us tend to be so preoccupied with what we see on the current scene we become utterly unaware of the differences between cultures and the transience of what appear to be facts.

Epidemic of Adolescent Pregnancies

The epidemic of adolescent pregnancies in the United States is in startling contrast to what appears to be much lower in rates in France. Whether this is because adolescent French mothers, or their obstetricians, or their statisticians are more successful in concealing the rates or whether they are really different is unclear. But surely if the Europeans are where the Americans would like to be, let them examine the American experience to determine what to avoid in order to minimize the problem. There is a great deal to be learned by this kind of cross-correlation.

Importance of Moral Development

One participant stressed the importance of studying moral development. One of the things that has characterized child psychiatry is the extent to which it attempts to emulate the sciences in their avoidance of the value issues, that is, moral issues. But in matters of human survival, value issues may indeed be the most crucial variable. The challenge is not the matter of studying the system of morals, which seems a less difficult task, but how to teach moral values, and the consequences, to young people living in a world in which it is fashionable to have a baby. How does one make that fashion unfashionable? Child psychiatrists in the United States are not well-equipped to face that problem.

When there was a concern about drug abuse in the 1960s, great emphasis was placed on education about drugs in the high schools. Studies of several apparently well-intentioned efforts at such education indicated that the children's behavior was sometimes worse rather than better after "education" had been provided. Giving something a noble name does not guarantee a noble outcome. What appears to be effective in the new systems of prevention is the use of fundamental psychological knowledge from the laboratory; namely, that inoculating people against false beliefs is more effective than giving them homilies about what they ought to do.

PARTICIPANTS

Samuel Berenberg, M.D.
Centre International de l'Enfance
Paris, France

Miss Maxine E. Bleich
Program Director
Josiah Macy, Jr. Foundation
New York, New York, U.S.A.

Dennis P. Cantwell, M.D.
Joseph Campbell Professor
   of Child Psychiatry
Neuropsychiatric Institute
Center for the Health Sciences
University of California,
   Los Angeles
Los Angeles, California, U.S.A.

Jean-Pierre Deschamps, M.D.
Professeur Agrégé
   de Santé Publique
Faculté de Médecine
Université de Nancy
Nancy, France

Felton Earls, M.D.
Assistant Professor
Department of Psychiatry
Harvard Medical School
Children's Hospital Medical Center
Boston, Massachusetts, U.S.A.

Leon Eisenberg, M.D.
Professor and Chairman
Department of Preventive
   and Social Medicine
Harvard Medical School
Boston, Massachusetts, U.S.A.

Alfred M. Freedman, M.D.
Professor and Chairman
Department of Psychiatry
New York Medical College
Valhalla, New York, U.S.A.

Philip J. Graham, M.D.,
   FRCPsych.
Walker Professor of
   Child Psychiatry
Department of Child Psychiatry
Institute of Child Health
University of London
The Hospital for Sick Children
London, England

Beatrix A. Hamburg, M.D.
Associate Professor of
   Psychiatry
Harvard Medical School
Children's Hospital
   Medical Center
Boston, Massachusetts, U.S.A.

Karen Hein, M.D.
Director
Division of Adolescent Medicine
Assistant Professor of Pediatrics
College of Physicians and Surgeons
Columbia University
New York, New York, U.S.A.

Margaret E. Hertzig, M.D.
Director
Child and Adolescent Psychiatry
    Outpatient Department
Payne Whitney Clinic
The New York Hospital—
    Cornell Medical Center
New York, New York, U.S.A.

Olivier Jeanneret, M.D.
Professeur de Médecine Sociale
Institut de Médecine
    Sociale et Préventive
Universite de Genève
Genève, Switzerland

Cyrille Koupernik, M.D.
Membre du Collège de Médecine
    des Hôpitaux de Paris
Paris, France

Michael Manciaux, M.D.
Director General
Centre International de l'Enfance
Paris, France

Mrs. Margaret E. R. Morrow,
    M.B.E.
Playgroup Organizer
National Society for the Prevention
    of Cruelty to Children
Belfast, Northern Ireland

Claude Olievenstein, M.D.
Médecin-Chef
Centre Médical Marmottan
Paris, France

Michel Péchevis, M.D.
Centre International de l'Enfance
Paris, France

Fritz Poustka, M.D.
Kinder- und Jugendpsychiatrische
    Klinik
Zentralinstitut für Seelische
    Gesundheit Mannheim
Mannheim, Federal Republic of
    Germany

Mrs. Elizabeth F. Purcell
Conference Director and Editor
Josiah Macy, Jr. Foundation
New York, New York, U.S.A.

Judith L. Rapoport, M.D.
Chief
Unit of Childhood Mental Illness
Alcohol, Drug Abuse, and Mental
    Health Administration
National Institute of Mental Health
National Institutes of Health
Bethesda, Maryland, U.S.A.

Lee N. Robins, Ph.D.
Professor of Sociology
    in Psychiatry
Department of Psychiatry
School of Medicine
Washington University
St. Louis, Missouri, U.S.A.

Roger Salbreux, M.D.
Director
Comité d'Étude de Soins et
   d'Action Permanente en
   Faveur des Déficients Mentaux
Siège Administratif
Paris, France

Mme. Henriette Taviani
Délégue
Haut Commissariat des Nations
   Unies pour les Réfugiés
   Délégation Française
Neuilly-sur-Seine, France

Eric Taylor, M.D.
Department of Child and
   Adolescent Psychiatry
Institute of Psychiatry
London, England

INDEX

368 PSYCHOPATHOLOGY OF CHILDREN AND YOUTH

World Health Organization (WHO),
  33, 45, 266, 293-94
  Expert Committee on Child Mental
  Health and Psychosocial
  Development, 42
  Expert Committee on Drug
  Dependence, 249

Yankelevich, N., 53*n*

Yates, A.J., 118
Yom Kippur War, 190, 193-95
Yule, W., 110, 147

Zafiropoulos, M., 53*n*
Zelnick, M., 303
Ziv, A.Z., 190, 191, 193
Zucman, E., 54